Volume 1
The Dental Patient

Clinical Dentistry
in health and disease

Volume 1: The Dental Patient Professor Crispian Scully

Volume 2: The Mouth and Perioral Tissues Professor Crispian Scully

Volume 3: The Dentition and Dental Care Professor Richard J. Elderton

Volume 4: Orthodontics and Occlusal Management Professor William C. Shaw

CLINICAL DENTISTRY
in health and disease

Co-ordinating Editor: Professor David K. Mason
Dean, Glasgow Dental Hospital
and School

Volume 1
The Dental Patient

Edited by

Crispian Scully,
BSc, BDS, PhD, FDSRCPS, MRCPath, MD

Professor, Head of Clinical Dental School and Head of Department,
University Department of Oral Medicine, Surgery and Pathology,
Bristol Dental School and Hospital

Heinemann Medical Books

Heinemann Medical Books
An imprint of Heinemann Professional Publishing Ltd
Halley Court, Jordan Hill, Oxford OX2 8EJ

OXFORD   LONDON   SINGAPORE   NAIROBI   IBADAN   KINGSTON

First published 1988

British Library Cataloguing in Publication Data
The Dental Patient.
   1. Dentistry. Therapy. Planning
   I. Scully, Crispian
   II. Series
   617.6

ISBN 0 433 00052 X

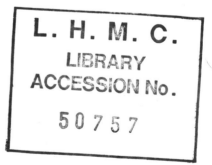
Filmset by Eta Services (Typesetters) Ltd, Beccles, Suffolk
and printed by Butler & Tanner Ltd, Frome

35.00

Contents

Contributors

Stephen Flint BDS MBBS FDSRCS
Lecturer and Honorary Senior Registrar
University Department of Oral Medicine, Surgery and Pathology, Bristol Dental School and Hospital, Lower Maudlin Street, Bristol

David A. McGowan MDS PhD FDSRCS FFDRCSI FDSRCPS
Professor, Consultant and Head of Department
Department of Oral Surgery, Glasgow Dental Hospital and School, 378 Sauchiehall Street, Glasgow

Robin W. Matthews BDS MDS PhD
Senior Lecturer and Honorary Associate Specialist
University Department of Oral Medicine, Surgery and Pathology, Bristol Dental School and Hospital, Lower Maudlin Street, Bristol

Robert Ord FDSRCPS FRCS
Consultant
Department of Oral and Maxillofacial Surgery, Sunderland District General Hospital, Kayll Road, Sunderland

Karen Porter BDS
Recognized Teacher and Honorary Registrar
University Department of Oral Medicine, Surgery and Pathology, Bristol Dental School and Hospital, Lower Maudlin Street, Bristol

Stephen R. Porter BSc BDS PhD FDSRCS FDSRCSE
Lecturer and Honorary Registrar
University Department of Oral Medicine, Surgery and Pathology, Bristol Dental School and Hospital, Lower Maudlin Street, Bristol

John Rayne FDSRCS DPhil DOrth
Consultant
Department of Oral Surgery, John Radcliffe Hospital, Headington, Oxford

J. Philip Rood MDS MBBS FDSRCS FRCS
Professor, Consultant and Head of Department
Department of Oral and Maxillofacial Surgery, Turner Dental School, Higher Cambridge Street, Manchester

Laksman Samaranayake BDS DDS MRCPath
Senior Lecturer and Consultant
University Department of Oral Medicine and Pathology, Glasgow Dental Hospital and School, Glasgow

Crispian Scully BSc BDS MBBS PhD FDSRCPS MRCPath MD
Professor, Consultant and Head of Department
University Department of Oral Medicine, Surgery and Pathology, Bristol Dental School and Hospital, Lower Maudlin Street, Bristol

Peter Ward-Booth BDS MBBS FDSRCS FRCS
Consultant
Department of Oral and Maxillofacial Surgery, Sunderland District General Hospital, Kayll Road, Sunderland

David Wiesenfeld MDSc FDSRCPS FRACDS (OMS)
Consultant
Lewis House, 766 Elizabeth Street, Melbourne, Australia

Preface

This volume covers general aspects of the diagnosis and management of the dental patient; more specific points are discussed in the other volumes in this series.

This is a synopsis of the subject that should give a foundation for further study. There is inevitably a degree of overlap between chapters and a minor degree of repetition where important points are being made. We hope there are no serious omissions; most apparent deficiencies are covered by sections in the other volumes. Medico-legal aspects of dentistry are not discussed herein, though of increasing importance, since excellent texts are already available.

This book is the product mainly of a number of younger workers in the field with whom the editor has personally worked or had close associations. They have a progressive approach to the teaching of dentistry and attempt here to give a contemporary and practical view, unrestricted by the somewhat artificial boundaries of the various disciplines within. Where possible, a symptomatic and clinical approach has been used since patients present in that way.

The book is designed to help mainly undergraduate students of dentistry but should be useful also to postgraduates.

The curriculum is now so full that one sympathizes with the vast amount of knowledge that undergraduates must assimilate. However, study and qualification at a postgraduate level are now accepted as essential for those who wish to work in one of the dental specialties and the realist accepts that vocational training is desirable even for those who wish to be 'generalists'.

The text aims mainly at those who have completed training in the basic sciences and human diseases, as well as pharmacology, and a degree of knowledge and understanding is assumed.

Acknowledgements

The encouragement of Professor David K. Mason has, as always, been most welcome. Dr Richard Barling has been an enthusiastic supporter and adviser whose pleasant and courteous approach has encouraged us to keep to schedule. I am always grateful to Professor R. A. Cawson for his frequent and stimulating discussions and his forebearance when I sometimes adopt and adapt his original ideas. I am also grateful to my various publishers, especially Wright PSG and British Dental Journal for their permission to adapt material. Finally, I am grateful to the contributors who tolerated any editing without complaint, to Hugh Levers for helping with reading the proofs, to Anthea Hardiman and Johh Bunn for help with Chapter 3, and to Ni Fathers.

C. Scully
Bristol
July 1988

Chapter

1

The dentist–patient relationship

A dental appointment is often an experience patients would rather avoid. Some 75% of patients experience a degree of anxiety before the encounter and 5–10% are so distraught that they avoid it. Such anxiety can be reduced somewhat by the establishment of a good dentist–patient relationship.

It is the duty of the practitioner to achieve the best professional relationship possible with the patient. Indeed, in general practice, such a relationship is the foundation of success. Of the 50% or so of the population who fail to seek regular dental care, about one-half do so because of fear and at least half of those who do attend but then leave their dentists, do so because of dissatisfaction or dislike. Patients often judge the dentist on the basis of the emotional support and alleviation of anxiety given, rather than on an objective assessment of his or her technical competence. Social skills are clearly important for the dentist.

THE 'GOOD DENTIST'

A recent survey of patients' attitudes confirmed the importance of the dentist's social skills in formulating their opinions (Table 1.1). Paramount appear to be the dentist's ability:

(a) to recognize and manage anxiety in the patient,
(b) to establish and maintain rapport, and
(c) to provide information and explanations about the various procedures, possible complications, etc.

Patients comprise, of course, a heterogeneous group and it was apparent from the results of the above survey that the dentist's social skills were more important to many more women and to irregular attenders and those receiving treatment on the health service than to men, regular attenders and those having private treatment. These last groups in general wanted professional skills most. Nevertheless, people tend to judge their dentist to a large extent by social skills both within and outside the surgery. A dentist who is polite and smartly turned out, befitting his role generally, has an easier relationship with his patient than does one who is unkempt or rude. Rightly or wrongly, patients tend to expect and demand the former presentation.

People are acutely aware of what is going on in the environment when awaiting or receiving treatment. Sounds of mirth or gossip from the staff are quite likely to be interpreted as an uncaring or slovenly attitude. The patient is at the surgery for treatment and expects to be seen promptly and efficiently by staff who are always courteous, happy, friendly and helpful. He will have little, if any, real sympathy for the dentist who is tired or irritable.

DISSATISFACTION WITH THE DENTIST: THE 'BAD DENTIST'

Interestingly, the majority of patients' complaints about dentists relate again to poor social skills rather than to lack of professional skills (Table 1.1). Furthermore, other health care professionals not infrequently complain that dentists appear not to be particularly approachable or sympathetic.

Those who are dissatisfied for any reason are less likely to keep appointments or to arrive on time and may by their attitudes arouse negative feelings in the dentist. This can make it difficult for the dentist to approach the relationship in a positive spirit—and a vicious circle can result.

THE ANXIETY RESPONSE

Anticipation of the discomfort presumed to be associated with a dental visit precedes the visit by minutes, hours,

Table 1.1
Attributes of 'good' and 'bad' dentists in order of descending importance in patients' opinions

Good dentists	Bad dentists
1. Professional skill	1. Charges too much (private treatment)
2. Reassuring attitude	2. Asks questions when patient's mouth is full of fingers/instruments
3. Cheerful and friendly approach	3. Does not explain procedures or give time for questions
4. Patience	
5. Good dental treatment	4. Takes too many x-rays
6. Carefulness	5. Does not give dental health education
7. Efficiency	6. Says it will not hurt when it does
8. Personal approach	7. Makes too many appointments
9. Explains treatment	8. Is impersonal and makes idle gossip
10. Cleanliness and hygiene	
11. Honesty and trustworthiness	
12. Gentleness	
13. Courtesy	

days or even longer. Anxiety will be heightened as patients approach and enter the surgery, especially when they meet the sounds and smells they associate with dentistry. The anxiety and apprehension result in a release of adrenaline and other hormones with a subsequent feeling of pounding of the heart and pulse, perhaps cold sweating of the palms, a feeling of nausea, dry mouth and an urge to urinate and/or defaecate (Table 1.2; Fig. 1.1).

The release of these hormones is centrally controlled via the hypothalamus which, in turn, is modulated by cerebral cortical activity and the arousal centres of the reticular formation. Increased sympathetic activity causes release of adrenaline and other catecholamines from the adrenal medulla and glucagon release from the pancreas—both hormones produce raised levels of blood sugar by mobilizing glycogen stores. There is also hypo-

Table 1.2
Typical presentation of the anxious dental patient

Tachycardia
Sometimes cardiac dysrhythmias
Often palpitations
Raised systolic blood pressure
Dry mouth
Nausea
Desire to defaecate
Sweating: cold clammy palms
Frequency of micturition
Headache (muscle tension)
Tremor
Dilated pupils

thalamic stimulation of the pituitary gland and release of a range of other hormones, including beta endorphins involved in pain modulation (see Chapter 6) and adrenocorticotrophic hormone (ACTH). ACTH stimulates release of corticosteroids from the adrenal cortex and a consequent rise in plasma steroid levels, a necessary feature of the reaction to 'stress'. The hormonal changes associated with the anxiety response together produce profound metabolic changes, with raised serum levels of free fatty acids, very low-density lipoproteins and cholesterol. Factors involved in haemostasis (factor VIII levels; platelet numbers and adhesiveness) all increase.

In essence, these 'stress' responses mobilize energy stores and prime the body to cope with potential assault.

The stress response, however, also includes a catabolic phase, with some conversion of fats and proteins to produce sugars, lasting up to 2 days. The cardiovascular sequelae include increased pulse rate and systolic blood pressure and increased skeletal muscle blood flow. In a few patients the autonomic activity, rather than being sympathetic, is mainly parasympathetic and thus vagal activity increases, causing bradycardia and a vasovagal attack or faint.

FACTORS IMPLICATED IN DENTAL ANXIETY

Factors implicated in dental anxiety include the following.

1. *Traumatic dental and/or medical experiences,* such as

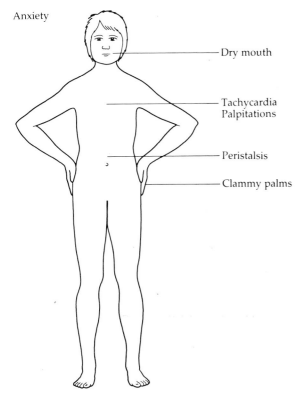

Anxiety

— Dry mouth

— Tachycardia
Palpitations

— Peristalsis

— Clammy palms

Fig. 1.1 *Features of an anxiety response.*

painful treatment procedures (particularly injections) and the use of noisy drills. Experiences such as these in childhood, and especially involving an unsympathetic dentist, may provoke anxiety in the future.

2. *Exposure to an anxiety-provoking environment* such as frightening instruments, strange odours, etc.

3. *Personal factors* that modify the level of anxiety in relation to any situation include the patient's age and sex, cultural, emotional, educational and ethnic backgrounds. For example, in general women tend to express anxiety more than men and those of Southern European descent tend to do so more than Anglo-Saxons.

4. *External influences,* such as those of peer groups, family and the media, modify the patient's level of anxiety. It is still a common joke that dental treatment is unpleasant. Comments about dental treatment such as 'it will not hurt' tend to lead people to expect pain rather than to reassure them.

5. *The dentist–patient relationship* is important in regard to anxiety experienced. Patient anxiety and dissatisfaction seem to some extent related to poor communication between dentist and patient. Fear and dislike of the dent-

ist, low confidence in him and a poor attitude of the dentist towards the patient all appear to cause people to be reluctant to visit the dentist. Some research workers have developed a Dental Visit Satisfaction Scale to assess patient satisfaction.

DENTAL PHOBIAS

Though most patients undergoing dentistry are anxious, this does not interfere with treatment. However, in some cases the anxiety is such an emotional stress as actually to force the patient to avoid seeking dental treatment. In a few patients a phobia develops which becomes quite overwhelming and totally inhibits any dental treatment. Psychiatrists have recognized this spectrum of anxiety, and they distinguish between so-called healthy anxiety and morbid anxiety. Many readers may find it difficult to believe that the awful sensation of anxiety which they feel before an examination, for example, is considered by psychiatrists as 'healthy'. Morbid anxiety is, of course, more distressing since the signs and symptoms of anxiety overwhelm the patient, are totally inappropriate to the event and interfere with normal activities. In fact, the event precipitating the anxiety may be entirely imaginary. The classic appearance of this morbid anxiety is frequently seen in some elderly people who become frightened to leave their houses or carry on a normal life. There is clearly no sharp divide between healthy anxiety and morbid anxiety, there being a whole spectrum and range of responses, depending on personality and age. The anxiety phobia is usually a conditioned or learnt response to previous distressing experiences, and certainly dentistry is included within these phobic states. Anxiety may also precede or be associated with acute depression.

MANAGEMENT OF DENTAL ANXIETY

Considerate care

The anxiety associated with the encounter with a dentist can be reduced by tender loving care (TLC)—a large proportion of the population prefer considerate and painless treatment to, for example, superb amalgams, though, of course, all really want both (see above). Communication should always take into consideration the educational and cultural background of the patient. The attitudes and behaviour of surgery assistant, receptionist and others, as well as of the dentist, will all influence the patient.

Pain avoidance and control (see also Chapters 6 and 9)

The careful and gentle handling of tissues and the efficient and judicious use of local analgesic injections, sedation, or general anaesthesia are by far the most important means of reassuring the patient and calming anxiety. They also imply that the operator will be equally careful with his operative work. Careful, but not over-detailed explanation of preoperative and operative procedures and postoperative complications will go a long way to avoiding untoward reactions from the patient. Some discomfort is almost inevitable and it is better to admit this rather than issue a false claim of painless treatment.

Drugs

For the few patients for whom further help is required to control anxiety there is a range of drugs available but, in practical terms, only two groups of drugs need be considered, the benzodiazepines and the beta blockers.

Drugs acting on the central nervous system are not as specific as either the drug manufacturers or the public would sometimes believe. Indeed, the terms anxiolytics, sedatives and tranquillizers are often confusing since they themselves are not specific. Some of the so-called tranquillizer drugs are, in fact, more appropriate to treating psychoses, although they, of course, will have some sedative effect as well.

The benzodiazepines are so effective in dentistry that it is important to consider them in some detail. Benzodiazepines act on the whole central nervous system but there are certain parts that seem particularly sensitive, especially the limbic system, which is physiologically central to arousal and emotional states. Destruction of the limbic system, or use of drugs acting on it such as the benzodiazepines, reduces the most aggressive raging animal to a docile, calm state.

The benzodiazepines also deplete levels of cerebral noradrenaline and serotonin (5-hydroxytryptamine, 5-HT), which may account for the initial drowsiness experienced as the drug is given. Benzodiazepines also produce an increase in the cerebral level of gamma-aminobutyric acid (GABA), which may well account for their anticonvulsant and other effects.

The benzodiazepines are particularly effective, therefore, in calming and reducing anxiety, in muscle relaxation and anticonvulsant activities, though these effects vary between different preparations (Table 1.3). It has been estimated that half of the prescriptions written in the Western World are now for benzodiazepines. This widespread use provides adequate evidence of the wide therapeutic range and relative safety of these drugs, though addiction is now well recognized, and they have now been added to the list of drugs controlled by criminal law in Britain (see Chapter 5).

The safety of benzodiazepines is remarkable. People have taken overdoses of chlordiazepoxide and of diazepam and have merely been sleepy and ataxic but rousable. Rapid intravenous injection, however, may cause respiratory arrest and has caused fatalities.

The two groups of patients for whom particular caution must be taken with the benzodiazepines are the old and the young. The elderly are particularly sensitive to benzodiazepines and should be monitored closely to ensure that respiratory depression is avoided. Young children may become somewhat more agitated and aggressive, rather than sedated, by benzodiazepines. This is particularly common when the drug is given intravenously but rarely occurs when given orally.

Clearly the side-effects of benzodiazepines of drowsiness and ataxia may be hazardous, and instructions (preferably printed) should be given to the patients to warn them to avoid using machinery, driving vehicles or making important decisions for at least 12 hours after receiving benzodiazepines (see Chapter 6).

There are many other anxiolytic or sedative drugs which are available but there seems little indication for

Table 1.3
Therapeutic role of benzodiazepines

Action	Proposed mechanism	Site of action
Anxiolytic	Affinity for glycine receptors	Mamillary body
Antegrade amnesia	Not known	Not known
Muscle relaxation	Affinity for glycine receptors	Spinal cord
Hypnotic	Gamma-aminobutyric acid (GABA)	Cerebral cortex
Anticonvulsant	May be GABA accumulation	Motor pathways

Table 1.4
Other drugs used in the past for 'sedation'

Drugs	Complication or contraindication
Barbiturates	Dependence, tolerance
Antipsychotic drugs	Not indicated for 'healthy' anxiety Widespread cholinergic side-effects (including dry mouth)
Opiates	Powerful analgesics Controlled drugs Respiratory depression

their use in preference to the benzodiazepines, since all cause significant adverse reactions (Table 1.4).

The benzodiazepines of greatest value in dentistry are diazepam and midazolam (see also Chapter 6), though newer compounds such as temazepam may prove to have advantages over these.

The use of oral benzodiazepines has recently become popular for adults. The recommendation is that 30–40 mg of a short-acting benzodiazepine such as Temazepam should be given as a premedication prior to the dentistry. A 30-minute interval should elapse prior to surgery. This preoperative sedation may be beneficial to the anxious patient. The sedation may not be so profound or readily increased as in intravenous (i.v.) techniques. The action of benzodiazepines can be at least partially reversed by flumazenil (p. 116).

Diazepam

Diazepam is well absorbed orally, giving a maximum blood level within 2 hours. Its value as a parenteral drug is, however, somewhat less than satisfactory, since it is not water soluble, causes pain if injected intramuscularly, and may produce thrombophlebitis when given intravenously. A preparation in a lipid emulsion (Diazemuls) has overcome the problem of thrombophlebitis. However, diazepam also has some other disadvantages in outpatient dentistry in that the main metabolite is also active and therefore the half-life is prolonged (see Chapter 6). A single intravenous dose of 10 mg still has significant sedative levels at 8 hours and measurable blood levels at 24 hours. If repeated doses are given, accumulation occurs (see p. 174).

Midazolam

Midazolam is one and a half times as potent as diazepam but has a number of advantages, particularly since it is

water soluble and none of its metabolites is pharmacologically active. Midazolam, therefore, does not accumulate and has a much shorter half-life than diazepam. A single bolus injection, of 7.5 mg midazolam intravenously, is eliminated within 12 hours (see p. 176).

Beta blockers

The main use of beta blockers (e.g. metoprolol), which block beta adrenergic receptors, is on the cardiovascular system, to maintain normal blood pressure in a hypertensive patient.

It has also been apparent for some time that these drugs can also reduce the signs and symptoms of anxiety. However, it is unfortunate that there is little demonstrable benefit from beta blockers for a normal patient facing an anxiety-provoking situation such as dental procedures. The main value of beta blockers is for the patient who is somewhat neurotic and anxious, in whom the relief of symptoms of anxiety may be beneficial.

Premedication (see also Chapter 9)

Premedication is a term used for medication given to a patient prior to treatment, usually when the treatment involves a general anaesthetic. Many of the drugs traditionally used for inpatient premedication, classically the opiates, should not be used for the outpatient. Others were used with particular types of general anaesthetic agent; for example scopolamine (hyoscine) was commonly used as a premedication for an ether anaesthetic.

Premedication with a short-acting drug such as diazepam or Temazepam is quite acceptable for the outpatient, but there does seem good evidence that the significant cardiac dysrhythmias which develop during exodontia under general anaesthesia can, and should be, reduced using a cardioselective beta blocker such as metoprolol premedication.

Behaviour therapies

The 5% or so of patients who are so fearful that they refuse all dental treatment may respond to management by the clinical psychologist. Behaviour therapies such as desensitization and modelling may be valuable.

Desensitization is a graded introduction to dental treatment building up from the least to the most stressful aspects of the exposure.

Modelling is the demonstration that another patient

(the model) can accept dental treatment without concern. Children, for example, can benefit by watching their parents' ready acceptance of treatment. Video can be useful.

Hypnosis (hypnosedation)

Hypnosis is a state of mind usually induced in one person by another, in which suggestions are more readily accepted and acted upon more powerfully than in the alert state. The depth of hypnosis is variable from person to person and is reduced if the subject is suspicious, anxious of losing control, or deliberately resists hypnosis. Hypnosis can, however, be useful either alone or in conjunction with sedation (see Chapter 9) for the management of anxious patients.

PSYCHOGENIC ASPECTS OF ORAL DISEASE

Facial pain in particular but also other oral complaints may have a psychogenic basis (Volume 2): there is even a 'syndrome of oral complaints'. Unfortunate life events such as bereavement, financial problems, chronic illness in the family, marital or work difficulties all appear to act as stress situations predisposing to orofacial psychogenic pain and other complaints.

Many dentists appear, perhaps because of their training with emphasis on mechanical techniques, to find difficulty in accepting that illness may have a psychogenic basis, but the facts are there, and they underline the need to treat the whole patient, not solely his mouth.

THE 'DIFFICULT PATIENT'

One of the most stressful aspects of dentistry, as seen from the dentist's point of view, is the 'difficult patient', namely the awkward, unco-operative, complaining or abusive patient. People with such characteristics will always exist, but it is remarkable how dentists with poor social skills seem to meet them with greater frequency than those who are socially skillful. Anxiety or a feeling that the dentist is being impersonal or uncommunicative often provokes this type of behaviour in patients who otherwise might be relatively co-operative and content. All patients expect to be treated courteously and with respect, even though only a minority become 'difficult' if not so managed.

FURTHER READING

Corah N. L., O'Shea R. M., Bissell G. D. (1986). The dentist–patient relationship: mutual perceptions and behaviour. *JADA,* **113**: 253–255.

Freeman R. E. (1985). Dental anxiety: a multifactoral aetiology. *Br. dent. J.,* **159**: 406–408.

Furnham A. (1983). Social skills and dentistry. *Br. dent. J.,* **154**: 404–408.

Giangrego E. (1986). Controlling anxiety in the dental office. *JADA,* **113**: 728–735.

Hall N., Edmondson H. D. (1983). The aetiology and psychology of dental fear. *Br. dent. J.,* **154**: 247–252.

O'Shea R. M., Corah N. L., Ayer W. A. (1986). Why patients change dentists: practitioners' views. *JADA,* **112**: 851–853.

Scott D., Hirschman R. (1982). Psychological aspects of dental anxiety in adults. *JADA,* **104**: 27–31.

Wardle J. (1982). Fear of dentistry. *Br. J. med. Psychol.,* **55**: 119–126.

Chapter 2 ✓

The history, diagnosis and treatment planning

Treatment of any condition can only be effective if an accurate diagnosis has been made, i.e. the nature of the disease has been established (Greek: *dia* = through; *gignoskein* = knowledge).

Diagnosis is made on the basis of the **history** of the complaint and also, in most cases, on the findings from **examination**. In some instances special **investigations** (such as radiographs) will help diagnosis and/or treatment planning or prognosis.

Prognosis is the prediction of the probable course of a disease in an individual and the chances of recovery. It is a prediction which should be based upon a sound knowledge and understanding of the disease and available treatments, and an assessment of the particular host response of the patient in question. Clearly an accurate diagnosis is a prerequisite for an effective treatment plan and accurate prognosis.

Treatment may be **medical** in nature (for example, antimicrobial therapy) or, often in dentistry, **surgical** in nature (for example, drainage of a fluctuant abscess), or may include a combination of methods. Unless a correct diagnosis has been made, treatment planning can only be empirical.

THE HISTORY

A history *must* be taken from every patient in order to make a diagnosis. Many conditions, such as facial pain, are often diagnosed on the basis of history alone. Nevertheless, even though, for example, in idiopathic trigeminal neuralgia there are no positive examination findings or useful positive investigations, an examination is always required to exclude organic disease, and some investigations may be warranted.

Taking a history is something of an art, based on a knowledge of disease processes, psychology, and experience. Students often find this difficult in the beginning since there should be a balance between encouraging patients to explain symptoms and medical history in their own words while at the same time ensuring that a basic set of questions is answered in sufficient depth and within a reasonably brief period of time. The history-taker has to act as a computer, sorting a jumble of facts into a semblance of order. Only practice makes perfect, but the following plan, which has very wide acceptance, should be followed in order to give structure to the interview (Table 2.1).

C.O. (complaining of). This should indicate, very concisely, the complaint, or complaints (e.g. facial pain).

H.P.C. (history of present complaint) or H.P.I. (history of present illness). Under this heading we need to know the duration of the illness; site of symptoms; character; exacerbating or relieving factors; any obvious precipitating event, etc. For example, in the case of facial pain, we should elicit:

The duration: when did the pain begin?
The site: where is the pain? Is it always in the same site?
The character: is the pain dull, sharp, or throbbing? Is it

Table 2.1
The history

Complaining of (C.O.)
History of present complaint (H.P.C.)
Past dental history (P.D.H.)
Social history (S.H.)
Family history (F.H.)
General medical history (G.M.H.)

---

persistent or intermittent? How long do episodes last? Does it occur at any particular time of day or night? Does it radiate elsewhere?

Exacerbating or relieving factors: is it worse with sweet foods? Is it worse with hot or cold? Is it worse on moving the head? Does anything else exacerbate it? Is it relieved by aspirin or paracetamol? Does anything else relieve it?

Any obvious precipitating event: did any obvious event precipitate the disease?

P.D.H. (past dental history). This may be relevant in terms of treatment planning especially. For example, the patient who has only attended previously when in pain and has then sought only extractions is hardly likely to want or be suitable for molar endodontics.

S.H. (social history). This should not be neglected since the needs and availability for treatment may differ quite substantially between an Antarctic explorer and a dental nurse. This aspect is especially important if the treatment or its sequelae are elective and likely to cause pain or swelling. For example, the surgical removal of wisdom teeth may best be deferred until the patient can arrange a suitable few days when his or her commitments and engagements can be cancelled or arrangements made to help care with children, dependent relatives, etc.

F.H. (family history). This may be relevant in some oral diseases (e.g. recurrent aphthae), and some systemic diseases that can affect dental treatment (e.g. haemophilia).

G.M.H. (general medical history) or *P.M.H. (past medical history)* or *R.M.H. (relevant medical history)*. With improvements in social and medical care, an increasing number of patients with fairly serious systemic disease now survive and need dental care. Systemic disease may influence dental treatment because of direct complications from the disease (e.g. a bleeding tendency will make surgical procedures hazardous), or because dental procedures or anaesthesia may need to be modified (e.g. general anaesthesia is a hazard in patients with heart disease), or because certain procedures are contraindicated (e.g. in pregnancy the use of drugs such as tetracyclines is contraindicated).

The most common important systemic problems that influence dental care are a bleeding tendency, cardiovascular and respiratory diseases, diabetes, epilepsy, immune defects, various infectious disorders and certain drugs. Some of the most serious difficulties arise when general anaesthesia is used and its use should therefore be fully justified, or an alternative used.

A medical history must be taken for every patient and it is prudent to recheck the history before any surgical procedure or the administration of general anaesthesia, since the patients' health may have changed since the history was taken.

Although patients must be encouraged to give the medical history in their own words, it must also be channelled so as to supply answers to certain particularly relevant points, viz:

Anaemia
Bleeding tendency
Cardiovascular and respiratory diseases
Drug treatment, drug addiction, drug allergies and reactions, and conditions with specific drug contraindications
Endocrine disorders
Fits and faints
Gastrointestinal disorders
Hospital admissions and operations
Infections
Jaundice or liver disease
Kidney disorders
Likelihood of pregnancy

Few patients give an absolutely clear and concise history, but it is the duty of the dentist to elicit the above points. Answers may be suggested indirectly, for example by drug treatment, e.g. patients with cardiac failure rarely know their diagnosis but they do know that they are on diuretics (or 'water pills'). Some patients carry cards or wear special bracelets warning of a relevant medical history (Figs. 2.1 and 2.2). It is the duty of the dentist to check with the patient's doctor if in any doubt. It is also the duty of the dentist to call for an interpreter if there are language difficulties.

The astute dentist will also observe his patient during the taking of the medical history, to detect any behavioural characteristics (anxiety, etc.) and any lesions obvious on face, neck or hands which might suggest systemic or local disease.

ANAEMIAS

Anaemia is a reduction in the haemoglobin level below the normal for age and sex.

Anaemia can:

(a) be a contraindication to general anaesthesia because the oxygen-carrying capacity of the blood is reduced;

(b) be a manifestation of a more serious disease, such as leukaemia;

(c) produce oral lesions.

Deficiency anaemias, such as due to deficiencies of iron, folic acid or vitamin B_{12}, may produce glossitis,

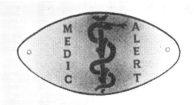

Front of disc, worn on stainless steel chain bracelet.

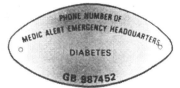

Reverse of disc, with engraving.

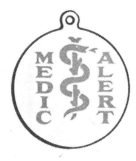

Front of disc worn on necklet chain.

Fig. 2.1 *Medic alert warning of relevant medical history. There are several other companies which run similar systems.*

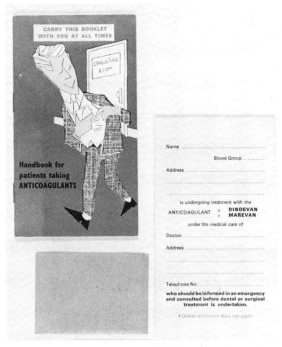

Fig. 2.2 *Warning card and handbook for patients on anti-coagulant treatment.*

angular stomatitis and mouth ulcers. In the early stages, where there is no true anaemia, patients with deficiency states may also complain of a sore or burning sensation, especially in the tongue. The cause of the deficiency state must be sought and, if the diet is adequate, clearly the patient is either not absorbing the iron or vitamins, or the body is failing to utilize them (Volume 2).

Diagnosis

Apart from the oral features mentioned, the patient may suffer the following.

1. *Pallor.* This is not usually obvious unless the haemoglobin level is very low; in contrast, many 'pale' persons prove not to be anaemic. Pallor is best checked in the nailbeds or palmar creases; inspection of conjunctiva for pallor can be misleading because conjunctivitis can confuse the diagnosis. Pallor can be difficult to detect in the oral mucosa.

2. *Breathlessness,* particularly on exercise.
3. *Tachycardia.*
4. *Palpitations.*
5. *Tiredness and lassitude.*

The following blood tests are required.

1. Haemoglobin estimation.
2. Red blood cell indices and blood film. Reduction in MCV (mean cell volume of red cells) is termed microcytosis, while an increase is termed macrocytosis. In the UK, the most common cause of microcytosis is iron deficiency due to chronic bleeding as in menorrhagia (heavy periods). Macrocytosis is usually caused by folic acid deficiency, alcoholism or vitamin B_{12} deficiency.

A blood film examination may show abnormalities in size and shape of red cells as well as white cell changes.

3. White cell count and differential. Anaemia is a feature of some white cell diseases, especially leukaemia, and therefore a total white cell count and differential count are required in the investigation of anaemia.

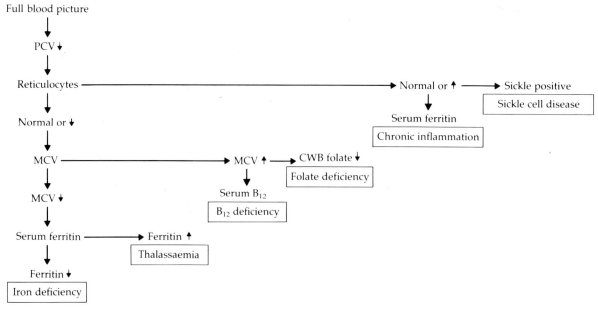

Fig. 2.3 *Diagnosis of anaemia. (PCV, packed cell volume; MCV, mean cell volume; CWB, corrected whole blood.)*

4. Other tests if sickle cell disease or another haemoglobinopathy is suspected (see below).

If anaemia is diagnosed, the type should then be established by other investigations (as shown in Fig. 2.3), and the *cause* of deficiency states should be sought before treatment is offered.

Most anaemia in the UK is caused by chronic bleeding in women who have heavy periods (menorrhagia) and who consequently become iron deficient. Deficiencies of folic acid and vitamin B_{12} are far less common. Folic acid deficiency in the UK is usually a result of a diet lacking green vegetables, often in elderly patients, or alcoholism. Vitamin B_{12} deficiency in the UK is usually caused by pernicious anaemia. Deficiency anaemias may cause a sore mouth or other oral lesions (see above and Volume 2).

Sickle cell disease

This is a hereditary condition found mainly but not exclusively in Blacks (Fig. 2.4). General anaesthesia is potentially dangerous in affected patients since not only is the oxygen-carrying capacity of the blood reduced but a haemolytic crisis may be precipitated if there is any hypoxia associated with general anaesthesia.

The haemoglobin in sickle cell disease is abnormal (haemoglobinopathy) so that erythrocytes alter shape to a sickle form if there is hypoxia, block small vessels to

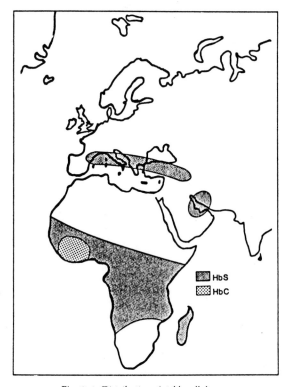

Fig. 2.4 *Distribution of sickle cell diseases.*

produce infarcts, and haemolyse. The homozygous sickle cell *anaemia* (in which there is no normal haemoglobin) is uncommon (occurring in less than 0.2% of UK Blacks), but is the anaemia causing the main danger in dentistry. It is rarely seen in the absence of severe anaemia. The heterozygous sickle cell *trait* is more common (in almost 9% of UK Blacks), but patients are not always anaemic, since they have some normal haemoglobin, and anaesthetic management is easier.

Diagnosis

1. Check the medical and family history for known sickle cell disease.

2. Screen all Black patients who have not already been tested with:

(a) full blood picture (haemoglobin: red blood cell indices and blood film),

(b) sickle screening test (Sickledex test: Fig. 2.5)

(c) haemoglobin electrophoresis in those positive in (b) above.

Haemoglobinopathy warning cards are now available.

Management in sickle cell anaemia or trait

Since even mild hypoxia can prove fatal in the homozygous sickle cell *anaemia, general anaesthesia must only be given by a specialist anaesthetist, in hospital.* Patients who have sickle cell haemoglobin together with another abnormal haemoglobin, especially those with sickle cell/haemoglobin C disease, are at similar risk during general anaesthesia (Fig. 2.6).

Most patients with sickle cell *trait*, provided that they have a normal haemoglobin level and no other haemoglobinopathy, can be given outpatient general anaesthesia as long as there is full oxygenation.

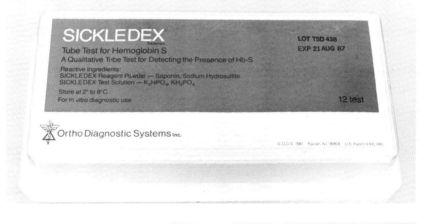

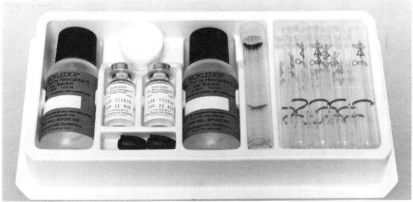

Fig. 2.5 *Sickledex test for haemoglobins.*

Sickle cell
anaemia

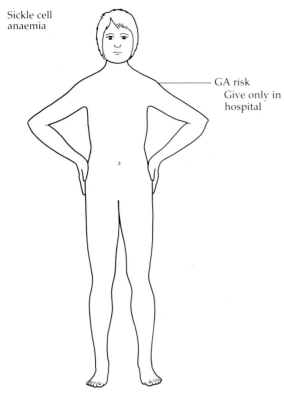

GA risk
Give only in
hospital

Fig. 2.6 *Main management problems in sickle cell anaemia.*

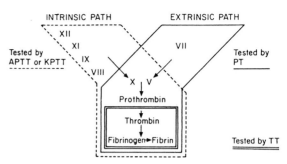

Fig. 2.7 *The blood clotting cascade. (APTT: activated partial thromboplastin time; KPTT: kaolin partial thromboplastin time; PT: prothrombin time; TT: thrombin time.)*

Local anaesthetics can be safely used either in sickle cell anaemia or trait.

Some suggest the need for an antimicrobial cover for surgery in patients with sickle cell anaemia since there is a slight immune defect and predisposition to infection.

Thalassaemia

Thalassaemia is a haemoglobinopathy especially common in Mediterranean peoples. Marrow expansion may lead to maxillary enlargement ('chipmunk facies'). Repeated transfusions used in the treatment of thalassaemia may predispose to bloodborne viral infections.

BLEEDING TENDENCY

Haemorrhage usually ceases because damaged blood vessels constrict and become plugged with platelets and the blood clots (Fig. 2.7). Most prolonged bleeding after oral surgical procedures is a consequence of local causes such as trauma (particularly to soft tissues) or interference with blood clot by tongue pushing, rinsing the mouth, etc. Therefore, after any oral surgical procedure where there has been bleeding, patients should be advised to eat on the other side of the mouth, avoid hot food or alcohol for the rest of the day, and not to interfere with the operation site.

The possibility of a systemic cause must be excluded if the history or features suggest a bleeding tendency, as follows.

1. Previous bleeding for more than 36 hours or bleeding restarting after 36 hours after operation, particularly if on more than one occasion.
2. Previous admission to hospital to arrest bleeding.
3. Previous blood transfusions for bleeding.
4. Spontaneous bleeding, for example into joints, from little obvious cause.
5. A convincing family history of one of the above, combined with a degree of personal history.
6. Current or recent treatment by drugs that produce a bleeding tendency, such as anticoagulants, aspirin, or sodium valproate (an anticonvulsant).
7. Systemic disease which may cause a bleeding tendency, such as any cause of platelet or clotting factor defects including leukaemia, AIDS, liver or kidney disease.
8. Warning cards carried by some patients (see Fig. 2.2).

The following features suggest a bleeding tendency.

1. Bruising or purpura of the skin (Fig. 2.8).
2. Oral purpura which may be seen anywhere but particularly in the soft palate. There may be spontaneous gingival bleeding.
3. Pallor or other signs of anaemia, if there is associated anaemia from blood loss or in leukaemia.

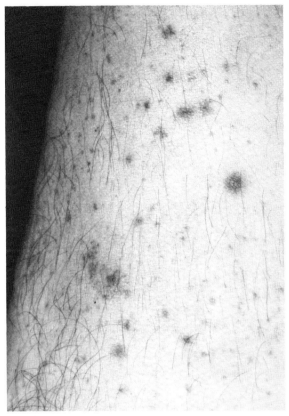

Fig. 2.8 *Purpura of the skin.*

Laboratory investigations if a systemic cause of bleeding tendency is suspected (Fig. 2.9)

Whole-blood clotting time is now obsolete and functional tests such as activated partial thromboplastin time (APTT) and prothrombin time (PT) are more useful. However, the tests required must be discussed first with the haematologist.

Basic tests include (Table 2.2):

(a) haemoglobin level,
(b) full blood picture,
(c) white cell count and differential,
(d) platelet count and possibly the 'bleeding time'.

Systemic causes of a bleeding tendency

A bleeding tendency results from defects in any of the three phases of haemostasis, viz:

(a) vascular,

(b) platelet,
(c) blood coagulation.

Vascular and platelet disorders give rise to purpura, the term given to bleeding beneath epithelium which produces ecchymoses (bruising) or petechiae (pin-point haemorrhages). There is commonly also spontaneous bleeding from the gingival margins. The easy bruisability of healthy young women is not unlike true purpura but is not usually associated with a bleeding tendency.

In the coagulation defects, bleeding typically is into deeper tissues such as joints or the muscles of the posterior abdominal wall, and only rarely is spontaneous oral haemorrhage.

Purpura

Purpura is characterized by:

(a) a bleeding tendency in which bleeding is continuous from the time of injury;
(b) spontaneous haemorrhage into skin and mucosa and from the gingival margins;
(c) a prolonged 'bleeding time';
(d) normal coagulation studies.

Petechiae may occur distal to the tourniquet of a sphygmomanometer cuff but this Hess test is of limited value only.

Purpura is usually caused by a reduced number of platelets (thrombocytopenia), but may be a result of defective platelet or vascular action.

1. *Acute leukaemia.* Thrombocytopenia is almost invariable in acute leukaemia.
2. *Idiopathic thrombocytopenic purpura* (ITP). This is an autoimmune disorder affecting young females predominantly. The thrombocytopenia may respond to corticosteroids and/or splenectomy.
3. *Drugs.* Various drugs, including aspirin and corticosteroids, induce purpura either by affecting the whole bone marrow or by inhibiting platelets alone.
4. *Other causes.* Connective tissue diseases, AIDS, old age, von Willebrand's disease, scurvy, and various vascular disorders may be responsible.

Dental management for platelet defects

Fresh platelet concentrates should be transfused before any surgical procedures if platelet counts are below 80×10^9/litre. Drugs capable of producing a bleeding tendency must be avoided (p. 12).

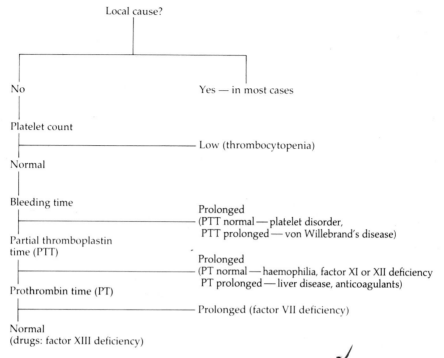

Fig. 2.9 *Investigation of postoperative bleeding.*

Table 2.2
Clinical and laboratory findings in bleeding disorders

	Clotting defect	Platelet defect
Sex affected	Males (inherited defects)	Either
Nature of bleeding	Delayed but then persistent	Early onset
Spontaneous bleeding into skin or mucosa, or from mucosa	Uncommon	Common
Deep bleeding	Common	Rare
Bleeding time	Normal	Prolonged
Platelet count	Normal	Often low
APTT	Prolonged in most defects	Normal
PT	Prolonged in patients on anticoagulants and in those with liver disease	Normal

APTT: activated partial thromboplastin time.
PT: prothrombin time.

Coagulation (clotting) defects

Clotting defects are characterized by the following (Table 2.2).

1. A bleeding tendency in which bleeding may appear to cease immediately after injury (since vascular and platelet phases of haemostasis are unaffected), only to recur after a short delay—and persist. Bleeding continues until treatment with the missing factors is instituted. Failure to recognize and treat the bleeding can lead to death of the patient.

2. Spontaneous haemorrhage into deeper tissues such as joints with consequent deformities. Bleeding into the fascial spaces of the neck (for example after a regional dental local anaesthetic injection—which is contraindicated) may obstruct the airway. After a head injury, intracranial bleeding may be fatal.

3. Normal 'bleeding time'.

4. Abnormal coagulation studies. In haemophiliacs, typical findings are:

   (a) prolonged APTT,
   (b) normal PT,
   (c) reduced level of specific clotting factors: reduced factor VIII in classic haemophilia (haemophilia A) and some patients with von Willebrand's disease; reduced factor IX in haemophilia B (Christmas disease).

In patients on anticoagulant drugs typical findings are:

   (a) normal APTT,
   (b) prolonged PT.

Causes of clotting defects include the following.

1. *Anticoagulant drugs*

Although heparin is injected to prevent deep vein thrombosis and thromboembolism at, and after, some operations, and is used during renal haemodialysis, oral drugs (particularly warfarin) are used in most other instances where anticoagulation is required. Heparin only acts for a few hours but oral anticoagulants persist for many hours.

Dental management of patients on anticoagulants

Anticoagulant drugs produce a liability to postoperative bleeding. Any drug such as aspirin that increases this tendency should therefore be avoided (see above). Minor oral surgery may be carried out if patients are orally anticoagulated only to usual therapeutic levels (prothrombin time of up to twice normal) and only a few teeth are to be extracted, with minimal trauma but careful suturing. Oral anticoagulant treatment is not usually reduced preoperatively as there is then a danger of rebound *hypercoagulability* and thrombosis. However, if more major surgery is needed, the physician must be consulted as a reduction in oral anticoagulation is almost invariably indicated for the perioperative period. Bleeding can also be controlled with vitamin K injections, plasma, or antifibrinolytic agents (e.g. tranexamic acid).

Heparin anticoagulation effect resolves within 6–9 hours of administration so that, in patients on heparin, oral surgery can be carried out after a delay of 6–9 hours from an injection of heparin.

2. *Liver disease*

Liver disease can cause a bleeding tendency because of:

   (a) failure of synthesis of clotting factors by the diseased liver;
   (b) malabsorption of vitamin K (needed for synthesis of clotting factors) because of obstruction to the flow of bile to the gut where bile salts are needed for the absorption of the fat-soluble vitamin K.

Dental management of patients with liver disease

Bleeding in liver disease can be difficult to control and, although vitamin K injections may help, can be persistent.

3. *Haemophilias*

Haemophilias A and B are inherited as sex-linked recessive characters and affect males only; von Willebrand's disease is inherited as an autosomal dominant condition and affects either sex.

Haemophilia A is some ten times more common than Christmas disease and is therefore discussed in some detail, but most of the comments apply to both disorders. Von Willebrand's disease has some of the features and problems of haemophilia plus those of purpura.

Problems affecting haemophiliacs (Fig. 2.10)

1. Bleeding tendency, leading to serious spontaneous and post-traumatic haemorrhage that can be fatal.

2. Consequences of repeated administration of blood or blood products, possibly including:

   (a) hepatitis B virus and delta agent infection (see below);
   (b) hepatitis non-A, non-B virus infections (see below);
   (c) infection with human immune deficiency virus—HIV—the AIDS virus (see below);

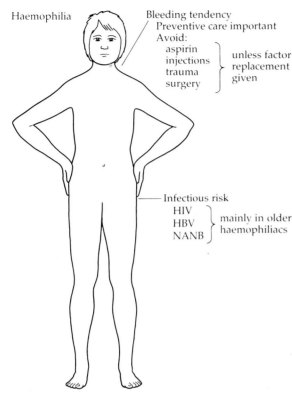

Haemophilia

Bleeding tendency
Preventive care important
Avoid:
  aspirin
  injections
  trauma
  surgery
} unless factor
  replacement
  given

Infectious risk
  HIV
  HBV
  NANB
} mainly in older
  haemophiliacs

Fig. 2.10 *Management problems in haemophilia A and B.*

(d) other viral infections;
(e) antibodies directed against factor VIII.

Dental management of patients with coagulation defects

It is extremely important to:

(a) prevent dental disease;
(b) plan treatment, particularly surgery, in order to re-duce the number of occasions when factor replacement has to be given, particularly to reduce the complications outlined above;
(c) control cross-infection.

Operative intervention

In general terms, intramuscular injections should be avoided. Trauma must be reduced to the very minimum and, when analgesics are needed, those such as aspirin that may enhance the bleeding tendency, or induce gas-tric bleeding, should be avoided. Paracetamol is a safe

alternative in this respect. Factor replacement and/or antifibrinolytics are required to prevent serious haemor-rhage if the patient has surgery. In a *few* instances, anti-fibrinolytics (e.g. tranexamic acid) or other drugs (e.g. DDAVP: desmopressin) alone are enough to aid haemo-stasis.

Anaesthesia

Regional local anaesthetic injections are best avoided unless the patient is receiving adequate factor replace-ment at the time, since there is a danger of bleeding into the fascial spaces of the neck, and hence obstruction of the airway. Intraligamentary or infiltration local anaesthe-sia may be used as an alternative.

Periodontal treatment

Scaling can be carried out in most mild cases using tranexamic acid as a cover. For severe haemophiliacs, or for any patient who requires periodontal surgery, factor replacement is needed.

Restorative treatment

Minor trauma such as may occur with the placement of matrix bands, or during endodontic treatment, can usually be adequately controlled by tranexamic acid cover.

Surgery of any kind

Before surgery, factor replacement is essential and patients should be treated in hospital, preferably in one with a haemophilia centre. Preoperatively, the following should be assessed.

1. Haemoglobin level.
2. Factor VIII assay.

The regime indicated depends on:

(a) the severity of operative trauma expected,
(b) the severity of the haemophilia.

Blood should be grouped and serum saved for cross-matching. Factor VIII replacement is usually given as fac-tor VIII concentrate. This may be supplemented with antifibrinolytic agents such as tranexamic acid, or occa-sionally, in mild haemophilia, with desmopressin (DDAVP).

Table 2.3 indicates the principles of factor replacement.

Table 2.3
Factor replacement for haemophiliacs requiring dental surgery

Operation	Factor VIII level required at operation	Immediately preoperatively give intravenous	Postoperative schedule
Minor oral surgery	Minimum of 50%	Factor VIII	Rest in-patient for 7 days; soft diet; penicillin V
Maxillofacial surgery	100% at operation	Factor VIII	Rest in-patient for 10 days; soft diet; twice-daily Factor VIII; penicillin V

A factor VIII level of 50%–75% is usually needed for surgery to be safely carried out and it is usual to give an antimicrobial (such as penicillin V 250 mg four times daily) postoperatively to help prevent infection and reduce the chance of secondary haemorrhage.

CARDIOVASCULAR DISEASE

Dentists are properly concerned to avoid cardiovascular collapse or deterioration in patients with pre-existing heart disease undergoing dental treatment, particularly under general anaesthesia, even though other forms of emotional or physical stress (or even exercise testing by physicians!) are likely to be as dangerous. The special risk of infective endocarditis arising from dental bacteraemia is important, but ischaemic heart disease and hypertension are much more common. While patients may volunteer a history of heart problems, inferences from the drug history may be the most useful source of information to the dentist.

Ischaemic heart disease and hypertension

The risk of harm from dental treatment generally arises more from inadequate control of anxiety and pain than from the treatment itself. 'Tender loving care' is of prime importance and a kind, confident and sympathetic approach is therapeutic in itself. Sedation with oral diazepam, or nitrous oxide and oxygen inhalation (relative analgesia) is safe, if needed, but intravenous agents should be used very cautiously and general anaesthesia should be avoided. Local analgesia using lignocaine 2%, with 1/80 000 adrenaline is safe and effective. Adrenaline-free local anaesthetic solutions are not effective, noradrenaline is unsafe, and prilocaine with felypressin produces less reliable anaesthesia than lignocaine with adrenaline (see Chapter 6).

Sensible management should include preventive dentistry, and treatment planning to avoid lengthy or difficult procedures. It is important to ensure that patients have taken their normal medication on the day of their visit to the surgery, and they should ideally be accompanied by a responsible adult. The surgery must of course be equipped for resuscitation and the staff trained to cope with any emergency which might arise (see Chapter 4).

Hypertensive patients do not bleed excessively after dental operations and should simply be treated as described. Anticoagulated patients are at risk of prolonged bleeding after oral surgery and they should ideally be tested in a hospital prothrombin clinic to determine their current level of anticoagulation (see above). The dentist must be available to provide control of bleeding by local methods in the first 24 hours, if required.

Patients with angina should bring their anti-anginal medication and keep it available during the dental appointment. Dental treatment in those with a recent heart attack (myocardial infarction) is probably best left until after 6 months, especially if general anaesthesia is needed.

Ultrasonic scalers, electric pulp testers, diathermy or electrosurgery, can upset pacemaker function, and this type of dental equipment should not be used for patients whose cardiac rhythm is controlled by a pacemaker.

Patients who have had coronary artery bypass grafts do not risk infective endocarditis following dental surgery and are usually fitter to withstand dental treatment after than they were before the cardiac operation.

Valvular and other heart disease predisposing to infective endocarditis

Valvular heart disease is usually either congenital or arises from rheumatic carditis following rheumatic fever (St Vitus' dance; Sydenham's chorea). It predisposes patients to infective endocarditis (Table 2.4). The bacter-

Table 2.4
Risk groups for infective endocarditis

Congenital heart disease
Rheumatic heart disease
Prosthetic heart valves
Previous history of endocarditis
Other less common conditions

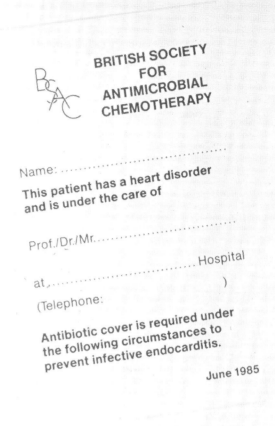

Fig. 2.11 *Warning card of need for antibiotic cover.*

aemia that occurs when a tooth is extracted, or when the periodontium is damaged in scaling or flap surgery etc., may result in oral micro-organisms settling upon, and infecting minute, transient vegetations on the already damaged valves (infective endocarditis). Oral organisms involved are usually streptococci of the viridans group, particularly *Strep. sanguis, S. mitior* or *S. mutans*.

Other uncommon but important risk groups, such as patients who have had valve-replacement surgery and those who have already suffered an attack of endocarditis, are important not so much in having enhanced susceptibility but in having a poor prognosis should they contract endocarditis. The hospital mortality for those 1 in 8 streptococcal cases associated with dentistry is quite low, but the figures conceal a considerable long-term morbidity (< 50% survival at 8 years).

Attempts to prevent the disease by avoiding, reducing or combating the effects of dental bacteraemia are therefore well worthwhile, despite the lack of convincing evidence of their success.

Identification of the patient at risk from infective endocarditis

The first step is identification of the patient at risk, and, while the highest risk groups have the clearest history, there is no doubt that patients with trivial heart murmurs and minor congenital heart defects can and do contract endocarditis. An uncertain history has to be taken as positive until further clarified by consultation with a physician. Some patients carry a warning card of the need for antibiotic cover (Fig. 2.11).

General treatment planning and preventive dentistry

Preventive dentistry is especially important for these patients. Comprehensive dental treatment planning, with

an assessment of the prognosis of the patient's whole mouth for life, is essential. Urgent risk-producing procedures should be accomplished first, and in one visit if possible. Periodontal disease with tooth mobility, periapical disease and pericoronitis must be eliminated. Root canal therapy is acceptable, provided a good prognosis can be assured. Maintenance of good oral hygiene is essential and, in some cases, is encouraged by the suggestion of dental clearance as an alternative. Diet counselling, fluoride supplementation and topical application, and fissure sealing may all have a role in preventing caries, especially in younger patients (Volume 3). All patients must be encouraged to attend for regular oral re-examination, ideally even if they have full dentures (endocarditis has occasionally occurred in wearers of full dentures).

Preoperative precautions

Extraction, scaling and surgery involving the gingival margin are the dental operations which often cause significant bacteraemia. The number of bacteria dispersed into the circulation can be greatly reduced by preoperative mouthwashes and gingival irrigation with an antiseptic such as 0.2% aqueous chlorhexidine. However, the effects of bacteraemia are best combated by giving an antibiotic that produces bactericidal levels in the blood during the period of bacteraemia. The antibiotic should only be given 1–2 hours preoperatively, since otherwise resistant organisms might arise; and should be effectively bactericidal for at least, say, 4 hours.

The correct choice of antibiotic for prophylaxis and the mode and timing of administration have long been controversial, but recent recommendations of a Working Party of the British Society for Antimicrobial Chemotherapy provide a commonsense approach to the problem, using oral amoxycillin, which is extremely well absorbed and gives high blood levels lasting 9–10 hours (see Chapter 7). There is some doubt about the efficacy of the recommended single 3-g oral dose of amoxycillin, and animal studies suggest that two 3-g doses may be more secure. The drug is marketed in the UK in a double 3-g sachet pack (Fig. 2.12), which is convenient for this purpose, one sachet being used for the preoperative dose and the second given to the patient to take about 6 hours later. The extra single oral dose on the same day is likely to be remembered and taken reliably.

The recommended antibiotic prophylaxis is therefore as follows:

Amoxycillin—3 g orally 1 hour before surgery and 3 g orally 6 hours after.
Or, when a penicillin is ruled out because of hypersensitivity or recent exposure:
erythromycin stearate—1.5 g orally 1 hour before treatment and 500 mg later.
Or, when there are other complicating factors, such as general anaesthesia or multiple drug allergies:
consult the BSAC Working Party Guidelines or seek hospital advice (Table 2.5).
And use local antisepsis in all cases (such as chlorhexidine).

Postoperative precautions

Since early diagnosis of endocarditis greatly promotes successful treatment, risk patients should be warned to report to the dentist or physician any symptoms which

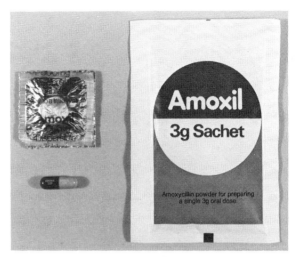

Fig. 2.12 *Amoxycillin preparations.*

occur in the month after dental treatment, however apparently minor and non-specific.

The study of this fascinating disease and its prevention have been greatly aided by the use of the rabbit experimental model. In animals whose valves and endocardium have been subjected to minor trauma from the passage of a plastic cannula, platelet/fibrin vegetations are formed. Following an inoculum of an appropriate micro-organism, the vegetations become infected and the animals develop an infective endocarditis which mimics the human condition closely. Studies of prophylaxis in this model are a valid guide to clinical practice, provided they are used to make comparisons between drugs and timings and not taken as absolute proof of efficacy.

RESPIRATORY DISEASE

Upper respiratory tract infections

The common cold

The common cold syndrome can be caused by many different viruses, usually a rhinovirus. The clinical features are of nasal discharge and obstruction, nasopharyngeal soreness and mild systemic upset. Earache may result from obstruction of the pharyngotympanic tube by oedema or, more seriously, by bacterial infection of the middle ear (otitis media). Sinusitis may develop and cause facial pain and tenderness.

Table 2.5
Antibiotic cover

General anaesthesia

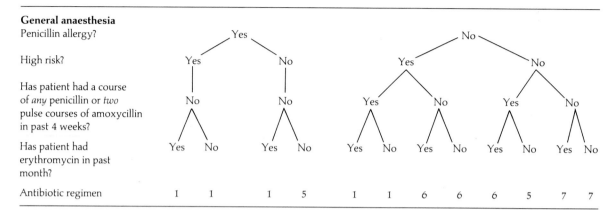

Penicillin allergy?			Yes					No			
High risk?		Yes		No		Yes			No		
Has patient had a course of *any* penicillin or *two* pulse courses of amoxycillin in past 4 weeks?		No		No		Yes		No		Yes	No
Has patient had erythromycin in past month?	Yes	No	Yes	No	Yes	No	Yes	No	Yes	No	Yes	No
Antibiotic regimen	1	1	1	5	1	1	6	6	6	5	7	7

1. *Intravenous* vancomycin 1 g by *slow* infusion over 1 hour followed by 120 mg gentamicin *i.v.* before operation.
5. *Oral* erythromycin 1.5 g (Stearate) *2 hours* preoperatively taken with *no more* than 10 ml water, *then* 500 mg orally 6 hours later.
6. *Intramuscular* ampicillin 1 g (in 2.5 ml 1% lignocaine) *plus* 120 mg gentamicin *i.m.* 30 minutes before operation, *then* 500 mg amoxycillin orally 6 hours later. (N.B. *Oral* amoxycillin 3 g may be given *2 hours* preoperatively in *no more* than 10 ml water with *i.m.* gentamicin.)
7. *Intramuscular* ampicillin 1 g in 2.5 ml 1% lignocaine 30 minutes preoperatively. (N.B. *Oral* amoxycillin 3 g may be given *2 hours* preoperatively in *no more* than 10 ml water.) *Then* 500 mg amoxycillin *orally* 6 hours later.

Children's dosages

Amoxycillin ⎱
Ampicillin ⎰ under 10 years—half adult dose.
Erythromycin ⎰ under 5 years—one-quarter adult dose.

Gentamicin: under 10 years—2 mg/kg body weight.

Vancomycin: 20 mg/kg body weight.

Pharyngitis and tonsillitis

Most cases of pharyngitis and tonsillitis are caused by viruses but other agents, especially *Streptococcus pyogenes, Mycoplasma pneumoniae, Epstein–Barr virus* infection or, rarely, *Corynebacterium diphtheriae,* may need to be considered in the differential diagnosis.

In streptococcal sore throat the throat is sore, with dysphagia and sometimes fever and conjunctivitis. Peritonsillar abscess (quinsy), scarlet fever, acute glomerulonephritis and rheumatic fever are rare complications. Therefore it is common practice to treat throat infections with an antimicrobial drug, often penicillin, even when the precise aetiological agent has not been identified.

Laryngotracheitis

Hoarseness, loss of voice and persistent cough are common in laryngotracheitis, which in children may also cause partial laryngeal obstruction by oedema, and may cause noisy inspiration (stridor or croup). A similar sound occurs if there is airway obstruction from a foreign body (see Chapter 4).

Dental management in upper respiratory tract infections

Most upper respiratory tract infections are innocuous and have no oral manifestations. Dental treatment is best de-

Table 2.5 (*continued*)
Antibiotic cover

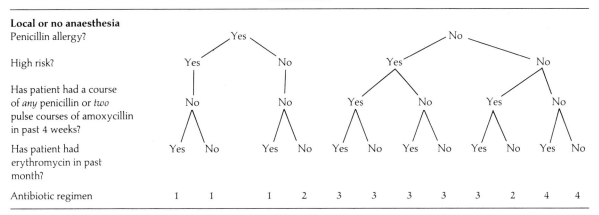

Local or no anaesthesia

Penicillin allergy?			Yes					No			
High risk?		Yes		No		Yes				No	
Has patient had a course of *any* penicillin or *two* pulse courses of amoxycillin in past 4 weeks?		No		No		Yes	No		Yes		No
Has patient had erythromycin in past month?	Yes	No	Yes	No	Yes	No	Yes	No	Yes	No	Yes	No
Antibiotic regimen	1	1	1	2	3	3	3	3	3	2	4	4

1. *Intravenous* vancomycin 1 g by *slow* infusion over 1 hour followed by 120 mg gentamicin *i.v.* before operation.
2. *Oral* erythromycin 1.5 g (Stearate) 1 hour before operation then 500 mg orally 6 hours later.
3. *Oral* amoxycillin 3 g 1 hour before operation *plus* 120 mg gentamicin *i.m.* 30 minutes before operation. *Then* 500 mg amoxycillin orally 6 hours later.
4. *Oral* amoxycillin 3 g 1 hour before operation.

Children's dosages

Amoxycillin ⎫
Ampicillin ⎬ under 10 years—half adult dose.
Erythromycin ⎭ under 5 years—one-quarter adult dose.

Gentamicin: under 10 years—2 mg/kg body weight.

Vancomycin: 20 mg/kg body weight.

ferred until recovery. General anaesthesia should usually be avoided since there is often a degree of respiratory obstruction, and infection can also be spread down to the lungs.

Sinusitis (see Volume 2)

Lower respiratory tract infections

Lower respiratory tract infections are frequently viral, although often complicated by bacterial infection.

Clinical features vary according to the part of the respiratory tract mainly affected. Bronchitis causes cough, wheezing and sometimes dyspnoea. Pneumonia is characterized by cough, fever, rapid respiration, breathlessness, chest pain, dyspnoea and shivering.

Pneumonia in a previously healthy individual is classed as primary (lobar pneumonia). Pneumonia (bronchopneumonia) may be secondary to some other disorder such as viral respiratory infections; aspiration of foreign material such as a tooth fragment; pre-existent lung disease, for example bronchiectasis or carcinoma; or depressed immunity, as a result, for example, of alcoholism. *Pneumocystis carinii* pneumonia is a typical feature in AIDS.

Dental management in lower respiratory tract infections

The majority of lower respiratory tract infections cause substantial incapacity and are contraindications to all but emergency dental treatment. Dental treatment should be deferred until recovery. General anaesthesia is absolutely contraindicated.

Chronic obstructive airways disease

Chronic bronchitis and emphysema are grouped together as chronic obstructive airways disease (COAD) or chronic obstructive pulmonary disease (COPD). Both are common in the UK, particularly in smokers. Severe COAD leads to respiratory failure and secondary cardiac failure (cor pulmonale).

Dental management

General anaesthesia (GA) and respiratory depressants such as diazepam or opiates are hazards to these patients. Local anaesthesia is the preferred form, although it may be feasible to give an outpatient GA if there is only mild COAD. Where a GA *must* be given, this should be in hospital. The patient should stop smoking at least one week before operation. Intravenous barbiturates are contraindicated in induction since laryngeal spasm may be precipitated and there can be severe respiratory depression. Postoperatively, chest physiotherapy and antimicrobials may be indicated.

Bronchial asthma

Bronchoconstriction, mucosal oedema and mucus hypersecretion impede breathing in asthma. Attacks can be precipitated by emotional stress, infections, some drugs (such as aspirin and mefenamic acid), and other factors. Avoidance of these may reduce the frequency of attacks but drug treatment with bronchodilators (e.g. salbutamol), corticosteroids or mast cell stabilizers (e.g. cromoglycate) is often required. Corticosteroid inhalers occasionally cause oropharyngeal candidosis (Volume 2).

Dental management of asthmatics

The asthmatic patient should be asked to bring his usual medication with him when he attends for dental care. Anxiety should be avoided as much as possible. Dental treatment is best carried out under local anaesthesia. Although relative analgesia *may* be given safely to mild asthmatics, GA must be avoided unless given in hospital and, in severe asthmatics, any treatment is best carried out in hospital. Allergies to penicillin and other drugs may be more frequent in asthmatics.

Emergencies are dealt with in Chapter 4.

Cystic fibrosis and bronchiectasis

Recurrent respiratory infections are common in cystic fibrosis. Bronchiectasis, in which bronchi became dilated, distorted and recurrently infected, may follow, and is also caused by other factors including various childhood infections.

Dental management in cystic fibrosis

Dental treatment should be carried out under local anaesthesia but, if GA is required, this is best given in hospital.

Pulmonary tuberculosis

Tuberculosis (TB) remains a relatively common disease in the UK, where it is a problem especially of immigrants from the Indian subcontinent, diabetics, alcoholics, vagrants and institutionalized patients and, increasingly, AIDS.

Pulmonary tuberculosis is usually contracted by the inhalation of *Mycobacterium tuberculosis* (or other mycobacteria) which cause lesions subpleurally and in the regional lymph nodes (primary complex). Haematogenous dissemination can lead to genitourinary, bone or joint lesions; the pulmonary lesions may extend and result in a pleural effusion; or lymph node tuberculosis may lead to pressure symptoms, for example on the bronchi. Miliary tuberculosis is characterized by widely disseminated lesions.

Post-primary tuberculosis usually follows the reactivation of an old primary pulmonary lesion and causes lesions ranging from a chronic fibrotic lesion to fulminating tuberculous pneumonia.

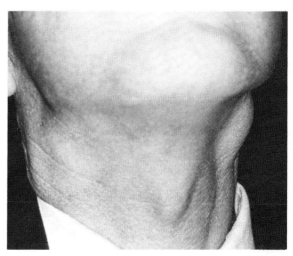

Fig. 2.13 *Cervical lymph node enlargement in tuberculosis.*

Tuberculosis formerly not infrequently involved the cervical lymph nodes, with chronic enlargement and caseation (scrofula). Bovine TB was often responsible but is now rare in the UK. Tuberculous cervical lymph nodes may still be seen, however, particularly in some immigrants (Fig. 2.13).

Dental staff are at risk from tuberculosis if treating patients with open pulmonary tuberculosis, who should be treated with precautions against cross-infection (see below and Chapter 7). Infected staff can also transmit TB to patients and a recent report showed transmission from a dentist to 15 patients!

General anaesthesia is contraindicated, since contamination of the anaesthetic apparatus is a hazard and pulmonary function may be impaired.

DRUG TREATMENT, ADDICTION, ALLERGIES AND REACTIONS

An increasing number of dental patients are receiving systemic medication from their physician, often with potent drugs.

Drug treatment can influence dental care in the following ways.

1. *The drugs may complicate operative intervention.* Anticoagulants and corticosteroids are the main drugs causing problems in dental treatment (see pp. 16 and 25).

2. *The drugs may cause oral complications.* Some drugs almost invariably cause oral side-effects, for example oral ulcers with some of the cytotoxic agents, while other drugs have few or no reported oral complications. The other most common drug-induced oral problems are candidosis, caused by tetracyclines, ampicillin or corticosteroids; gingival hyperplasia, induced by phenytoin, cyclosporin and nifedipine; and dry mouth, caused by many drugs with an atropinic action. Some of the drugs that may occasionally cause oral complications are shown in Table 2.6.

3. *The drugs may interact with drugs given during dental treatment.* Antihypertensive drugs may interact with general anaesthetics to produce severe hypotension, but other drug interactions are rare in general dental practice. If, however, GA is used, drug interactions are more likely. They are also more common in the elderly or medically handicapped patient. Some possible drug interactions are shown in Table 2.7.

4. *The patient may have additional medical problems.* Drug addicts, for example, may be hepatitis B, non-A, non-B, or HIV positive (see p. 37).

5. *The patient may be allergic to drugs.* Allergies must be

Table 2.6
Some oral side-effects of drug use

Teeth	
Discoloration	Chlorhexidine
	Iron
	Tetracyclines
Mucosa	
Candidosis	Tetracyclines
	Corticosteroids
Ulcers	Cytotoxic drugs
Lichenoid lesions	Non-steroidal anti-inflammatory agents
	Gold
	Methyldopa
Erythema multiforme	Sulphonamides
	Barbiturates
Gingiva	
Hyperplasia	Phenytoin
	Cyclosporin
	Nifedipine
Salivary glands	
Dry mouth	Anticholinergics
	Sympathomimetics
Hypersalivation	Anticholinesterases
Swelling	Chlorhexidine

identified since there is a danger of anaphylaxis if the offending drug is given. Penicillin and intravenous general anaesthetic agents are the most dangerous of the drugs used in dentistry in this respect, but even aspirin may be implicated.

6. *The patient may have a medical condition that precludes the use of certain drugs used in dentistry.* This applies especially to liver disease, when drug metabolism is impaired, and is a problem mainly when general anaesthesia is used.

Significance of commonly used drugs

Analgesics

Aspirin can produce two main adverse reactions: a bleeding tendency and gastric erosion. Aspirin therefore should not be given to patients who:

   (a) have a bleeding tendency,
   (b) have gastric lesions such as peptic ulcer,

Table 2.7
*Some drug interactions in dentistry**

Adrenaline	Halothane	Dysrhythmias
Antibiotics	Contraceptive pill	Reduced contraceptive effect
Aspirin	Alcohol ⎫ Corticosteroids ⎬	Increased risk of gastric bleeding
Codeine	Monoamine oxidase inhibitors	Coma
Diazepam and midazolam	Any CNS depressant	CNS depression
Metronidazole	Cimetidine Alcohol	Increased benzodiazepine effect Disulfiram-type (Antabuse-type) reaction

* For GA agents see Chapter 6.

(c) are on other drugs likely to cause peptic ulceration (e.g. corticosteroids) or a bleeding tendency (e.g. anticoagulants).

Aspirin *occasionally* produces allergic reactions or precipitates an asthmatic attack. Aspirin is contraindicated for children because of the rare possibility of producing a type of liver disease (Reye's syndrome).

Anticoagulants

These cause a bleeding tendency (see p. 16).

Antidepressants

Antidepressants can produce a dry mouth. Tricyclics and monoamine oxidase inhibitors do *not*, however, cause a serious interaction with adrenaline in local anaesthetic solutions. Monoamine oxidase inhibitors may produce serious interactions with ephedrine or with pethidine or opiates, as well as with various wines and foods such as cheese, bananas and yoghurt.

Antihypertensive drugs

These may produce a dry mouth but, more seriously, potentiate the hypotensive effect of general anaesthetic agents. Nifedipine may cause gingival hyperplasia.

Antimicrobials

Antimicrobials cause relatively little concern in dental care though they may predispose to oral candidosis. Metronidazole may cause an 'Antabuse' (disulfiram) reac-

tion with alcohol (see p. 231). Tetracyclines should not be given to pregnant or lactating mothers or to children under the age of 8 years since they can produce tooth discoloration. Antibiotics may, to some extent, interfere with the efficacy of the contraceptive pill.

Contraceptive pill

The oral contraceptive may predispose to venous thromboembolism in patients having operations, but usually patients are left on the 'pill' during operation unless there is a particular liability to thromboembolism.

Corticosteroids

The most important effect of corticosteroids absorbed systemically is to suppress the hypothalamo–pituitary–adrenal axis (Fig. 2.14) such that the patient fails to respond adequately to the 'stress' of trauma, general anaesthesia or infection, and consequently may collapse during or after operation unless given an adequate steroid cover. Patients should carry a blue warning card giving details of the steroid used and precautions to be taken (Fig. 2.15).

Adrenocortical suppression follows the use of systemic corticosteroids, even for a course as brief as one week. Occasionally, adrenocortical suppression may also follow the prolonged use of steroid skin ointments. *Patients currently taking steroids, or those who have been on them during the previous year, may be at risk of collapse if not given steroid cover before operation or if traumatised.*

Guidelines for the dental treatment of patients who are or have been on steroids are shown in Table 2.8. Non-surgical treatment under local anaesthesia may require no steroid cover but, if there is any suggestion of collapse or

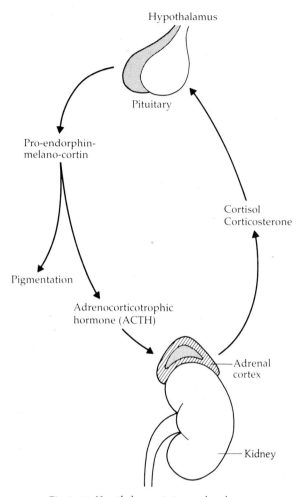

Fig. 2.14 *Hypothalamo–pituitary–adrenal axis.*

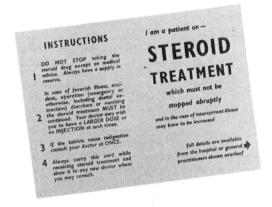

Fig. 2.15 *Corticosteroid warning card.*

falling blood pressure, intravenous hydrocortisone hemisuccinate 200 mg should be given immediately, the patient laid flat with the airway kept patent, and medical assistance sought.

Minor surgical treatment under local anaesthesia must be covered with steroids, 200 mg hydrocortisone hemisuccinate given intravenously, 30 minutes preoperatively.

Major oral surgery must be carried out in hospital and under steroid cover. Any general anaesthetic must only be administered under steroid cover and is best given only in hospital.

All patients should be kept under observation, and blood pressure monitored, for *at least* one hour postoperatively (see also 'Immunosuppressive drugs').

Immunosuppressive drugs

Corticosteroids and other immunosuppressive drugs such as azathioprine and cyclosporin predispose to oral infections and postoperative infections and therefore antibiotics may be indicated to cover surgical procedures. Cyclosporin may cause gingival hyperplasia.

Cytotoxic drugs

These may cause mouth ulcers (Volume 2).

Insulin

This is discussed under Diabetes (see p. 33).

Hypnotics, sedatives and tranquillizers

These may potentiate general anaesthetics and also each other. Some are drugs of abuse.

Table 2.8
Management of dental patients with history of systemic corticosteroid therapy

	No steroids for previous 12 months	Steroids taken during previous 12 months	On steroids currently
Minor surgery	No cover required	Give hydrocortisone 200 mg orally,* i.m.† or i.v.†	Give hydrocortisone 200 mg orally,* i.m.† or i.v. preoperatively **or** increase the dose of oral steroid (by 100% on day of operation; 50% on day 2; 25% on day 3)
Intermediate surgery	Consider cover if large doses of steroid were given	Give hydrocortisone† 200 mg i.v. preoperatively and i.m. 6-hourly for 24 h	Give hydrocortisone 200 mg i.v. preoperatively and i.m. 6-hourly for 24 h, then continue normal medication
Major surgery or trauma	Cover if large doses of steroid were given	Give hydrocortisone† 200 mg i.v. preoperatively and i.m. 6-hourly for 72 h	Give hydrocortisone† 200 mg i.v. preoperatively and i.m. 6-hourly for 72 h, then continue normal medication

* Hydrocortisone given orally 2 hours preoperatively.
† Hydrocortisone sodium succinate (e.g. E$_f$-Cortelan soluble) or phosphate (e.g. E$_f$Cortesol) given 30 min preoperatively.
Monitor blood pressure half-hourly for at least 2 hours if a GA has been given.

Drug dependence and abuse

Compulsive drug use is what is generally known as dependence or addiction: the drug is taken in the absence of any medical indication and despite adverse medical and social consequences. Numerous drugs and chemicals are abused, including alcohol, tobacco, barbiturates, narcotics (opiates and opioids), amphetamines, cocaine, psychodelics (LSD, phencyclidine, etc.), cannabis, solvents and others.

Behavioural disorders, drug resistance or interactions, social problems, or infections such as viral hepatitis, AIDS or other sexually transmitted and blood-transmitted disorders may cause management problems in dental practice (Fig. 2.16).

Alcohol

Many diseases can be caused or aggravated by alcohol. There is a high incidence of alcohol-associated accidents and disease, and up to 30% of those attending accident and emergency departments, including those with facial injuries, may be intoxicated.

Complications of alcohol abuse include the following (Fig. 2.17).

1. *Injuries.* Alcohol is frequently an important, if not the main, causal factor in road traffic accidents and also in many other accidents or assaults. Many patients with maxillofacial or head injuries have been drinking alcohol.

2. *Social problems.* Common social problems in alcoholics include marital difficulties, aggressive behaviour, crime, absenteeism and financial embarrassment. Alcohol is often also a factor in violent or sexual crimes and suicides.

3. *Medical complications.* Common medical problems of chronic alcoholism include liver disease, malnutrition, neurological complications, tuberculosis and pneumonia.

Recognition of the alcohol-intoxicated patient

No social class or profession is immune to alcoholism. Signs or symptoms of excessive drinking include slurred speech, smell of alcohol on the breath, self-neglect, an evasive, truculent, over-boisterous or facetious manner, indigestion, anxiety, or tremor of the hands. Later there may be palpitations and signs of liver disease or malnutrition.

Laboratory investigations that may be helpful in the diagnosis include raised blood levels of alcohol and 'liver

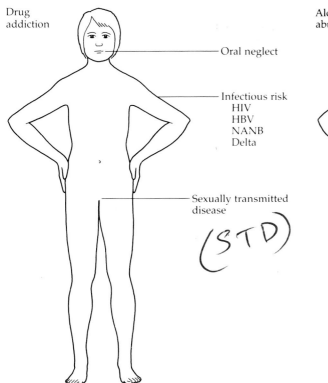

Drug addiction

— Oral neglect

— Infectious risk
HIV
HBV
NANB
Delta

— Sexually transmitted disease
(STD)

Fig. 2.16 Management problems in drug addicts.

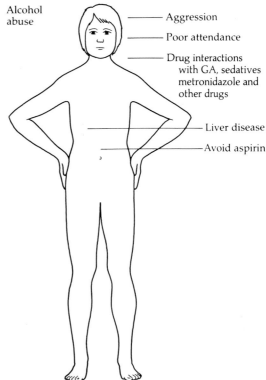

Alcohol abuse

— Aggression
— Poor attendance
— Drug interactions
with GA, sedatives
metronidazole and
other drugs

— Liver disease
— Avoid aspirin

Fig. 2.17 Complications of alcohol abuse.

enzymes' such as gamma glutamyl transpeptidase. Folate deficiency of no obvious cause, macrocytosis alone, or macrocytic anaemia, should also lead to the suspicion of alcoholism.

Dental management of alcoholics

Many alcoholics present no dental management problems, but the following complications may arise.

1. Erratic attendance.
2. Aggressive behaviour.
3. Liver disease.
4. Drug interactions, especially with general anaesthetic agents, sedatives or hypnotics which have an additive effect with alcohol, although heavy drinkers become tolerant. Once liver disease develops, the position is reversed and drug metabolism is then impaired and drugs have a disproportionately greater effect.

General anaesthesia is best avoided—especially if the patient has premedicated himself with more alcohol,

which increases the risk of vomiting and the potentially lethal inhalation of vomit.

Aspirin should be avoided since it is more likely in the alcoholic patient to cause gastric erosion and to precipitate bleeding.

Metronidazole and alcohol interact to cause nausea, vomiting, sweating and palpitations—symptoms which are unpleasant but rarely dangerous.

5. Oral manifestations. Caries and periodontal disease are common. There may be folate deficiency or other anaemia, with glossitis and sometimes angular cheilitis or recurrent aphthae. Alcoholic cirrhosis may rarely cause bilateral painless swelling of the parotids or other major salivary glands (sialosis).

Spirit drinking was thought to be a cause of leukoplakia (see Volume 2) but this may have applied to the nineteenth century when alcohol was heavily adulterated, or to associated factors prevalent at that time. Whether the carcinogenic effect is directly caused by carcinogens in the preparation or indirectly by impairing host defences, such as by causing liver cirrhosis, is unclear.

Tobacco

Smoking may cause mucosal keratinization. Smoker's keratosis, in which there is diffuse hyperkeratosis of the palate, is typically caused by pipe smoking. The hyperkeratosis itself is benign and rapidly reversible, even after many years of pipe smoking. There is some epidemiological evidence of an association between pipe smoking and oral cancer but when cancer develops in a pipe smoker it is likely to be in the lower retromolar region and not in the area of keratosis. Increased cigarette smoking has been associated with an overall decline in the incidence of cancer in the mouth in the UK (Volume 2), though there is very recent evidence of an increase in tongue cancer.

A new problem that has arrived from the USA is that of the intraoral use of tobacco and snuff. Children are now placing pouches of tobacco or snuff in the oral vestibule. Whether this habit will predispose to oral cancer, as do tobacco-chewing habits elsewhere in the world, is unclear, but the habit does cause mucosal lesions (Volume 2).

Cigarette smoking is the most common cause of extrinsic staining of teeth.

Stopping smoking may bring other problems. Aggravation or the onset of recurrent aphthae is noted by some, while others take to eating sweets as a substitute for smoking and may then have increased caries activity, or put on weight.

Dental management of smokers

Problems in dental management may include particularly:

    (a) chronic obstructive airways disease,
    (b) heart disease.

Intravenous drug abuse

Abuse of narcotics (especially heroin) in the UK is mainly seen in urban areas, particularly the larger cities and new towns, and is rapidly increasing.

Complications of intravenous drug abuse

Complications of intravenous drug abuse can be serious and include the following.

1. Behavioural disturbances including the faking of dental pain in order to obtain drugs.
2. Hepatitis B virus; hepatitis non-A, non-B virus; delta agent (see p. 37) infection and liver disease.
3. AIDS and related disease.
4. Sexually transmitted disease.
5. Maxillofacial injuries, head injuries and epilepsy.
6. Infective endocarditis and other infections.
7. Tetanus.

Intravenous drugs used by addicts are often adulterated, or suspended in non-sterile water, syringes and needles are often re-used or shared by several addicts and infective complications such as septicaemia, pneumonia, endocarditis and viral infections can be fatal or leave substantial damage. In some areas addicts comprise the group at greatest risk for various forms of viral hepatitis and HIV infection (see p. 37).

Recognition of the intravenous drug abuser

Early signs of drug abuse can be difficult to detect but lack of concentration, poor performance at work, irritability, desire to be left alone, absenteeism or self-neglect may all be indications. Loss of weight and emaciation, bizarre behaviour, needle marks and pupil constriction are more obvious guides. The narcotic addict is a 'depressed introvert with pin-point pupils'.

Dental management of intravenous drug abusers

In the established untreated addict, non-narcotic analgesics may fail to control dental pain. Large doses of narcotic analgesics may have to be given but not without first seeking expert advice. Pentazocine, being a narcotic antagonist, may precipitate a withdrawal syndrome and is therefore contraindicated. Local anaesthesia is often of little value and general anaesthesia may therefore be preferred unless there are other medical contraindications.

If the patient is under treatment for narcotic addiction, narcotics must be avoided. Local anaesthesia is preferred at this time.

Other drugs of abuse

Amphetamines

Amphetamines are the main central nervous system stimulants, characterized by their ability to elevate mood. Amphetamines are taken orally or intravenously ('speed'). Chronic toxicity causes restlessness, hyperactivity, loss of appetite and weight, tremor, repetitive movements and picking at the face and extremities. Eventually, with large doses, a paranoid psychosis may develop. Addicts may be resistant to GA.

Cocaine

Cocaine and the recently introduced 'crack' (a purified form of cocaine) are usually taken as snuff or hypodermically. The cocaine addict is garrulous, witty and the 'life and soul of the party'—a 'sexed-up extrovert with dilated pupils'. There are no specific dental problems but oral neglect is common.

Cannabis

Cannabis (marijuana) can be taken by many routes but is often smoked as a 'reefer' ('joint'). The effects resemble those associated with alcohol. Abuse of hard drugs may follow. Bronchitis, possibly impaired fertility, and a tendency to tachycardias may occur. There are no specific dental problems.

Psychodelic drugs

Psychodelic drugs may induce enhanced clarity of senses, higher awareness of sensory input and altered perception. They include lysergic acid diethylamide (LSD), psilocybin, mescaline and phencyclidine (PCP). New 'designer' drugs such as 'Ecstasy' are constantly appearing.

Grossly abnormal behaviour can follow abuse of psychodelics but there are no significant dental problems.

Solvent sniffing

Sniffers are usually male teenagers who predominantly use glue (glue-sniffers), petrol or other organic liquids or aerosol sprays. An effect somewhere between that of alcohol and a psychodelic results. Toxic effects include hypoxia, cardiac arrhythmias, liver damage, neurological damage and death.

A rash around the nose and/or mouth may be the most obvious sign of solvent abuse.

Anaesthetic abuse

Nitrous oxide produces impairment of consciousness with a sense of dissociation and often of exhilaration ('laughing gas'). Addiction to nitrous oxide is an occupational hazard of anaesthetists and dental surgeons, and can lead to a neuropathy and, occasionally, death (Chapter 10).

Drug allergies and reactions

Any suggestion of previous drug reactions or allergy, and particularly any adverse reaction during anaesthesia, should be taken seriously and an alternative given (see Table 6.1). Patients with allergy to one drug and those who suffer from atopic disease (eczema, asthma or hay fever) are particularly liable to drug allergies.

Allergies to penicillin and to sticking plaster (Elastoplast) are the most common problems encountered, and alternatives (such as erythromycin and micropore tape respectively) should therefore be used.

In contrast, complaints of 'allergies' to various dental materials and drugs are common but evidence for such 'allergies' is often lacking. True allergic reactions to some of the impression materials and resins (such as epoxy resins) may occur, but allergies to polymethyl methacrylate (acrylic), lignocaine, or mercury in amalgams are *extremely rare. Few, if any, practitioners will encounter even one patient in a lifetime with a genuine allergic reaction to these materials.*

Hypersensitivity to penicillins

The common reactions are rashes, usually urticarial ('hives'), or angioedema. The most dangerous is anaphylaxis, which can be fatal (see Chapter 4).

Allergic reactions are more likely after injections of a penicillin than after oral administration. Patients allergic to one penicillin will also be allergic to others, including ampicillin, amoxycillin, flucloxacillin, etc. A history must always be taken and, if there is any suggestion of allergy, an alternative (such as erythromycin) used.

Hypersensitivity to intravenous anaesthetic agents (see also Chapter 6)

Hypersensitivity to various anaesthetic agents (e.g. Althesin, propanidid) has been serious enough to result in their withdrawal from the market. However, any agent can cause reactions such as bronchospasm, flushing of the skin and acute hypotension but this is not a problem with sedative agents such as diazepam or midazolam.

Hypersensitivity to local anaesthetic agents (see also Chapter 6)

Lignocaine is a very safe local anaesthetic agent. True allergic reactions are *very rare* indeed.

Allergy to other local anaesthetics has sometimes been caused by the preservative (often para-aminobenzoic acid—parabens), and 'parabens-free' local anaesthetics are now available.

However, fainting, rather than hypersensitivity, is the main 'reaction' of patients given LA. (For other reactions, see Chapters 4 and 6.)

Suxamethonium sensitivity (Scoline sensitivity)

Suxamethonium is a muscle relaxant used during the induction of GA, whose effect is eventually terminated by plasma cholinesterase. Reduced levels of cholinesterase are found in liver disease and an autosomal recessive trait known as suxamethonium (Scoline: Anectine) sensitivity. If given suxamethonium, such individuals will remain paralysed for several hours, unable to breathe.

Management

Patients with suspected or known suxamethonium sensitivity must not be given suxamethonium.

Porphyria

Hepatic porphyria is a rare inborn error of metabolism, most common in South Africans of Afrikaaner descent. Affected patients may develop acute neuropsychiatric and cardiovascular disturbances, or convulsions, if given barbiturates, pentazocine, sulphonamides, or some other drugs.

Malignant hyperthermia (malignant hyperpyrexia)

Malignant hyperthermia is a rare inherited disorder characterized by an acute onset of fever after the administration of a general anaesthetic (particularly halothane and enflurane) or muscle relaxant (suxamethonium or curare).

Reactions are rare following the use of nitrous oxide, local anaesthetics, or intravenous anaesthetics.

Management

It is important to ask all patients about the course of previous anaesthetics and any relevant family history.

Dantrolene is a prophylactic agent which, together with other measures, enables patients with malignant hyperthermia to be treated safely, General anaesthetics should not be given in dental practice.

Halothane 'hepatitis' (see also p. 161)

Transient impairment of liver function appears to follow the administration of any GA, but in the obese patient, or when GA is repeated after intervals of less than a month, halothane may, rarely, predispose to 'hepatitis', manifesting as pyrexia and jaundice appearing 1–3 weeks after administration. Enflurane may be less prone to cause this reaction.

Repeated halothane anaesthetics should not, therefore, be given (Chapter 6).

Other systemic conditions affecting the use of drugs in dentistry

Drug metabolism and excretion may be impaired, particularly in the elderly and in:

(a) liver disease (see p. 47),
(b) renal disease (see p. 48).

Many other medical conditions may be relative or absolute contraindications to various drugs (Table 2.9) and enquiry should be made if patients present for treatment having unusual conditions about which the practitioner has hazy or no knowledge. *This is especially important if any form of general anaesthesia or intravenous sedation is to be used.*

ENDOCRINE DISORDERS

Endocrinopathies that influence dental care include mainly:

(a) adrenocortical hypofunction,
(b) diabetes mellitus,
(c) hyperparathyroidism.

Patients with other endocrinopathies usually only attend for dental treatment when the endocrinopathy is under control; they may be at risk from general anaesthesia but, in general, dental care is otherwise relatively uncomplicated.

Adrenocortical hypofunction

Adrenocortical hypofunction is usually a consequence of systemic corticosteroid treatment (see p. 24), and occasionally a consequence of Addison's disease.

Addison's disease is usually an autoimmune disorder in which there is adrenocortical atrophy and consequent weakness, loss of weight, hypotension, nausea and vomiting, and hyperpigmentation (Volume 2).

The hypothalamo–pituitary–adrenal axis is stimulated by the feedback of low levels of plasma cortisol which induce increased secretion of adrenocorticotrophic hormone (ACTH) from the pituitary gland (see Fig. 2.14). Part of the ACTH molecule is similar to the melanocyte-stimulating hormone, and the high levels of ACTH stimulate an increase in pigmentation in both normally pigmented areas (e.g. genitals) and also the skin and

Table 2.9
Contraindications to drugs used in dentistry

Drug	Possible contraindications	Possible reaction
Adrenaline	Hypertension	Hypertension
	Hyperthyroidism	Arrhythmias
	Ischaemic heart disease	Arrhythmias
	Phaeochromocytoma	Hypertension
	Liver disease	Althesin potentiated
Ampicillin (or amoxycillin or derivatives	Allergy to penicillin	Anaphylaxis
	Chronic lymphocytic leukaemia	Rash
	Gout	Rash
	Infectious mononucleosis	Rash
	Oral contraceptive	Reduced contraceptive effect
Aspirin	Allergy to aspirin including aspirin-induced asthma	Anaphylaxis
	Bleeding disorders	Gastric bleeding
	Children	Reye's syndrome
	Glucose 6-phosphate-dehydrogenase deficiency	Haemolysis
	Gout	Gout worse
	Liver disease	Bleeding tendency
	Peptic ulcer	Gastric bleeding
	Pregnancy	Haemorrhage
	Renal disease	Fluid retention and gastric bleeding
Atropine	Glaucoma	Raised intraocular pressure
	Hyperthyroidism	Tachycardias
	The elderly	Confusion: urine retention
	Urinary retention or prostatic hypertrophy	Urinary retention
Chloral hydrate	Cardiovascular disease	Fluid retention
	Gastritis	Gastric irritation
	Liver disease	Coma
	Renal disease	CNS depression
Codeine	Colonic disease	Constipation
	Liver disease	Respiratory depression
	Hypothyroidism	Coma
Corticosteroids	Diabetes mellitus	Diabetes worsened
	Hypertension	Increased hypertension
	Peptic ulcer	Perforation
	Tuberculosis	Possible dissemination
Dextropropoxyphene	Liver disease	Potentiated
	Respiratory disease	Respiratory depression
	Pregnancy	Fetal depression
Diazepam and midazolam	Cerebrovascular disease	Cerebral ischaemia
	Chronic obstructive airways disease	Respiratory depression
	Cimetidine	Increased diazepam effect
	Glaucoma	Increased ocular pressure
	Hypothyroidism	Coma
	Neuromuscular disorders	Condition deteriorates
	Porphyria	Acute porphyria
	Pregnancy	Fetal hypoxia
	Severe kidney disease	Increased diazepam effect
	Severe liver disease	Increased diazepam effect
	The elderly	Cerebral ischaemia

(continued)

Table 2.9   (*continued*)

Drug	Possible contraindications	Possible reaction
Dihydrocodeine	Hypothyroidism	Coma
	Renal disease	Increased toxicity
	Respiratory disease	Respiratory depression
	The elderly	Increased toxicity
Halothane	Cardiac arrhythmias	Increased arrhythmias
	Halothane hepatitis	Hepatitis
	Malignant hyperpyrexia	Pyrexia
	Recent anaesthesia with halothane	Hepatitis
Mefenamic acid	Asthma	Bronchospasm
	Diarrhoea	Diarrhoea worse
	Peptic ulcer	Bleeding
	Pregnancy and lactation	Teratogenic
	Renal disease	Renal disease worse
Methohexitone	Addison's disease	Coma
	Allergies	Anaphylaxis
	Barbiturate sensitivity	Anaphylaxis
	Cardiovascular disease	Cardiovascular depression
	Dystrophia myotonica	Increased weakness
	Epilepsy	Epileptogenic
	Hypothyroidism	Coma
	Liver disease	Increased anaesthesia
	Myasthenia gravis	Increased weakness
	Porphyria	Acute porphyria
	Postnasal drip	Laryngeal spasm
	Respiratory disease	Respiratory depression
Midazolam	See diazepam	
Metronidazole	Blood dyscrasias	Leucopenia
	CNS disease	Neuropathy
	Renal disease	Increased drug effect
	Pregnancy (first trimester)	Teratogenic
Paracetamol	Liver disease	Hepatotoxicity
	Renal disease	Nephrotoxicity
Penicillins	Allergy to penicillin	Anaphylaxis
	Renal disease	Hyperkalaemia with i.m. benzyl penicillin
Pentazocine	Hypertension	Hypertension
	Liver disease	Enhanced activity
	Myocardial infarct (recent)	Cardiac arrest
	Narcotic addict	Withdrawal syndrome
	Pregnancy	Fetal depression
Tetracyclines	After gastrointestinal surgery	Enterocolitis
	Children under 8	Tooth staining
	Myasthenia gravis	Increased muscle weakness
	Pregnancy/lactating mother	Tooth staining (child)
	Renal disease	Nephrotoxicity
	Systemic lupus erythematosus	Photosensitivity
Thiopentone	Addison's disease	Coma
	Barbiturate sensitivity	Anaphylaxis
	Cardiovascular disease	Cardiovascular depression

(*continued*)

Table 2.9   *(continued)*

Drug	Possible contraindications	Possible reaction
Thiopentone *(continued)*	Dystrophia myotonica	Increased weakness
	Hypothyroidism	Coma
	Liver disease	Increased anaesthesia
	Myasthenia gravis	Increased weakness
	Porphyria	Acute porphyria
	Postnasal drip	Laryngeal spasm
	Respiratory disease	Respiratory depression

mucosa. Oral pigmentation is usually patchy brown or black, affecting the gingiva, lips and buccal mucosa predominantly.

Management

Patients with Addison's disease, even if already on steroid replacement therapy, may collapse under the stress of trauma, general anaesthesia or infection and must therefore receive steroid cover during dental treatment similar to that described under 'Corticosteroids' (p. 24).

Diabetes mellitus

Diabetes is common; up to 4% of the population are affected. It is characterized by an inability to transfer glucose from the blood into cells for metabolism because of a deficiency of, or resistance to, insulin. There are two main types of diabetic.

Juvenile-onset diabetes is a serious disease of acute onset in children or adolescents, with thirst, hunger, loss of weight, polyuria and susceptibility to infections. Insulin injections as well as dietary control are normally required for management.

Maturity-onset diabetes is often less serious and is of insidious onset in the middle-aged or elderly. The patients are often obese and may complain of polyuria, thirst, fatigue and failing vision (diabetic retinopathy or cataracts), or may be asymptomatic. They may be controlled by diet, with or without hypoglycaemic drugs.

Diabetes is diagnosed from the clinical features, glycosuria and a raised fasting blood glucose level or abnormal glucose tolerance test.

Complications of diabetes are protean but include especially cardiovascular (atherosclerosis, gangrene), ocular (retinopathy, cataracts), renal (polyuria, renal failure), and neurological (peripheral and autonomic neuropathies) aspects.

Management

Accelerated periodontitis may be a complication of poorly controlled diabetes, as may be other uncommon oral manifestations (Volume 2).

The major concern in the dental treatment of diabetics is to avoid *hypoglycaemia* since, if this occurs, not only

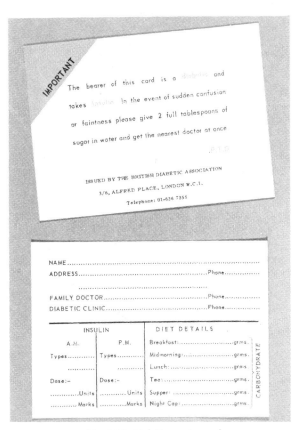

Fig. 2.18 Diabetic warning card.

will the patient collapse and rapidly go into coma, but he or she may also suffer from irreversible brain damage. Collapse in a diabetic should be regarded as caused by hypoglycaemia until proved otherwise (see p. 106) and glucose should be given. Some patients carry a warning card (Fig. 2.18). Patients with juvenile-onset diabetes are most at risk during dental treatment. General anaesthesia should be avoided where possible; treatment under local anaesthesia is far safer (Fig. 2.19).

In the case of minor surgery under local anaesthesia, treatment is best carried out early in the morning after the patient has had breakfast and his usual insulin injection so that he should be able to resume eating at lunchtime, and thus avoid hypoglycaemia.

If general anaesthesia is needed, except in exceptional circumstances such as a mild well-controlled maturity-onset diabetic having simple extractions, this should be given in hospital. The patient should be admitted a day or so preoperatively, such that the diabetes can be controlled with soluble insulin. During and after operation, the blood glucose level is monitored and controlled by use of intravenous glucose and insulin, until the patient is able to resume normal diet and medication. Since diabetics may be prone to infections, antibiotics may be warranted to prevent infection of surgical wounds.

Hyperparathyroidism

Hyperparathyroidism is usually primary, caused by parathyroid hyperplasia or adenoma, but may be secondary to renal disease or malabsorption. Bone lesions may present in the jaws or with oral swellings (Volume 2). Dental management in hyperparathyroidism is relatively uncomplicated.

FITS AND FAINTS (see also Chapter 4)

Syncope

Syncope is a transient loss of consciousness caused by a sudden decrease in blood flow to the brain.

Vasovagal syncope

Vasovagal syncope (fainting) is a reflex mediated by parasympathetic autonomic nerves, especially the vagus, in which there is vasodilatation and pooling of blood in the lower extremities, bradycardia and subsequent collapse. Fainting can be precipitated by psychological factors such as fear at the sight of an injection needle or blood, or pain. Few patients faint in the waiting room—most who faint do so in relation to the administration of a local anaesthetic.

Fainting may also be caused by postural changes, anoxia or the carotid sinus syndrome. The latter is usually seen in elderly patients in whom mild pressure on the neck causes syncope with bradycardia or cardiac arrest—a vagal effect.

Management

The best course is prevention where possible: giving local anaesthetic injections with confidence, painlessly and with the patient laid flat (at least not upright) will prevent many fainting episodes. Syncope is dangerous if the patient is not laid flat, since cerebral hypoxia can result and the patient may then have a convulsion and suffer from brain damage (Chapter 4).

Febrile convulsions

Febrile convulsions result from high fever, usually in young children, a few of whom go on in later life to de-

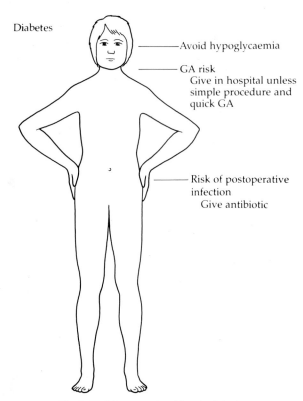

Diabetes

—Avoid hypoglycaemia

—GA risk
    Give in hospital unless simple procedure and quick GA

—Risk of postoperative infection
    Give antibiotic

Fig. 2.19 *Management problems in diabetics.*

velop epilepsy. Severe febrile convulsions can cause brain damage and can be an early sign of meningitis.

Children who develop high fevers (above 38°C) should be put in a cool environment, sponged with tepid water and given paracetamol elixir.

Epilepsy

Epilepsy is a disorder of brain function which causes episodic disturbances of consciousness and usually of motor function. It affects over 1% of the general population.

The cause of epilepsy is usually not identifiable (**idiopathic** epilepsy) but epilepsy may be secondary to brain disease, drug addiction or metabolic disorders (**symptomatic** epilepsy). Epilepsy is more prevalent in the young, in the mentally or physically handicapped and after head injuries.

The main type of epilepsy is grand mal or major epilepsy, but there are also minor or focal convulsions and many variants.

Grand mal epilepsy (major epilepsy)

A grand mal seizure typically begins with a warning (aura) followed by loss of consciousness, tonic and then clonic convulsions and finally recovery.

The aura may consist of a mood change, hallucination or headache and is followed by total body tonic spasm and loss of consciousness when the patient falls and may damage himself (tonic phase). Initially the head and spine are thrown into extension (opisthotonus), and glottic and respiratory muscle spasm may cause a brief cry and cyanosis. There may also be incontinence, and biting of the tongue or lips.

After less than a minute the clonic phase begins, with

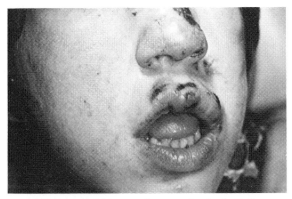

Fig. 2.20 *Facial trauma after a grand mal epileptic fit.*

repetitive jerking movements of trunk, limbs, tongue and lips and sometimes salivation, tongue-biting and vomiting. Clonus is followed by flaccid semicoma for a further 10–15 minutes. Confusion and headaches are then common and the patient may sleep for up to 12 hours before full recovery.

Most seizures end without mishap, but major convulsions can cause trauma, asphyxia and brain damage, or, if lasting more than 5 minutes or starting again after apparently ceasing, become **status epilepticus**, in which the tonic and clonic phases alternate repeatedly without consciousness being regained. Brain damage due to cerebral hypoxia may result from laryngospasm or inhalation of vomit or saliva.

Management

As consciousness is lost, the patient falls and may injure his face, mouth, teeth or jaws. Lacerations, haematomas and fractures of the facial skeleton (especially of the zygomatic complex, nasal bones and mandible) are well-recognized complications (Fig. 2.20). Fractures, subluxation, or dislocation of the maxillary incisors are also common.

It is important to find any broken tooth fragments lest they be inhaled. Chest radiographs in two planes at right-angles are necessary if fragments cannot be located. Because of the probability of future injuries, restorative materials should be radio-opaque to allow localization if the prosthesis is swallowed or inhaled. In some instances prostheses are contraindicated.

Epilepsy is controlled mainly with anticonvulsants such as phenytoin, sodium valproate or barbiturates.

The main oral side-effect of phenytoin, in nearly 50% of users, is gingival hyperplasia in which the papillae may enlarge to such an extent that they meet and form vertical pseudoclefts (Volumes 2 and 3). The effect is more severe in the young and when oral hygiene is poor. The main problem is aesthetic. Removal of the excess gingival tissue by gingivoplasty is often followed by recurrence in the young or if oral hygiene is poor. If the patient is stabilized, the anticonvulsant regimen should not be changed but the physician may agree to modify it if hyperplasia is exceptionally severe. Sodium valproate may cause a slight bleeding tendency.

Epileptics have good and bad phases. Dental treatment should preferably be carried out in a good phase. A substantial mouth prop should be kept in position and the oral cavity kept as free as possible of debris. As much apparatus as possible should be kept away from the area around the patient. Methohexitone, enflurane, ketamine,

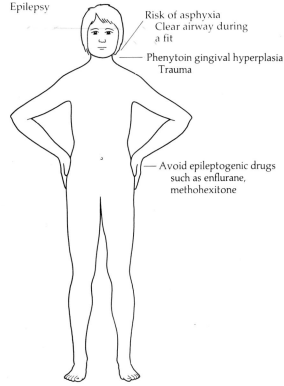

Epilepsy

Risk of asphyxia
Clear airway during
a fit

Phenytoin gingival hyperplasia
Trauma

Avoid epileptogenic drugs
such as enflurane,
methohexitone

Fig. 2.21 *Management problems in epilepsy.*

chlorpromazine and tricyclics should be avoided as they may precipitate fits (Fig. 2.21).

For details of the management of a fit in the dental surgery, see Chapter 4.

Other forms of epilepsy

Petit mal (minor epilepsy) is restricted to children and consists of transient arrests of movement, attention and speech ('absences') which may be precipitated by over-breathing. Petit mal can be controlled with ethosuximide or sodium valproate.

Temporal lobe epilepsy (psychomotor epilepsy) is characterized by hallucinations, illusions of taste, smell, sight and hearing, disorientation, confusion and amnesia. It is controlled by many of the anticonvulsants used in major epilepsy.

Ictal facial pain is a type that appears to have an 'epileptic' aetiology. It is an unusual manifestation of sensory epilepsy which predominantly affects women of late middle age. It consists of a throbbing, diffuse facial pain

which may be associated with muscle twitches or generalized convulsions. It is controlled with phenytoin.

Localized motor seizures (focal motor epilepsy) may take the form of clonic movements which may spread (march) to adjacent muscles on the same side of the body (Jacksonian epilepsy). They are controlled with phenytoin.

GASTROINTESTINAL DISEASE

Gastrointestinal disorders that predispose to vomiting may be a risk during the induction of general anaesthesia because of the danger of inhalation of gastric juices which may choke or even kill the patient, or later produce serious inflammation of the lung (Mendelsohn's syndrome).

Diseases of the small intestine, such as coeliac disease or Crohn's disease, predispose to malabsorption and consequent deficiency states or anaemia that may precipitate a sore mouth and, in some patients, oral ulcers, glossitis, and angular cheilitis (Volume 2).

Peutz–Jegher's syndrome of 'circumoral melanosis with intestinal polyposis' consists of melanotic macules on the lips and elsewhere, with small intestine polyps that may lead to intussusception and obstruction.

Gardner's syndrome consists of osteomas (sometimes of the jaws), desmoid tumours, and polyps in the large intestine that may undergo malignant transformation.

HOSPITAL ADMISSIONS AND OPERATIONS

A history of admission to hospital for medical or surgical treatment may reveal a systemic disease of relevance to dentistry. Conversely, if a patient has previously tolerated a general anaesthetic, and surgery, without untoward effect, it is unlikely that he has an inherited bleeding tendency or anaesthetic drug sensitivity.

If the patient has been given blood or blood products, the possibility of infection with hepatitis B virus, non-A, non-B virus, or HIV should be borne in mind.

INFECTIONS (AND CROSS-INFECTION)

Body fluids—especially blood—are potentially infected by micro-organisms, particularly certain viruses that can cause significant morbidity and, indeed, mortality. Transmission of these infections is predominantly by needle-stick injuries, administration of blood and blood products, or sexually. The dentist is morally and legally obliged to prevent cross-infection during the course of his or her practice.

Viruses

Many viruses can be transmitted but those of main concern in dentistry are the agents causing hepatitis B, non-A, non-B hepatitis (NANB), the delta agent, and human immunodeficiency virus (HIV—AIDS virus), since they can be transmitted during dental treatment if appropriate measures against cross-infection are not followed, and may cause significant morbidity and mortality.

Hepatitis B

The hepatitis B virus (HBV) is a DNA virus found, as the Dane particle, in the serum of patients with hepatitis B. It consists of a central core containing DNA, the enzyme DNA polymerase (DNA-P) and a core antigen (hepatitis B core antigen—HBcAg), and an outer protein shell of surface antigen (hepatitis B surface antigen—HBsAg). Also present in the serum are spherical and tubular particles of HBsAg which are non-infectious. HBcAg is not present in serum but its breakdown product, termed e antigen (hepatitis B e antigen—HBeAg), may be found (Figs. 2.22 and 2.23, and see below).

Some 50% of HBV infections are subclinical and do not cause jaundice (i.e. they are anicteric). Other persons infected with HBV develop acute hepatitis with anorexia, malaise, nausea, and the appearance of jaundice, pale fatty

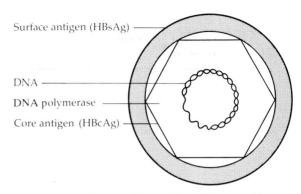

Fig. 2.23 *Structure of hepatitis B virus (Dane particle).*

stools and dark urine. The liver tends to enlarge and become tender. Liver enzymes (transaminases) appear in the serum, along with raised levels of bilirubin and often of alkaline phosphatase. Evidence of HBV infection (HBsAg; see below) is present for a variable period from 1 to 6 months, following which there remains serological evidence of previous HBV infection in the form of antibodies to the various viral antigens (see below).

The early mortality rate in HBV infection is low, about 1%. Most patients with acute hepatitis B recover spontaneously within a few weeks with no sequelae, but a much higher mortality has been recorded in some outbreaks, particularly where there has also been infection with the delta agent (see below). There may be late complications of HBV infection, particularly chronic hepatitis, cirrhosis and liver cancer (hepatocellular carcinoma).

Carrier state

Some 5% of patients become chronic carriers characterized by persistence of HBV antigens (HBsAg) in the serum. This state more frequently follows anicteric infection than acute hepatitis.

About 1 in 1000 of the indigenous UK population are carriers, but there are a number of patients who are far more likely to be HBsAg positive—especially those who have been exposed to blood or blood products, are sexually promiscuous or are from the Far East (see high risk groups in Table 2.10). Most carriers constitute a low infective risk: only 1 in 4 of HBsAg carriers are also HBeAg positive and 'high risk' (see below).

Serological markers of hepatitis B virus infection

The various serological markers are discussed below (Table 2.11).

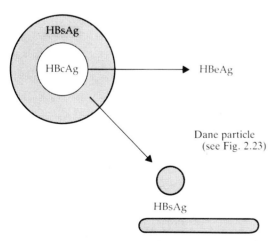

Fig. 2.22 *Serum particles found in patients infected with hepatitis B virus (HBV).*

Table 2.10
High-risk groups for hepatitis B, non-A, non-B hepatitis and/or delta agent infection

Recent or past history of hepatitis

Intravenous drug abusers

Male homosexuals

Patients receiving increased blood or blood products, e.g. some haemophiliacs

Patients from the Third World, especially S.E. Asia

Patients and staff of long-stay mentally handicapped or custodial institutions

Sexually promiscuous

Table 2.11
Serological markers of hepatitis B virus

Marker	Significance
HBsAg	Present or previous infection with HBV (may or may not be infective risk)
anti-HBs	Previous infection or vaccination (immunity)
HBeAg	Infection with HBV (infective risk)
anti-HBe	Recovery from HBV infection (not an infective risk)
anti-HBc	Present or previous infection with HBV (may or may not be infective risk)

1. *HBsAg.* The presence of HBsAg implies that the patient is or has been infected with HBV. However, in as many as half of the individuals with subclinical HBV infection, HBsAg never reaches detectable levels in the serum; HBV infection in these cases can be detected by the appearance of antibodies to surface (anti-HBs) and core (anti-HBc) antigens. Conversely, as indicated above, HBsAg may be positive in some individuals who have actually cleared HBV infection; if these patients are HBeAg negative they usually are not infectious.

2. *Anti-HBs (HBsAb).* Antibody to the surface antigen begins to appear in the serum as the patient with HBV infection starts to recover. Anti-HBs also appears after immunization with hepatitis B vaccine since this consists of inactive HBsAg (see below). Anti-HBs frequently is long lived and is detectable for many years.

In a few patients with previous HBV infection, anti-HBs is undetectable. Antibody to core antigen (anti-HBc) may detect such patients (see below).

3. *HBcAg.* This antigen is *not* present in serum.

4. *Anti-HBc (HBcAb).* In contrast to surface antibody, anti-HBc appears at the onset of disease and rises quickly in titre to remain for many years as an indicator of previous HBV infection. Anti-HBc in high titres may indicate a chronic carrier state and is then found in the absence of anti-HBs.

5. *HBeAg.* This antigen appears in the serum simultaneously with HBsAg but disappears before it during recovery. HBeAg is an indicator of high infectivity since e antigen is closely associated with viral DNA, DNA-P and Dane particles. Absence of HBeAg implies very low, if any, infectivity. Carriers of HBsAg who have HBeAg present are more likely to develop chronic active hepatitis, serious complications, and to transmit infection.

6. *Anti-HBe (HBeAb).* Antibody to e antigen appears in the serum soon after the appearance of HBeAg in most patients and heralds recovery.

7. *DNA-P.* DNA polymerase in the serum is, like HBeAg, an indicator of high infectivity.

Sources of infection and mode of transmission of hepatitis B virus

Blood and blood products appear to be the fluids most likely to be involved in cross-infection, and minute quantities, far less than 0.0001 ml, have transmitted the disease. Needlestick injuries, injections and blood transfusion may transmit infection, but, as discussed above, the risk from HBeAg-negative blood is substantially lower than that from HBeAg-positive blood. Saliva from HBeAg-positive patients may be infective but the risk is much lower than from blood.

Hepatitis B infection is more likely, therefore, in individuals who, for one reason or another, are exposed frequently to blood, blood products or to other infected individuals, *but this is mainly if the exposure is intimate or involves close contact with body fluids.*

These individuals form a high-risk group (Table 2.10). Many of these categories, particularly male homosexuals and abusers of intravenous drugs, are also high-risk groups for other infections such as HIV and other sexually transmitted diseases.

Transmission of hepatitis B virus in the dental surgery

The suggestion that hepatitis could be transmitted in dentistry was made over 35 years ago and it is obvious that there is ample opportunity for cross-infection if there is any lapse in sterilization procedures or if there is transmission of infected body fluids, especially blood, to patients.

Risk of transmission to dental surgeons

There is a risk to dental and ancillary personnel of contracting HBV infection. This risk is above that in the general population but, with increasing awareness and subsequent precautions, it is falling. For dental surgeons, the routine use of gloves has been associated with a lower incidence of HBV infection and some recent surveys have now shown little risk above that in the general population.

As might be expected, the risk of contracting hepatitis B in dentistry increases with age and with duration in practice. It relates to the intensity of exposure to blood and tissue fluids (i.e. it is higher in surgeons and periodontologists), and is higher in urban areas, particularly in large metropolitan hospitals and in the USA, than in rural areas or in the UK or Scandinavia.

Risk of transmission from operator to patient

Overall, about 1% of dentists are HBsAg positive, but transmission of HBV infection to patients must be rare, though infection has been shown to have been transmitted to patients by health-care workers and dentists. In one study, an HBsAg-positive doctor transmitted HBV infection to his patients until he instituted simple measures such as hand-washing before examination of patients—a practice that has always been routine for dentists.

Identification of the patient who may be HBsAg positive

The procedure for screening patients is outlined below but it must be borne in mind that:

(a) absence of HBsAg does not *always* indicate absence of HBV;

(b) there are infective risks in practice other than HBV, often in the same group of patients (e.g. non-A, non-B hepatitis; HIV infection);

(c) the risk from HBeAg-negative patients is extremely low;

(d) most carriers of HBsAg have had anicteric infections and there will always be some who are outside an at-risk group; therefore, some will always escape suspicion;

(e) dentists have for years been treating (unknown) antigen-positive patients with few sequelae;

(f) simple precautions such as wearing gloves, glasses and mask, and avoiding needle pricks, if used for **all** dental patients irrespective of their antigen status, are

most likely to be effective. *There are other very good reasons for adopting such precautions.*

Screening patients for hepatitis B

If there is a risk of the patient carrying HBV, a blood sample, taken with special precautions laid down for high-risk patients, can be sent to the appropriate special laboratory for HBsAg screening. This test takes about 30 minutes but, until a report has been received, no further blood tests should be carried out unless they are very urgent and the situation has been discussed with the pathologists. If the screening test is negative, no further special precautions are indicated unless there is some other infective risk such as HIV.

Patients positive for HBsAg must be treated at this stage as an infective risk and HBeAg should be assayed in order to establish the level of risk. Those negative for HBeAg (and positive for anti-HBe) are regarded as low risk.

Those who are HBsAg positive should again be screened at 3 months and thereafter until negative; those positive at 9 months are 'chronic carriers'.

For details of the management of high-risk patients, see page 44.

Delta agent

The delta agent is an RNA virus that will only replicate in the presence of HBsAg—i.e. it is a 'defective' virus (Fig. 2.24). Delta infection is only transmitted parenterally, similarly to HBV, and it is becoming a major problem in abusers of intravenous drugs and haemophiliacs. The delta agent produces acute hepatitis which may precipitate fulminant liver disease, although there is resolution in most cases.

Vaccine against hepatitis B virus

The first vaccine against HBV was produced by the extensive preparation of HBsAg particles which are immu-

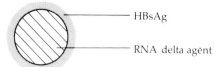

Fig. 2.24 *Structure of delta agent.*

nogenic and induce protection against HBV infection but are not themselves infectious. The vaccine appears safe and does not transmit any other infection.

The vaccine produces high titres of HBsAb with concurrent protection lasting at least 6 years. It is given as an initial immunization with subsequent doses 1 month later and then after 6 months and is associated with few if any side-effects apart from mild soreness at the site of injection and occasional mild fever or malaise.

New recombinant vaccines are now available.

There is every reason for dental staff, particularly those in surgical specialties or treating high-risk groups, to consider seriously immunization against hepatitis B, since it protects against both HBV and (indirectly) delta agent.

Non-A, non-B hepatitis

Non-A, non-B hepatitis (NANB) affects a similar group to those infected by HBV—especially intravenous drug addicts. By definition, there was until recently no diagnostic test to detect this infection, which is transmitted by and may carry much the same implications as HBV infection, except that chronic hepatitis is more common.

Acquired immune deficiency syndrome

Acquired immune deficiency syndrome (AIDS) is the name given to a group of disorders characterized by various infections and malignant neoplasms and associated with profound defects in T lymphocytes. RNA retroviruses, the human T cell lymphotropic viruses (HTLV-III and HTLV-IV and possibly others), now known as human immunodeficiency viruses (HIV), appear to be the causal

agents (Fig. 2.25) which infect and damage macrophages, T lymphocytes and some brain cells.

Clinical features

The incubation period appears to range up to at least 7 years. As with most viral infections, many of the patients infected with HIV are asymptomatic (subclinical infection), at least initially.

Those patients who go on to develop symptoms have a prodromal stage of malaise, low-grade fever, weight loss, generalized lymph node enlargement, and nonproductive cough in a glandular fever type of syndrome. Some 30%–90% or more of patients with the prodrome progress to full-blown AIDS (Fig. 2.26). Some develop a range of syndromes (Table 2.12) including progressive brain damage.

The full-blown syndrome of AIDS is characterized by infections with organisms that, in the normal host, are commensals (opportunistic infections; Table 2.12), and/or malignant neoplasms. Some 60% of patients develop pneumonia caused by a parasite, *Pneumocystis carinii*, and about 25% develop a malignant endothelial tumour, Kaposi's sarcoma. Of the several other malignant neoplasms that may appear in AIDS, primary lymphoma of the brain is most common. Dementia and other neurological damage is common.

AIDS-related complexes

Patients in high-risk groups with clinical features related to AIDS but without full-blown AIDS fall into a group with disorders termed AIDS-related complex (Table 2.13). Persistent generalized lymphadenopathy (PGL)—also known as lymphadenopathy syndrome (LAS)—is defined as lymph node enlargement of more than 3 months' duration, involving two or more extra-inguinal sites.

It is quite unclear how many will develop full-blown AIDS, but the outlook seems to worsen as patients are followed up for longer periods.

Epidemiology

The two main modes of transmission of HIV are via:

(a) intimate sexual contact,
(b) blood and blood products, e.g. intravenous drug abusers and some haemophiliacs.

The risk groups are shown in Table 2.14. The major risk groups are still homosexual or bisexual men in the

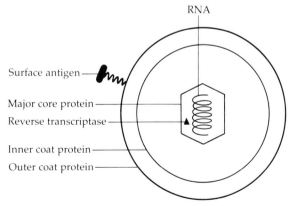

RNA

Surface antigen

Major core protein
Reverse transcriptase

Inner coat protein
Outer coat protein

Fig. 2.25 *Structure of human immune deficiency virus (HIV). HIV$_1$ and HIV$_2$ have now been described.*

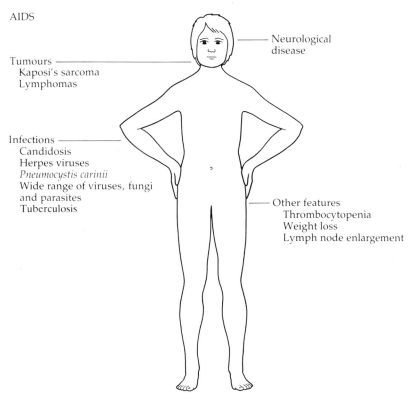

Fig. 2.26 *Features of acquired immune deficiency (AIDS).*

AIDS

Tumours
  Kaposi's sarcoma
  Lymphomas

Infections
  Candidosis
  Herpes viruses
  Pneumocystis carinii
  Wide range of viruses, fungi
  and parasites
  Tuberculosis

Neurological
disease

Other features
  Thrombocytopenia
  Weight loss
  Lymph node enlargement

Table 2.12
Main features of HIV infection

Opportunistic infections	Malignant neoplasms	Neurological disease	Autoimmune phenomena
Fungi: candidosis	Kaposi's sarcoma	Dementia	Bleeding tendency (thrombocytopenia)
Viruses: herpes viruses	Lymphomas		
Mycobacteria: TB			
Parasites: *Pneumocystis carinii*			

West, but in Africa there is strong evidence of heterosexual transmission. In any society, female consorts of infected individuals are at risk and infection *can* be sexually transmitted between females and males, and from mothers to their unborn children.

AIDS appears to be very prevalent in central Africa. It is possible that connections with Haiti and Belgium, together with increasing air travel, have been responsible for the suggested spread of AIDS from Africa to the USA, Western Europe and other areas.

The number of AIDS cases is rapidly rising, but full-blown AIDS almost certainly represents only the tip of

Table 2.13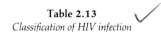
Classification of HIV infection

Asymptomatic HIV infection

↓

AIDS-related complexes
(e.g. persistent generalized lymphadenopathy: PGL)

↓

AIDS
(full-blown acquired immune deficiency syndrome)

Table 2.14
High-risk groups for HIV infection

Male homosexuals or bisexuals

Intravenous drug abusers

Recipients of unscreened blood or blood products (e.g. older haemophiliacs)

Prostitutes

Patients from Central Africa and areas of high prevalence such as California and New York

Consorts of the above

Children of HIV-positive mothers

the iceberg in relation to the number of infected individuals.

Immunology

AIDS is characterized by widespread immunological abnormalities that are amongst the most profound and persistent known. In full-blown AIDS there is a striking lymphopenia with a uniquely severe reduction in T inducer–helper lymphocytes (T4 or CD4 cells) and apparently irreversible abnormalities of those remaining. The reduction in T4 cells leads to an irreversible fall in the ratio of helper (T4) to suppressor (T8) cells.

Infection with HIV usually leads to an antibody response. Patients with HIV antibodies (HTLV-III or HIV-positive patients) at present are regarded as infectious.

Prognosis and management

There is still no effective treatment for the underlying immune defect in AIDS and therapy is limited to antimicro-

bial and supportive treatment, though there is some hope from agents such as AZT (azidothymidine).

Mortality in full-blown AIDS approaches 100%. Long-term morbidity from HIV infection again is unclear, particularly now that brain disorders are appearing as complications.

Oral manifestations (Volume 2)

At least 50% of patients with AIDS have head and neck manifestations, predominantly cervical lymph node enlargement, candidosis, hairy leukoplakia and Kaposi's sarcoma.

Transmission of HIV in the dental surgery

Transmission of HIV is blood borne; saliva is not known to transmit infection. HIV appears to be much less transmissible than hepatitis B virus and although there is clear evidence of transmission of HIV by blood and blood products, of the very many medical, paramedical and

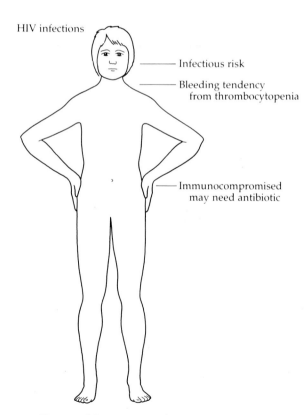

Fig. 2.27 *Management complications in HIV infection.*

dental staff treating AIDS victims, there are very few established cases who have been proven to have contracted AIDS in this way.

Close contact of mucosal surfaces, particularly through sexual intercourse, appears to be the only type of social contact likely to predispose to transmission of HIV infection.

AIDS and related disorders may also cause management difficulties because of:

(a) a bleeding tendency (see p. 13).
(b) immunosuppression (Fig. 2.27).

Since there may be a risk from infection, immunocompromised dental staff (e.g. those on systemic corticosteroids) should not be involved in treating AIDS patients since they may be more at risk from serious complications of HIV or other infections.

Respiratory viruses

Viral respiratory tract infections such as the common cold can readily be transmitted in the surgery (see p. 19). Epstein–Barr virus is shed into saliva and can be transmitted by kissing (Volume 2). Herpes simplex virus can be transmitted from infected saliva or vesicle fluid to cause primary herpetic stomatitis or herpetic whitlow in non-immune individuals (Fig. 2.28; Volume 2).

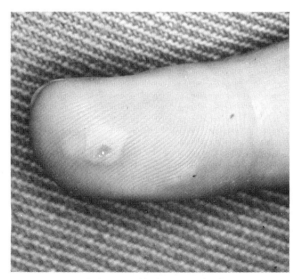

Fig. 2.28 *Whitlow caused by herpes simplex virus infection, in a dentist not wearing operating gloves.*

Other viruses

Cytomegalovirus and others are profusely excreted by some immunocompromised patients (Volume 2).

Bacteria

There is little evidence that oral commensal organisms cause particular harm if transmitted to other normal individuals though there is clear evidence for transmission of various organisms to close social contacts. However, pyogenic organisms that cause impetigo, such as *Staphylococcus aureus* and *Streptococcus pyogenes*, are readily transmitted from skin lesions. Human bites occasionally result in fusospirochaetal infections.

Tuberculosis can and has been transmitted in the dental surgery. One dental surgeon infected at least 15 patient contacts, and dental staff have contracted TB from patients with pulmonary tuberculosis who cough infected sputum. Vagrants, alcoholics, patients with AIDS, and immigrants from Ireland and some Asian countries are among the high-risk groups at present (Volume 2).

Syphilis is increasing in prevalence, and oral lesions of primary and secondary stages can present an infective risk to dental staff (Volume 2). Oral gonorrhoea appears to pose little, if any, infective risk to dental staff (Volume 2).

Legionella pneumoniae, the cause of respiratory disease affecting particularly the elderly (Legionnaires disease), is classically transmitted through water humidifiers and air-conditioning systems. There is some concern that it might also be transmitted in the water sprays and cooling systems in dental units but, as yet, there is little evidence for this.

Prevention of cross-infection (see Chapter 9)

Identification of high-risk patients

The medical history, directed specific questions as to lifestyle, and clinical examination will detect some but not all high-risk patients. High-risk individuals include mainly those in Tables 2.10 and 2.14.

Screening tests are widely available for HBV but not for delta and non-A, non-B hepatitis. The antibody response to HIV infection can be detected by serum assay, but not all infected patients have a positive result, and screening should never be carried out without appropriate counselling and consent of the patient in view of the serious implications of a positive result.

Dental treatment of any patient

Since the majority of patients infected with hepatitis B virus (HBV) or the AIDS virus (HIV) are asymptomatic and may not have been identified as infected, *the only safe approach is to assume that any dental patient may be a carrier of an infectious agent, and to follow good cross-infection control always.*

Personal hygiene

It goes without saying that all dental staff should have the highest possible standards of personal hygiene.

Vaccination

All dental health-care workers, including hygienists and dental surgery assistants, should be vaccinated against the childhood infections, tuberculosis and hepatitis B. Following HBV vaccination it is recommended that an antibody test is performed within a year to ensure protection.

Gloves

Operating gloves should be worn routinely by all clinical staff when touching blood, saliva or mucous membranes, or contaminated instruments and ideally changed or, failing that, washed with hot water and soap or appropriate handwashing agents between patients (Fig. 2.29). An antimicrobial handscrub, such as a chlorhexidine-containing preparation, should be used before surgical procedures. Any cuts or abrasions should be covered (under gloves). Damaged gloves should be changed immediately and discarded. Hands should be washed after gloves are removed.

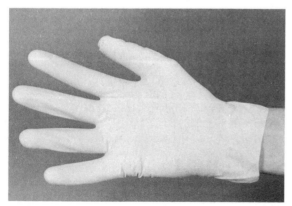

Fig. 2.29 *Disposable rubber gloves (essential for all clinical dentistry).*

Protection against airborne infection

Rubber dam should be used wherever feasible as this will prevent infective aerosols. Protective glasses and masks should be worn when using high-speed machinery such as air rotor or ultrasonic scaler, where aerosol spray or

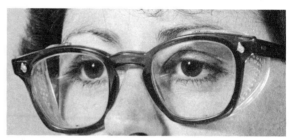

Fig. 2.30 *Protective eye wear should be worn during all operative procedures. These glasses have a side screen as well.*

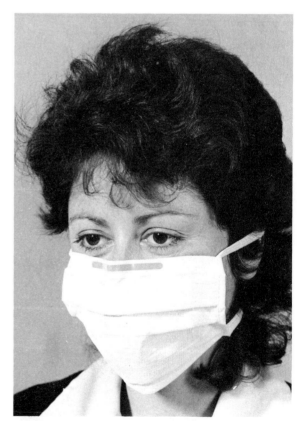

Fig. 2.31 *Although there is no evidence of aerosol transmission of many agents, it is prudent to wear a mask if aerosols are created and to prevent transmission of infection from operator to patient.*

splashing is likely (Figs. 2.30 and 2.31). High-volume aspirators are required and should be exhausted externally, with good ventilation in the surgery.

Cleaning and sterilizing instruments (see also Chapter 9)

Use disposable equipment wherever possible and do not re-use this. Non-disposable items should be cleaned thoroughly with a disinfectant such as 2% glutaraldehyde before sterilization (Table 2.15, Fig. 2.32). Ultrasonic

Table 2.15
Chemical disinfection (see Table 9.6)

Chemical	Disinfectant	Sterilant
Sodium hypochlorite	Dilute 1 in 10 to 1 in 100; leave for 10–30 min	—
Glutaraldehyde		
2% alkaline	Full strength, leave for 10 min	Full strength, leave for 10 h
2% alkaline with phenolic buffer	Dilute 1 in 16, leave for 10 min	Full strength, leave for 7 h
2% neutral	Full strength, leave for 10 min	Full strength, leave for 10 h

cleaners are recommended for cleaning small instruments before sterilization. Boiling water is inadequate for sterilization since it will not reliably destroy the hepatitis B virus and other agents, and so instruments should be autoclaved at 134°C for a minimum of 3 minutes (Table 2.15; see also p. 210).

Where possible, use disposable trays or covers such as plastic film on surfaces, and clean work surfaces with alcohol or 500 ppm hypochlorite (1 in 100 dilution domestic bleach), even if they appear clean. However, where visible blood is present, the surface should be cleaned with a disposable cloth using 5000 ppm (1 in 10 dilution) hypochlorite solution (or glutaraldehyde if the surface is metal, since hypochlorite is corrosive) (Table 9.6).

Waste disposal

Sharps should *always* be placed in rigid 'safe' containers (Fig. 2.33). This is especially important since refuse disposal officers and others might harm themselves. Other items should be disposed of in stout plastic bags, sealed and incinerated.

Impressions and appliances

Impressions and appliances should be rinsed thoroughly in running water before being sent to the laboratory, and technicians should wear gloves when handling impressions (see also Chapters 7 and 10).

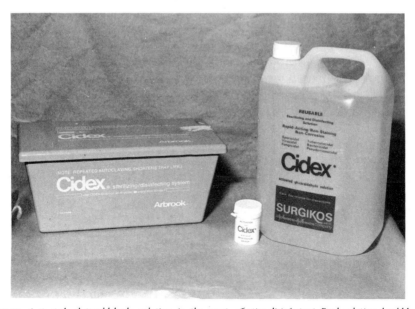

Fig. 2.32 *Activated glutaraldehyde solution is the most effective disinfectant. Fresh solution should be made up.*

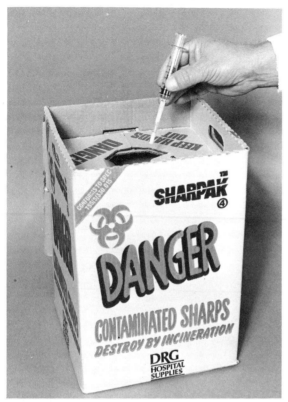

Fig. 2.33 *Needlestick injuries are the most likely means of contracting infection. All sharps should be disposed of into a rigid 'sharps bin'.*

Training of staff (see also Chapters 7 and 10)

All staff should be thoroughly trained to understand policies adopted to prevent cross-infection and procedures should be reviewed regularly to ensure they are being carried out correctly. The Health and Safety at Work Act regulates this aspect.

Care of ultrasonic scalers, 3-in-1 syringe, handpieces and dental units

Although sterilization of scalers, 3-in-1 syringe, handpieces and other instruments is highly desirable, not all can be sterilized. However, all items that *can* be autoclaved should be; others should be cleaned with 2% glutaraldehyde between patients and then rinsed with sterile water since glutaraldehyde can otherwise cause chemical burns.

It is impossible to ensure a supply of sterile water through water lines on the dental unit and the best that

can be done is to flush the system through for about 30 seconds first thing in the morning and after completing the use on each patient. This should at least physically remove gross contaminants.

However, where surgical procedures are carried out, *sterile* saline must be used as a coolant/irrigator.

Dental treatment of the known high-risk patient (see also Chapter 7)

The dental surgeon in charge of the patient, or his delegated member of staff, should inform the nurse in charge of the surgery or theatre (and in hospital also the Control of Infection Officer) of the 'at-risk' patient. Staff must be educated about the risks. The patient's notes, and operation list, should be clearly marked as IR ('infective risk'), with the date of the test result, if any.

All staff involved with the patient should be made aware of the risk and those with cuts on their hands and pregnant staff are best not to be involved.

The following guidelines should be observed.

1. Make the appointment at the end of the day.
2. Wear gowns, gloves, mask, protective glasses and overshoes throughout treatment. Change gloves if they perforate.
3. Use disposable instruments wherever possible. Cover surfaces with plastic film.
4. Sterilize all other instruments and handpieces: autoclave/fresh 2% glutaraldehyde solution—soak for 1 hour, then 3 hours in *fresh* solution.
5. Do not use ultrasonic scalers, airturbine or 3-in-1 syringe if the patient is HBeAg positive (i.e. highly infectious) unless there is rubber dam, adequate surgery ventilation and staff are vaccinated against HBV. There is, however, no evidence of risk from aerosols if the patient is HIV positive.
6. Use high-volume aspiration to minimize aerosol.
7. Surfaces and any contaminated areas (floor, walls, chair) should be cleaned with hypochlorite solution, which should be left on for 30 minutes and then rinsed and dried (if metal, glutaraldehyde for 3 hours).
8. Flush the aspirator with 2% glutaraldehyde and leave the solution in the system collector for 3 hours.
9. Take impressions in silicone material (which shows best dimensional stability and has the least water absorbance) and soak in glutaraldehyde for 1 hour before sending to the laboratory, where they should be soaked for a further 3 hours.
10. Avoid needlestick injuries.

Aspirated fluids should have one-tenth volume of

10 000 ppm hypochlorite (1-in-5 dilution of household bleach) added and should be left for at least 30 minutes before disposal. Metal instruments should be immersed for 30 minutes in fresh 2% glutaraldehyde (see Fig. 2.32) before autoclaving or despatch to CSSD. Sharps must be discarded into appropriate rigid 'sharps' containers (Fig. 2.33). Disposable items should be suitably discarded into special bags. Non-disposable clothing etc. should be sealed into special coloured bags for sterilization. Sterilization requires the use of the autoclaves, not boiling water. Suitable disinfectants for cold 'sterilization' are shown in Table 2.15, but this is disinfection rather than sterilization.

After all traces of blood have been removed by wiping with 2% glutaraldehyde, surfaces should be thoroughly cleaned with hypochlorite, then detergent and water before any further patients are treated in the room.

Procedure in the event of accidental injury involving a high-risk patient (needlestick injuries)

The risk to the wounded person from HBV infection is greatest if he is anti-HBs negative and if the infected blood is HBeAg positive. The risk from HIV infection is unclear but is much lower. The risks from non-A, non-B viruses and delta agent are unclear.

First, rinse the wound in running water and ensure that the accident is not repeated, by discarding sharps, etc. The HBsAg and anti-HB, and HBeAg and anti-HBe status of both parties should then be established and, if there is a risk of transfer of infection by the accident, the appropriate microbiologist should be consulted.

Two main courses are open with regard to HBV or delta infection: passive immunization with hepatitis B immunoglobulin (which should be given as soon as possible and in any event not later than 48 hours after the injury), and vaccination. Immune globulin may be useful if there has been exposure to non-A, non-B virus.

With respect to HIV infection, there is currently no prophylaxis but zidovudine may help.

JAUNDICE AND LIVER DISEASE

Most jaundice is caused by liver or biliary-related disease. Dental management may be complicated by:

(a) infective problems such as viral hepatitis (see p. 37),
(b) bleeding tendency (p. 12),
(c) impaired drug metabolism.

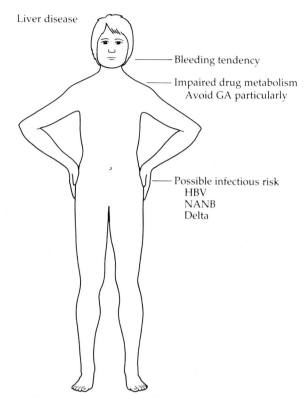

Fig. 2.34 *Management problems in patients with liver disease.*

The liver is the main route for the metabolism of most drugs, and liver disease, therefore, often causes drug effects to be potentiated and prolonged. In dentistry the greatest danger is when GA is used, but the dose of sedatives (such as diazepam or midazolam), hypnotics and analgesics should also be reduced and sometimes the drugs are absolutely contraindicated in patients with liver disease (see Table 2.9; Fig. 2.34).

The responsible physician should always be consulted before medication is given to a hospital patient with liver disease.

Postoperative jaundice

Postoperative jaundice is uncommon but may be a sign of serious complications. Causes include:

(a) haemolysis from incompatible blood transfusion;
(b) liver disease:
    (i) viral hepatitis (p. 37)
    (ii) sepsis

(iii) halothane hepatitis (p. 30)

(iv) Gilbert's syndrome—a benign disorder in which jaundice only arises if the patient has a GA, starves or takes alcohol. It is a congenital defect of bilirubin metabolism but has no serious connotations. Apart from occasional jaundice, the patients are otherwise quite well.

KIDNEY DISEASE

Of all patients with renal disease, it is those with chronic renal failure and those who have renal transplant grafts who pose the greatest problems to the dentist in terms of oral manifestations and management complications (Fig. 2.35).

Chronic renal failure

Chronic renal failure (CRF) manifests with a reduced glomerular filtration rate and nocturia, polyuria, anorexia,

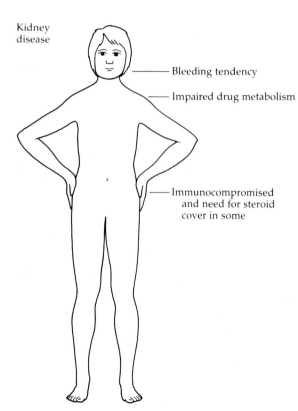

Kidney disease

Bleeding tendency

Impaired drug metabolism

Immunocompromised and need for steroid cover in some

Fig. 2.35 *Management problems in patients with kidney disease.*

anaemia, hypertension, bleeding tendency, liability to infections and disordered bone metabolism. In children with CRF, growth is often retarded. Patients are often on corticosteroid or other immunosuppressive treatment. There may be enamel hypoplasia and retarded tooth eruption in children but fewer caries and less periodontal disease.

Oral candidosis and mixed bacterial plaques may appear and there is a predisposition to keratotic lesions and viral infections. A bleeding tendency may produce mucosal bleeding or purpura. Bone lesions include loss of lamina dura, osteoporosis and osteolytic lesions (renal osteodystrophy) and sometimes lesions of secondary hyperparathyroidism (Volume 2).

Dental management

Patients with CRF may present problems related to:

(a) bleeding tendency (p. 12),

(b) hepatitis B carriage (p. 37),

(c) corticosteroid or other immunosuppressive treatment (p. 30),

(d) impaired drug excretion (see Table 2.9).

LIKELIHOOD OF PREGNANCY

Pregnancy is an ideal opportunity for dental education of the mother in relation to herself and the child.

There is no evidence for tooth demineralization or increased caries during pregnancy but, in the absence of good oral hygiene, a very hyperaemic gingivitis (pregnancy gingivitis) may result. Occasionally a proliferative pyogenic granuloma (pregnancy epulis: Fig. 2.36; Volume 2) occurs. This usually requires no treatment because it regresses spontaneously at parturition, but it may need to be excised if especially unaesthetic, or interfering with occlusion.

Dental treatment is best avoided during the first trimester (3 months) of pregnancy and GA in particular is best avoided since it is at this time that spontaneous abortions are most likely. However, it should be borne in mind that women are not always aware that they are pregnant during the first trimester, and therefore *all* prescription of drugs should be cautious for women of childbearing age. Conversely, in the last trimester the mother may find physical difficulty in sitting or lying in the dental chair: indeed lying may cause the fetus to impede venous return to the heart by pressure on the inferior vena cava. This may cause the mother to faint (supine hypotensive syndrome). Vomiting is likely at the first trimester and GA is therefore best avoided.

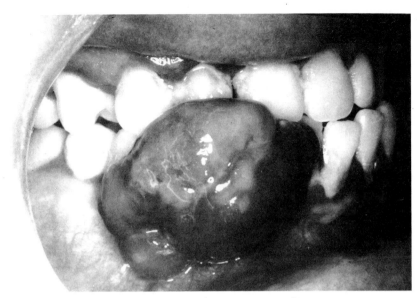

Fig. 2.36 *Pregnancy epulis (an extreme example).*

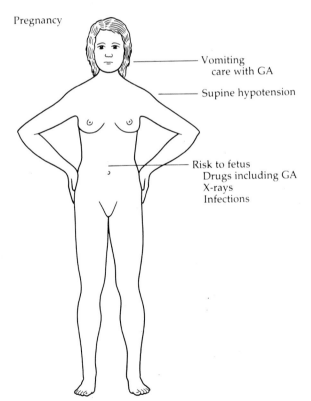

Pregnancy

— Vomiting
  care with GA

— Supine hypotension

— Risk to fetus
  Drugs including GA
  X-rays
  Infections

Fig. 2.37 *Management problems in pregnancy.*

Dental treatment is therefore best carried out during the second trimester. Exposure of the pregnant person to infections, irradiation, general anaesthetic gases and drugs should be kept to a minimum—this applies to patients and staff. (Fig. 2.37; see Chapter 10).

There is no absolute assurance of the safety of any drug in pregnancy. Therefore the safest course of action is to prescribe no drugs, particularly during the first trimester. This is not always practicable, but tetracyclines *must* be avoided and also, if possible, drugs that may be teratogenic, such as cotrimoxazole, metronidazole, aspirin and non-steroidal anti-inflammatory agents, and tranquillizers or sedatives should be avoided (Table 2.16).

Breast-feeding

Since drugs may pass in the milk to the infant, some, such as tetracyclines, are contraindicated. Penicillin may cause candidosis or diarrhoea in the child. Aspirin may cause a bleeding tendency. Benzodiazepines may produce lethargy and reluctance to feed (Table 2.17).

CHILDREN

Although children can occasionally suffer from oral diseases more common in adults, including malignant oral lesions, certain conditions are more specific to childhood.

Table 2.16 ✓
Drug use in pregnancy

Drugs that should be avoided	Use
Aspirin	Paracetamol
Mefenamic acid	
Dextropropoxyphene	
Pentazocine	
Tetracyclines ⎫	⎧ Penicillin
Metronidazole ⎪	⎪ Erythromycin
Aminoglycosides ⎬	⎨ Cephalosporins
Co-trimoxazole ⎪	⎪ Sulphisoxazole
Sulphonamides ⎪	⎩
Rifampicin ⎭	
Benzodiazepines (unless short acting)	Temazepam
Opiates (and related compounds)	
Barbiturates	Nitrous oxide
	Halothane
Povidone iodine	
Etretinate	
Antidepressants	
Corticosteroids	
Danazol	

Table 2.17 ✓
Drug use in breast-feeding mothers

May be contraindicated		Use
Analgesics	Aspirin (high dose)	Aspirin (low dose)
	Dextropropoxyphene	Paracetamol
		Codeine
		Mefenamic acid
Antimicrobials	Tetracyclines	Penicillins
	Co-trimoxazole	Erythromycin
	Metronidazole	Rifampicin
	Sulphonamides	Cephalosporins
	Aminoglycosides	
Premedication	Atropine	Benzodiazepines (low dose)
	Chloral hydrate	Phenothiazines (low dose)
	Beta blockers	
Others	Antidepressants	
	Etretinate	
	Carbamazepine	
	Corticosteroids (high dose)	Corticosteroids (low dose)

Mucosal disorders

Teething

Teething is the discomfort experienced by children associated with the eruption of deciduous teeth. Teething is a purely local phenomenon without malaise or fever and, if the child is unwell at the same time, this is due either to a systemic disease or some other oral disease.

The main treatment for teething is reassurance of the parents, and possibly the use of teething gels for the child.

Viral infections

Herpetic stomatitis, chickenpox, herpangina and hand, foot and mouth disease are infections predominantly of childhood (Volume 2).

Candidosis

Thrush may be seen in healthy neonates who have not yet become immune, but is rare in other children unless they are immunocompromised or have severe xerostomia (Volume 2).

White sponge naevus (Volume 2)

Erythema migrans (Volume 2)

Recurrent aphthae (Volume 2)

Aphthae usually start in childhood.

Diseases in or close to bone and joints

1. *Congenital epulis* is a swelling on the anterior maxillary ridge, which is present at birth. This rare benign lesion is histologically identical to granular cell tumour (Volume 2) and does not recur if excised.

2. *Pigmented neuroectodermal tumour* also affects the anterior maxilla but appears slightly later in infancy. Again rare and benign, it consists of a mixture of small, darkly staining cells and larger paler cells that contain melanin, and does not usually recur if excised (Volume 2).

3. *Cherubism* is an autosomal dominant bilateral condition of the jaws, otherwise resembling fibrous dysplasia in its histology and behaviour (Volume 2).

4. *Condylar hyperplasia* (see Volume 2).

5. *Juvenile rheumatoid arthritis* (see Volume 2).

6. *Burkitt's lymphoma* (see Volume 2).

Cleft palate and lip (see Volume 4)

Salivary gland disorders

1. *Mumps* (see Volume 2).
2. *Recurrent parotitis* (see Volume 2).

Neurological disorders

Moebius' syndrome of congenital facial palsy is a rare disorder in which cranial nerves VI and VII are affected.

The neck

Cystic hygroma is a rare developmental anomaly of the lymphatics that usually presents at birth and almost invariably by the age of 2 years. It presents as a fluctuant swelling of the side of the neck and may extend into the mediastinum. Some children also have lymphangioma of the tongue. Cystic hygroma is usually surgically removed since not only is it unaesthetic, but liable to spontaneous haemorrhage and spontaneous infection (Volume 2).

Dental treatment of children

The prevention and management of disorders of the teeth and periodontium are discussed in the other volumes in this series (Volumes 2 and 3).

Although in some ways children can be treated similarly to adults and are often more resilient, certain general differences should be borne in mind. Children tend to become ill much more rapidly and dramatically than adults, yet they also tend to recover more rapidly. Fevers tend to be higher than in adults and, since there may be a liability to febrile convulsions, antipyretics such as paracetamol are often indicated. Aspirin should be avoided since, rarely, it can produce liver damage (Reye's syndrome: fatty liver with central nervous system damage). Children lose fluid rapidly, especially if they are febrile: this, in young children, can lead to potentially lethal dehydration. Therefore, it is vital to ensure that ill children are given adequate fluids: food is far less important.

Children must be given smaller drug doses not only because of their lower body weight but also because they are often particularly sensitive to drug toxicity. Doses are best calculated from body surface area. Children may react to drugs differently to the way that adults react. Diazepam, for example, does not necessarily always sedate children but may cause hyperactivity. Tetracyclines are contraindicated under the age of 8 years in view of the likelihood of tooth discoloration.

Drugs are best given orally and are more acceptable as

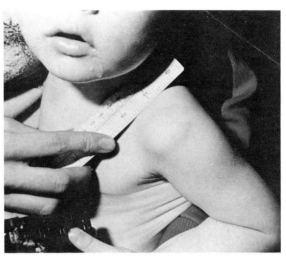

Fig. 2.38 *Child abuse (battered baby syndrome): a bite on the shoulder (courtesy of Mr M Midda).*

liquid preparations or suspensions. Sucrose-based preparations should be avoided if long-term administration is likely, because of the risk of caries. Drugs should not be mixed with milk or other drinks since the contents may react and absorption be impaired.

Child abuse

Child abuse is increasingly common. The children, who are usually under the age of 3 years, are deliberately injured, usually by a parent or guardian. There is a 60% chance of recurrent abuse and a 10% eventual fatality.

Injuries often involve the orofacial region, with lacerations especially of the upper labial fraenum and mucosa, bruising, bite marks or burns (Fig. 2.38). Skull and facial fractures are not uncommon.

Child abuse can most readily be recognized by an inexplicable delay in seeking treatment or a discrepancy between injuries and the history given. The injuries should be carefully recorded, with radiographs and photographs, and the Social Services Department contacted so that the child is returned to his environment only when he is safe from further abuse.

THE HANDICAPPED

Any condition that impairs mobility or communication can cause management problems, and these are compounded if there are behavioural disturbances or complicating medical disease. Unfortunately, it is a sad trick of nature that if one handicap is present the patient frequently has, or develops, further problems. A good example of this is the cleft palate deformity: most people are aware of the defect but less appreciated are the other possible complications involving, for example, the heart.

Mentally or physically handicapped patients may be at risk if they develop dental or oral disease, or if they require operative intervention especially with a general anaesthetic.

Management

Patients handicapped for various reasons have many oral problems in common with each other. These common problems are discussed here and points specific to the various categories of handicap are outlined later.

Oral hygiene

Oral hygiene is often poor because of physical defects such as hemiplegia, or the intellectual deficits of the mentally handicapped. Oral hygiene procedures and preventive dentistry are therefore more important in handicapped than in other patients. Automatic toothbrushes can be of more use for these than for any other patients. Chlorhexidine is a useful adjunct to the maintenance of oral hygiene but will not remove existing plaque.

Access to the dental surgery

Sometimes the only problem for handicapped patients is the difficulty of travelling to the surgery, or of getting into the dental chair. This difficulty may be physical, as in the chairbound patient; mental, as in the mentally handicapped; or, in some instances, psychological. The problem worsens as the patient's parents or guardians, who often manage well while the patient is young, become elderly themselves and find increasing difficulty in bringing the patient for treatment. Should public transport be needed, the difficulties are compounded, as they are if access to the surgery involves climbing stairs. Although, in these instances, social services may need to be involved and the patient may need transporting by ambulance or by the hospital car service or may require the assistance of a domiciliary attendant, some patients prefer, and manage to retain, their independence.

Treatment of the handicapped can be most rewarding and is not necessarily so time consuming as to result in financial loss. Communication with the medical practitioner often helps to outline any potential management problems and can allay unnecessary fears in the mind of the dental surgeon. Handicapped patients appreciate the care and attention that come from sympathetic handling and explanation of treatment procedures.

The dental surgery assistant can be invaluable in helping the handicapped patient both physically and psychologically, and it may be easier for the patient to convey anxieties or fears about dental treatment through the DSA.

Referral of patients

The GDP can refer patients who need specialist attention to the community dental service, the hospital service or occasionally to colleagues who have a special interest in the handicapped.

Mental handicap

By convention, persons with an intelligence quotient (IQ) below 70 are usually regarded as mentally handicapped ('subnormal' or 'retarded'). There are many causes of the brain damage that leads to mental handicap, but among the more common identifiable causes are congenital disorders such as Down's syndrome (mongolism) and acquired defects such as may occur with cerebral hypoxia, infection or trauma.

Few situations can be more distressing than the occurrence of brain damage such as from meningitis or after a head injury in a previously healthy person. The effects of mental handicap on the lives of the patient and relatives, as well as the implications for the community at large, are profound.

Although most mentally handicapped patients are otherwise well and indeed few appear distressed at their plight, they may have additional handicaps—particularly epilepsy, cerebral palsy and defects of hearing and sight. Some have associated craniofacial or other malformations which may increase the social handicaps and the prejudices of the public and even of some health-care professionals. Neglect of health care, including oral health, is therefore common since not only is the patient unaware of the need but if often lacking the manual dexterity required to maintain oral hygiene and may also receive less professional attention than 'normal' persons.

Down's syndrome

About 1 in 700 live births in the UK are of children with Down's syndrome. Usually the cause is abnormal meiosis in the mother's oocyte resulting in unequal separation of chromosomes into daughter cells (non-disjunction) such that one cell contains one extra chromosome 21—hence the term trisomy 21. Non-disjunction becomes increasingly common with age and thus most children with Down's syndrome are born to mothers over the age of 35–40 years.

Characteristic features

Mental handicap is almost invariable, though many patients are happy, friendly individuals. Short stature, a broad neck and a mongoloid facial appearance characterize Down's syndrome, but virtually all tissues are abnormal, especially:

1. immune defects and liability to infections, including hepatitis B and respiratory infections;
2. congenital cardiac defects in up to 40% of patients.

Orofacial features

1. The eyes have a mongoloid appearance and there is midface hypoplasia with mandibular prognathism (Fig. 2.39).
2. The tongue tends to be large and fissured (Fig. 2.40).

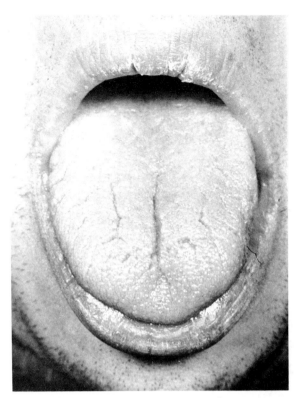

Fig. 2.40 *Large tongue in Down's syndrome.*

3. The dentition is liable to:
   late eruption
   hypodontia
   microdontia—particularly the tooth roots are short
   morphological anomalies.
4. There is no predisposition to dental caries.
5. There is a predisposition to rapidly destructive periodontal disease which, together with shortness of the roots, frequently leads to early tooth loss, particularly from the lower anterior region (Fig. 2.41).

Management

Special precautions may be required because of hepatitis B carriage (p. 33) or a cardiac defect (p. 17) though the latter tends to be an atrial septal defect not particularly liable to infective endocarditis.

Physical handicap

Although there are many different physical handicaps,

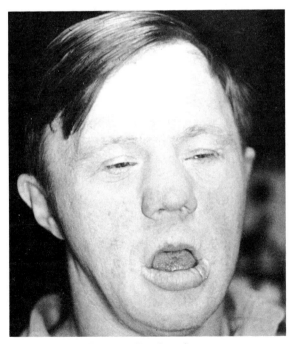

Fig. 2.39 *Down's syndrome.*

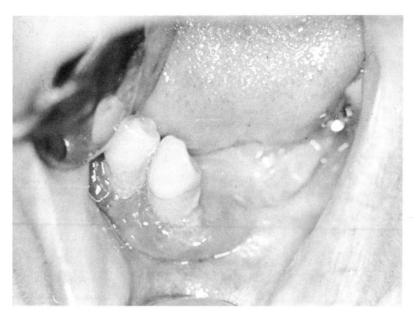

Fig. 2.41 *Periodontal disease causing premature tooth loss in Down's syndrome.*

perhaps the most obvious of the congenital ones is cerebral palsy (spasticity), and of the acquired ones traumatic paraplegia, stroke, and Parkinsonism.

Patients with severe physical handicap frequently are disadvantaged by the difficulties they have in mobility because they are bed-bound, chairbound or simply because access (for example to the dental surgery) is difficult. Some have additional problems such as epilepsy and/or mental handicap or communication handicaps (hearing, speech or sight) and it is unfortunate that many who are intelligent individuals are unjustifiably regarded as retarded, simply because of speech or hearing problems.

Cerebral palsy (spasticity)

Several different kinds of paralysis may follow brain damage, including:

(a) hemiplegia: paralysis of one side of the body;
(b) monoplegia: paralysis of one limb (usually the arm);
(c) quadriplegia: paralysis of most of the body below the neck;
(d) choreoathetosis: involuntary writhing movements with extreme incoordination (often associated with deafness and caused by congenital rubella or haemolytic disease of the newborn).

General features

Increased tone and spasticity characterize cerebral palsy and, if untreated, can result in permanent limb deformities (Fig. 2.42).

Orofacial features

Most have a perfectly normal facial appearance and any abnormalities are related to altered (usually increased) muscle tone. Speech is abnormal and there may be unusual jaw movements and bruxism (grinding and gnashing of the teeth).

Management

The main problems are:

(a) communication difficulties,
(b) involuntary movements,
(c) associated epilepsy.

Spinal cord lesions

Spinal cord damage is usually caused by congenital anomalies (spina bifida), trauma or infection. There may be severe handicap, the clinical effects depending on the level of the lesion. When paraplegia (paralysis below the

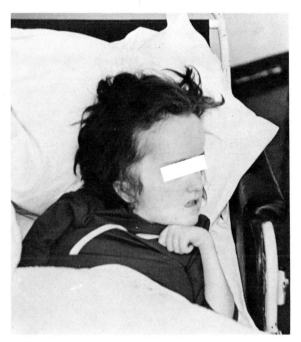

Fig. 2.42 *Cerebral palsy in a patient with hydrocephalus, showing wasted and flexed deformity of arm and hand.*

waist) is present it causes mobility problems, muscle wasting, urinary and faecal incontinence and urinary infections. High level lesions can also cause respiratory embarrassment or death. Patients with congenital spinal defects, such as spina bifida, may have additional problems such as epilepsy, mental handicap or renal disorders.

Management

The main dental management problems relate to impaired mobility. In early post-traumatic paraplegia, the possibility of postural hypotension may necessitate treatment in the supine position, but such patients are unlikely to be seen in dental practice. Quadriplegics are also rarely seen by the GDP and since they are at risk from respiratory infections secondary to impaired respiration, general anaesthesia is hazardous.

Autism

Autism is an unusual disorder in which there is a failure to develop interpersonal relationships, delayed speech, a profound desire to be alone and to retain the status quo of the environment, and ritualistic or compulsive phenomena. The disorder usually becomes apparent during the first two years of life when the child fails to respond emotionally to stimuli such as being picked up by the parents, and seems to wander about aimlessly, apparently oblivious of others.

Management

Many autistics have a minor degree of mental handicap but there are no specific medical complications that influence dental care.

Autistics insist on strict routine and strongly resist changes. It is, therefore, most important that the same GDP and ancillary staff continue to care for the autistic patient and that he or she is not subjected to new places or faces. Dental treatment can be most difficult to carry out as it may seem impossible to gain the child's attention. General anaesthesia or relative analgesia may well be required.

Visual defects

Impaired vision can have many causes but is always a severe handicap. Although dental treatment can usually be carried out by the GDP without complication, consideration of the cause of the visual defect is always necessary, for example to exclude diabetes mellitus. Clearly the patient with a visual defect is dependent on others to communicate so that surprise and fear are minimized. Patients must be reassured about dental treatment by a careful explanation and warning before instruments are used, especially if noisy apparatus is to be turned on.

Hearing defects

Deafness is a common problem which also causes severe communication difficulties but is uncommonly associated with medical complications. The GDP may need extreme patience in managing the hard-of-hearing. A few GDPs can manage sign language but, failing this, slow, deliberate pronunciation or the writing of notes can be useful. Some deaf patients may be unduly sensitive to vibration and dislike, for example, automatic amalgam condensers.

THE ELDERLY

The elderly can suffer any oral condition affecting other adults but some are more common in this group (Figs. 2.43 and 2.44). These are summarized in Tables 2.18–2.21; more details are outlined in Volumes 2 and 3.

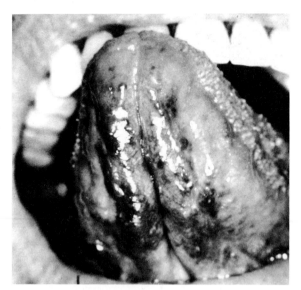

Fig. 2.43 *Lingual varices in an elderly patient.*

Table 2.18
Oral mucosal diseases in the elderly

Lingual varicosities are large tortuous veins on the ventrum of the tongue, of no consequence, which may become more prominent in the elderly (see Fig. 2.43)

Foliate papillae may appear large or inflamed and can be mistaken for a neoplasm

Mucosal atrophy may occur with age, the thin fragile mucosa appearing less resistant to trauma, for example from dentures

Denture-induced stomatitis (Volume 2)

Burning mouth (oral dysaesthesia) (Volume 2)

Vesiculobullous disorders—especially pemphigoid and pemphigus (Volume 2)

Lichen planus ⎫
Keratosis ⎬ (Volume 2)
Erythroplakia ⎪
Carcinoma ⎭

Management

Specific dental needs of the elderly are discussed elsewhere in this series (Volumes 2, 3 and 4). In general, however, the elderly require more patience and time for their treatment and they may be less resilient. Most are conservative in outlook and may well dislike lying flat in the

Table 2.19
Bone and joint diseases in the elderly

Gross alveolar atrophy can occur in edentulous jaws and there may be changes of osteoporosis. Anatomical structures such as the mylohyoid ridge, genial and mental tubercles remain and may become prominent and cause pain from pressure of overlying dentures. The mental nerve may come to lie beneath the lower denture, causing pain (see Fig. 2.44)

Osteoarthrosis of the temporomandibular joint is not a common problem

Paget's disease (Volume 2)

Table 2.20
Salivary gland diseases in the elderly
(see also Volume 2)

Dry mouth (especially due to drug use)

Sjogren's syndrome

Neoplasms

Table 2.21
Neurological diseases in the elderly
(see also Volume 2)

Herpes zoster

Trigeminal neuralgia

Giant cell arteritis

Facial palsy (caused by a stroke)

Parkinsonism

dental chair or various other 'new-fangled' ideas. Even a simple dental appointment can be a fairly major event in their lives. A few kind words can be most reassuring but an impatient brusque manner can be most hurtful.

Elderly patients may have multiple pathology and there may be deteriorating hearing, vision and mobility, all of which need to be considered in relation to dental treatment.

Lower drug doses are usually required in the elderly. The elderly are especially sensitive to the effects of sedatives and tranquillizers, whose dose should be reduced. Patient compliance is often poor and mistakes in drugs taken common because of the patient's senility, blindness or bewilderment. Elderly patients often have medical problems and receive multiple drugs—facts that compound the problem.

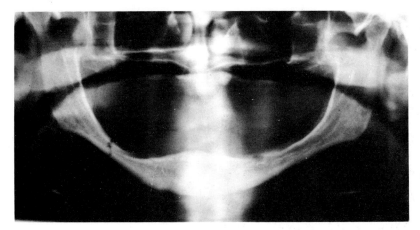

Fig. 2.44 *Extreme alveolar atrophy in an elderly patient. The mental foraminae lie on the crest of the ridge and the body of the mandible fractured spontaneously on the right side of the patient.*

The elderly do not necessarily manifest disease in the same way as younger adults. Infective conditions do not necessarily cause significant fever, rather the fact that the patient is ill may become apparent more by behavioural changes.

PSYCHIATRIC PATIENTS

The psychogenic reactions experienced by many persons in relation to dental treatment are discussed in Chapter 1, and the psychogenic bases to some orofacial pain and other lesions discussed in Chapter 1 and Volume 2. Psychogenic disorders merge into psychiatric disease when the disorder extends beyond the bounds of 'normality' and causes problems to others in the environment. A good example of this relates to obsessions and compulsions. Many normal persons have an obsessional nature—especially many dentists, for whom it is often regarded as a desirable trait. Persons with such personalities are prone to psychogenic reactions such as anxiety and/or depression if they cannot live up to the standards they set themselves and may mildly irritate those in the work/family environment. If, however, the obsession is such that it totally disrupts these environments, e.g. compulsive handwashing, such that every time someone washes his hands he is compelled to wash them again because he is obsessed that they are still dirty, and so on, then this can be regarded as a psychiatric disease.

Psychiatric patients can present management problems in dentistry because of behavioural problems, or because the effects of the drugs used in management interfere with routine dental treatment procedures or cause oral disease.

Orofacial manifestations in psychogenic and psychiatric disease

These include the following, especially if there are multiple complaints (Table 2.22); further details can be found in Volume 2.

Table 2.22
Oral features of psychogenic disorders

Dry mouth

Sore or burning mouth

Bad taste or disturbed taste

Atypical facial pain

Atypical odontalgia

Paraesthesia and anaesthesia

Mandibular pain-dysfunction syndrome

Non-existent discharges

'Gripping' dentures

Vomiting or nausea caused by dentures

Supposed sialorrhoea

Non-existent lumps

Factitious (self-induced) injuries (including lip-chewing)

Bruxism

Occlusal line keratatosis

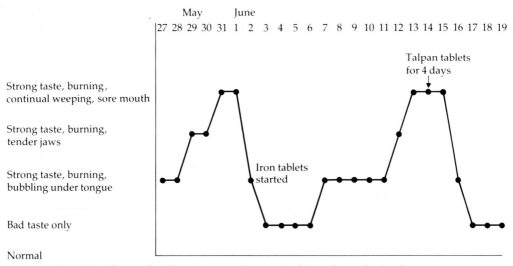

Fig. 2.45 *Chart produced by a patient with multiple oral complaints related to depression.*

Some patients will graphically describe their problems (Fig. 2.45) and others write screeds of notes about their symptoms (maladie du petit papier).

Drug treatment of psychiatric disease may cause dry mouth (mainly caused by antidepressants and lithium) and facial dyskinesias (mainly caused by tranquillizers).

Oral neglect and subsequent caries and periodontal disease are not uncommon in psychotic patients. Depressed neurotic patients may occasionally also neglect themselves to the extent of developing such poor oral hygiene as to fall prone to oral disease. Patients with anorexia nervosa (who have a pathological desire to lose weight) or bulimia (who vomit to lose weight) may develop tooth erosion because of repeated regurgitation of gastric contents. Hypochondriac patients may be preoccupied with the fear of having serious disease: some (Munchausen's syndrome) repeatedly submit themselves to unnecessary investigations or operations.

Management

The main management difficulties involve patients who have phobias about treatment, who are hysterical, who are depressed, paranoid or schizophrenic, or who are intoxicated or disorientated.

Phobias

Phobias are persistent and irrational fears that result in a compelling desire to avoid the dreaded object, activity or situation. Psychiatric treatment with or without drugs or techniques such as hypnosis may well be required to enable these patients to cope with dental treatment (Chapter 1).

Hysteria

Hysteria is a sudden inexplicable temporary loss or alteration of motor behaviour in the absence of organic disease. Patients are usually adult females who may behave bizarrely in relation to dental treatment, often feigning a faint and hyperventilating. Care should be taken to ensure no organic emergency is occurring (Chapter 4) and the patient should be calmly but firmly reassured. Because hyperventilation may blow off carbon dioxide, causing alkalosis, rebreathing expired air (for example from a paper bag) may facilitate recovery.

Depression

Apart from the apathy and negative attitudes that characterize depression, the main treatment complication is related to drug therapy. Pethidine and sympathomimetic amines such as ephedrine and noradrenaline can, by releasing endogenous catecholamines, cause dangerous hypertension in patients taking monoamine oxidase inhibitors (MAOI). Local anaesthetics, even if containing adrenaline, appear to be safe in these patients but GA may be contraindicated. The tricyclic antidepressants are **not** now thought to contraindicate the use of local anaesthesia, even if the solution contains adrenaline.

Paranoia and other types of schizophrenia

Persistent persecutory delusions or delusional jealousy characterize paranoia. These, with delusions, hallucinations and disturbed thought processes or behaviour, characterize schizophrenia. Such patients need psychiatric care and treatment with major tranquillizers such as phenothiazines.

Intoxicated or disorientated patients

It is unwise to carry out routine dental treatment in intoxicated patients. Medical advice should be urgently sought. Many patients attending accident and emergency units are intoxicated or have been using alcohol or drugs, but disturbed behaviour may also be due to organic disease (e.g. diabetes, head injury).

Patients may be disorientated because of organic disease (e.g. hypoglycaemia in diabetics who miss a meal often causes disorientation); intoxication; or psychiatric disease. The elderly may become disorientated if ill or given CNS-active drugs, or because of dementia. No drugs should be administered; medical assistance should be sought.

The Mental Health Acts give powers for admission or detention of people in hospital against their will provided certain conditions apply. A medical practitioner is needed to implement most of these compulsory procedures (Sections: p. 112) though, in emergency, a police officer may remove a patient who appears to be mentally disordered in a place to which the public have access (under Section 136 of the Mental Health Act, 1983, or Section 104 of the Mental Health Act, Scotland, 1960).

IMMUNOCOMPROMISED PATIENTS

There is an increasing number of patients who have immune defects, mainly acquired because of infection with human immunodeficiency virus (HIV), or immunosuppressive drugs (usually corticosteroids, azathioprine and/or cyclosporin). Immunological disorders such as leukaemia and lymphoma are also associated with immune defects. Congenital immune defects are rare.

Orofacial manifestations

These are discussed in Volume 2.

In general terms, immunocompromised patients are prone to develop the following orofacial problems.

1. Fungal infections—especially candidosis

2. Viral infections—especially herpes simplex and zoster

3. Neoplasms—especially lymphomas and Kaposi's sarcoma

Management

Immunocompromised patients have, by definition, impaired resistance to infection and, therefore, surgical procedures must be carried out as far as possible aseptically, atraumatically, and under antibiotic cover.

Patients may have additional problems such as the following.

1. Cross-infective risk to staff/other patients. Many immunocompromised patients excrete and shed a range of micro-organisms—mainly various herpes viruses including herpes simplex, cytomegalovirus and Epstein–Barr virus (Volume 2). There may be an infective risk in HIV infection (p. 40).

2. Bleeding tendency:
   in leukaemia
   in HIV infection
   in patients on cytotoxic drugs.

3. Adrenocortical suppression in patients on systemic corticosteroids (p. 24).

PATIENTS UNDERGOING TREATMENT FOR CANCER

Surgical treatment of cancer in the head and neck can be disfiguring, while radiotherapy involving the mouth and salivary glands can lead to a range of complications—especially mucositis and dry mouth (Table 2.23; see also Volume 2). Cytotoxic chemotherapy can also cause mouth ulcers and other complications.

Table 2.23
Oral complications of cancer treatment

Teeth	Caries
Mucosa	Mucositis
	Ulcers
	Candidosis
Gingiva	Inflammation
Salivary gland	Dry mouth
Others	Trismus
	Loss of taste
	Osteoradionecrosis

Mucositis invariably occurs over the first 2–4 weeks after radiotherapy and responds best to oral hygiene and local antiseptic mouth baths. Xerostomia is far more persistent and normal salivation may never return. Dry mouth is in itself unpleasant, causing dysphagia (difficulty in swallowing), dysarthria (difficulty in articulating words) and loss of taste sensation, but also predisposes to caries and other infections such as candidosis. Preventive dentistry and salivary substitutes are indicated (Volumes 2 and 3).

The obstruction of blood vessels and reduced vascularity (endarteritis obliterans) induced by radiotherapy can lead to fibrosis in the masticatory muscles—with increasing limitation of jaw opening—and can reduce the vascularity of the jaw bones. The latter predisposes to osteoradionecrosis (Fig. 2.46) and, therefore, extractions should be carried out before, or shortly after, radiotherapy (Volume 2).

Cytotoxic chemotherapy is only of minimal value in the treatment of oral cancer but is valuable in the treatment of other malignant neoplasms such as lymphomas and leukaemias. These agents commonly cause oral ulceration. Folinic acid may be used to reduce the ulcers associated with methotrexate therapy but, in general, chlorhexidine mouthwashes and analgesics are of more use.

In any of the patients undergoing treatment for cancer there may be a predisposition to infections and therefore surgery should only be undertaken under antibiotic cover. Prophylactic antifungals and antiviral agents are often given because patients, especially leukaemics, are predisposed particularly to oral candidosis and herpes virus infections. Cytotoxic drugs may cause thrombocytopenia and a bleeding tendency (p. 13).

PATIENTS WITH PROSTHESES OR TRANSPLANTS

Prostheses are now fairly commonplace, particularly cardiac valvular prostheses, prosthetic joints, and ventriculoatrial shunts (for hydrocephalus).

Cardiac prostheses and pacemakers

Patients with cardiac prostheses and those with pacemakers clearly have or have had underlying cardiac disorders which may be a contraindication to general anaesthesia. Patients with prostheses have additional problems in relation to bleeding tendency (anticoagulants: p. 15) and infective endocarditis (p. 17). Patients with pacemakers may be at danger in relation to the use of equipment that can interfere with their pacemaker, such as diathermy, electrosurgery, ultrasonic scalers, and pulp testers (p. 17).

Prosthetic joints

There is no good evidence for infection of these prostheses arising from oral sepsis. However, since there is perhaps a theoretical risk that the bacteraemia associated with tooth extraction might lead to metastatic infection, it seems reasonable to give an antimicrobial cover if the orthopaedic surgeon wishes.

Ventriculoatrial shunts

The complications of infection of these valves (e.g. the Spitz–Holter valve) used in the management of hydrocephalus are so serious that, although there is little evidence for an oral source, again it seems reasonable to give an antimicrobial cover if the responsible neurosurgeon so wishes.

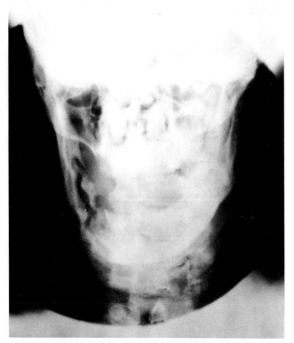

Fig. 2.46 *Osteoradionecrosis of the mandible following radiotherapy.*

Organ transplants

Organ transplants are commonplace today, particularly renal transplants. Patients with transplants are, particularly during the postoperative period, liable to present a number of complications to dental treatment, especially a liability to infection (they are immunosuppressed), a bleeding tendency (if on anticoagulants) and a need for a corticosteroid cover (if on corticosteroids).

Dental treatment should be carried out in close consultation with the physicians/surgeons responsible for the patient and, in many instances, would be better performed preoperatively. Oral health is important in these patients, who are particularly liable to the fungal and viral infections and other complications seen in immunocompromised patients on chemotherapy for malignant disease (p. 59).

SEXUALLY PROMISCUOUS PATIENTS

Sexually promiscuous patients may present with orofacial manifestations of sexually transmitted diseases such as syphilis, gonorrhoea (Volume 2) or AIDS, and may present a cross-infection risk, including that of infection with HIV or hepatitis viruses (p. 37). Multiple infections, or a series of infections with different agents, are not uncommon. Although patients who are promiscuous cannot necessarily be identified, certain obvious occupations, such as prostitution, and groups, such as drug abusers, are predisposed to sexually transmitted diseases.

PATIENTS OF DIFFERENT ETHNIC GROUPS

Management problems may relate to ethnic genetic background, to the environment from which patients have emigrated, or to cultural or environmental factors. Black patients, for example, comprise the main group in which sickle cell disease is found. Thalassaemia and Behçet's syndrome (Volume 2) are most common in those from the Mediterranean area and South East Asia. Oral cancer is a major neoplasm in India and Pakistan and other parts of South East Asia. Recent immigrants from Asia, Africa and Vietnam have a high carriage rate of hepatitis B virus, but this is not the case in second-generation immigrants in the UK. AIDS is rife in Central Africa. Drug abuse, especially with cannabis, is prevalent in some black cultures in the UK (e.g. Rastafarians). Other rare disorders are prevalent in certain ethnic groups: pernicious anaemia

Table 2.24
Some medical problems more common in immigrant populations

Ethnic group	Relevant medical problems
Asians	Hepatitis B Tuberculosis
African Blacks	Haemoglobinopathies Hepatitis B HIV infection
Greeks	Thalassaemia
Indo-Chinese	α-thalassaemia Hepatitis B Tuberculosis
Jews	Factor XI deficiency Pemphigus
South African Boers	Porphyria

appears more common in Northern Europeans, pemphigus in Jews, and porphyria in Afrikaaners (Table 2.24).

OTHER RELEVANT MEDICAL PROBLEMS

Hereditary angioedema

Angioedema caused by an allergic reaction has been discussed above (p. 23).

Hereditary angioedema (HANE) is a rare autosomal dominant condition in which even mild trauma (such as dental procedures) can precipitate angioedema with the consequent danger of airway obstruction and asphyxia. The essential cause is a defect in control of the complement pathway (Volume 2) in which the C1 esterase inhibitor is lacking. This can be confirmed by testing the serum, and C4 and C2 levels may also be low. Stanozolol, an androgenic steroid, must be given prophylactically to prevent these dangerous attacks.

FURTHER READING

Dunne S. M., Clark C. G. (1985). The identification of the medically compromised patient in dental practice. *J. Dent.*, **12**: 45–51.

Hurlen B., Jonsen J., Aas E. (1980). Viral hepatitis in dentists in Norway. *Acta Odontologica Scandinavica*, **38**: 321–324.

Jacobsen P. L., Murray W. (1980). Prophylactic coverage of dental patients with artificial joints: a retrospective analysis of 33 infections in hip prostheses. *Oral Surg., Oral Med., Oral Path.*, **50**: 130–133.

Reingold A. L. *et al.* (1982). Transmission of hepatitis B by an oral surgeon. *J. inf. Dis.*, **145**: 262–268.

Ross J. W., Clarke S. K. R. (1981). Hepatitis B in dentistry: the current position. *Br. dent. J.*, **150**: 89–91.

Rothstein S. S., Goldman H. S., Arcomano A. (1981). Methods of hepatitis B virus transfer in oral surgery. *J. oral Surg.*, **39**: 754–756.

Scully C. (1980). Examination of the head and neck (3 parts). *Student Update*, **2**: 159; 197; 228.

Scully C. (1985). *The hospital dental surgeon's guide.* London: British Dental Association.

Scully C. (1988). Infectious diseases. In *World Workshop on Oral Medicine* (Millard D., Mason D., eds.). Michigan: University of Michigan Press (in press).

Scully C., Cawson R. A. (1987). *Medical problems in dentistry*, 2nd edn. Bristol: Wright.

Smith J. M., Sheiham A. (1980). Dental treatment needs and demands of an elderly population in England. *Com. Dent. Oral Epidemiol.*, **8**: 360–364.

Chapter

3 ✓ *Investigations*

It is sometimes not possible to diagnose an oral disorder by history and clinical examination alone—although these are the most important means of making a diagnosis. This chapter details additional investigative procedures employed to enable a correct diagnosis to be made.

VITALITY TESTING OF TEETH

When investigating dental pain, cystic bone lesions, and assessing patients with facial bone fractures, it is often necessary to know if the teeth are vital.

Tooth vitality can be assessed by thermal or electrical means.

Thermal tests

Warm gutta percha, or a cotton-wool pledget cooled in ethyl chloride, is applied to the intact, dried surface of an isolated tooth. If the tooth is vital, the stimulus evokes a sensation of mild pain or paraesthesia, but if it is non-vital no sensation is perceived. If the pulp is hyperaemic, these tests can provoke severe pain lasting several minutes.

Electrical tests

Electric pulp testers (Fig. 3.1) deliver a constant-current electrical stimulus. In a healthy tooth, the threshold of pulpal nerves is less than 100 µamps, whereas nerves of the periodontal ligament are stimulated by a threshold current of 200 µamps. Since an electric pulp tester can deliver a maximum of 150 µamps, it only detects pulpal responses.

In order to assess the vitality of a tooth, the moistened tip of the active electrode is applied with light pressure to the dried, intact surface of an isolated tooth. To ensure a circuit between the operator and tooth is completed, a metal instrument is held in the clinician's ungloved hand against the patient's buccal mucosa. Recently an adaptor has become available to enable the operator to wear gloves yet complete an electric circuit. The dial of the tester is gradually turned to increase the test current until the patient feels a paraesthesia-like sensation in the tooth. The tooth is likely to be non-vital if the patient repeatedly reports no pain even when the maximum electrical stimulus is applied.

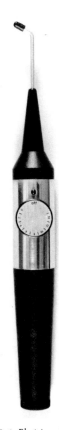

Fig. 3.1 *Electric pulp tester.*

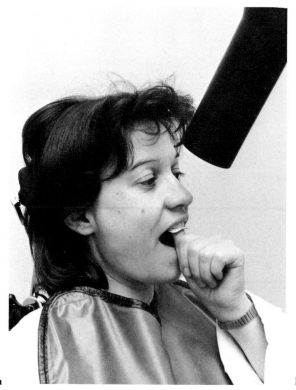
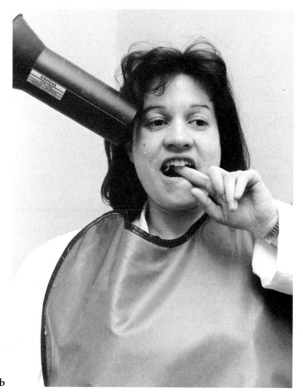

a   b

Fig. 3.2 *Positioning for periapical views of the: (a) upper central incisors, (b) upper right premolars, (c) lower central incisors, and (d) lower right premolar region.*

With both thermal and electrical pulp testing techniques, adjacent, opposing or contralateral teeth should also be tested, thus acting as controls. The method of testing must be the same for each tooth and, whenever possible, the same tooth surface used.

Vitality testing is quick, simple, relatively cheap and non-invasive but prone to both false positive and negative results. False positive results are usually due to inadvertent stimulation of adjacent mucosa or expansion of gas within necrotic pulpal tissue. False negative reactions are often a result of secondary dentine deposition in teeth heavily restored or with marked attrition. The responses of very young patients are often unreliable, and testing recently traumatized teeth may be of limited diagnostic value, since trauma more readily disrupts the pulpal nerve supply than the blood supply. A traumatized tooth may therefore have a vital pulp although it is unable to respond to thermal or electrical stimuli.

RADIOGRAPHIC INVESTIGATION

Radiographs can be valuable in confirming clinical diagnoses of oral diseases—mainly those with dental or osseous involvement—and may be the only means of diagnosing some lesions. However, radiographs only give a two-dimensional view: thus, when trying to localize a lesion, two radiographic views at 90° to each other must be taken.

Due to the cumulative effect of radiation, radiographic investigations should only be undertaken when deemed essential (Chapter 10). Whenever possible, investigations in women of child-bearing age should be restricted to the 10 days following the start of menstruation (the 10 day rule). Pregnant women must not be x-rayed, especially during the first trimester—when the fetus is especially vulnerable—unless radiographs are absolutely necessary. Radiation is also especially damaging to the gonads, thyroid gland and eyes.

Facial views whereby x-ray beams are directed anteroposteriorly should be avoided in all patients where possible, due to the radiosensitivity of the lens of the eye.

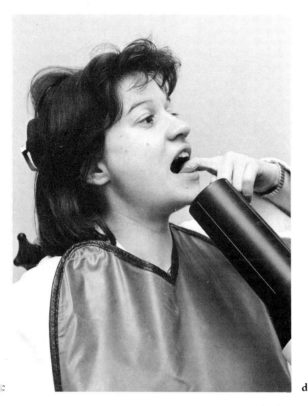
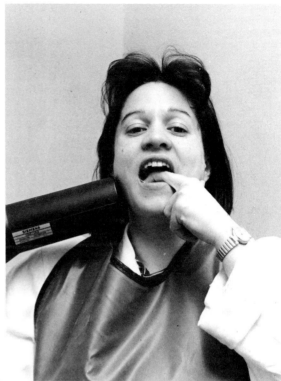

d

Intra-oral radiography

Intra-oral radiographs are obtained using a dental x-ray unit, with the radiographic film in the patient's mouth. Radiographs are taken using either the short-cone bisecting angle technique, or the long-cone paralleling method. The mechanics and the relative merits of each technique are outside the scope of this text (see Further reading).

Intra-oral views consist of the following.

Periapical views, which demonstrate the longitudinal features of teeth and adjacent alveolar bone. They are required when periapical pathology is suspected (Figs. 3.2 and 3.3).

Bitewings show the crowns of teeth and the adjacent alveolar crest. Periodontal disease and interstitial caries can be investigated using this type of radiographic view (Figs. 3.4 and 3.5).

Occlusal views show the axial relationship of teeth, alveolar bone and any adjacent radio-opaque structures. When used in conjunction with views taken in other planes, they are particularly useful in demonstrating the presence and position of unerupted teeth, submandibular calculi, bone cysts, and fragments of compound and comminuted mandibular fractures (Figs. 3.6 and 3.7).

Parallax, which determines the relative position of two structures, is commonly used to assess the relation of unerupted teeth to the dental arch. Two periapical views which differ only in the horizontal angulation of the x-ray beam are taken. When comparing the radiographs, apparent movement of the tooth in the same direction as the x-ray beam implies that its position is palatal to the arch; if movement is in the opposite direction, then it is buccally placed.

Extra-oral radiography

Radiography of the facial skeleton

Radiographs of the facial bones are taken using a specifically designed craniostat. The following two planes serve as useful guides when positioning patients for extra-oral radiographic projections.

The *radiographic baseline*—which extends posteriorly from the outer (lateral) canthus of the eye to the centre of

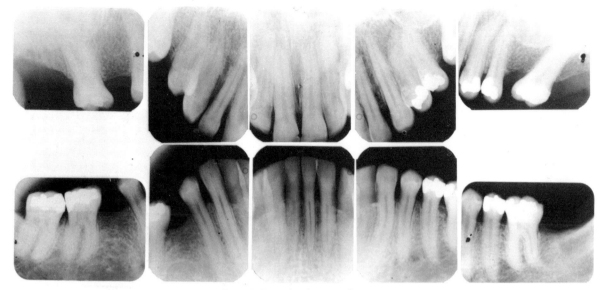

Fig. 3.3 Examples of periapical views.

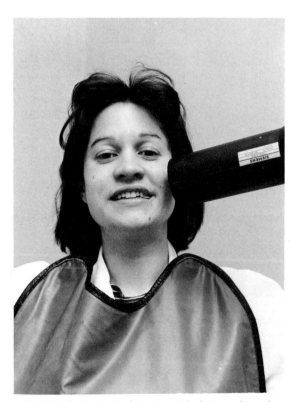

Fig. 3.4 Positioning for bitewings of the left premolar and molar regions.

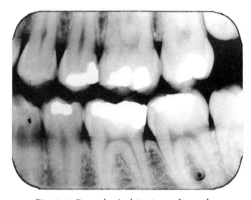

Fig. 3.5 Example of a bitewing radiograph.

the external auditory meatus and is sometimes referred to as the *orbital–meatal plane*.

The *interpupillary line*—which extends between the centre of the two orbits (i.e. the centre of the two pupils when the patient is looking straight ahead).

Common radiographic views of the head

Occipitomental (OM)

The occipitomental views are especially useful for demonstrating lesions in the maxillary antra and orbits,

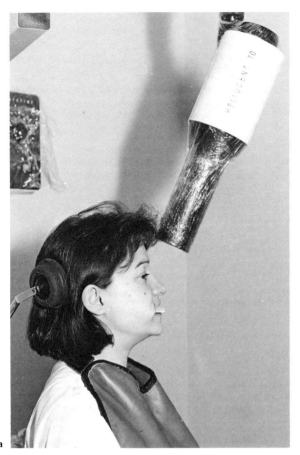

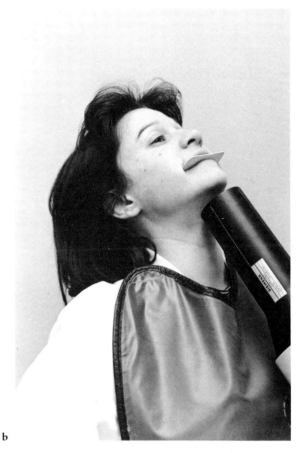

Fig. 3.6 *Positioning for occlusal views of the (a) upper and (b) lower anterior regions.*

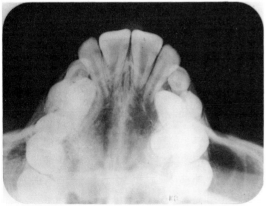

Fig. 3.7 *Occlusal view of the upper anterior region of the palate.*

e.g. maxillary sinusitis, or fractures involving the middle third of the face (Figs. 3.8 and 3.9). Occipitomental views are taken as shown in Figure 3.10.

Several occipitomental views can be taken; these are summarized in Table 3.1.

Submentovertex (SMV)

Submentovertex views are taken with the patient's head tipped back such that the radiographic baseline is perpendicular to the horizontal and the interpupillary line horizontal. The x-ray tube is angled 5° upwards from the horizontal and directed towards the symphyseal region (Fig. 3.11).

Submentovertex views show the zygomatic arches well (Figs. 3.12 and 3.13) and are used to evaluate the degree of depression in cases of suspected fracture of these structures.

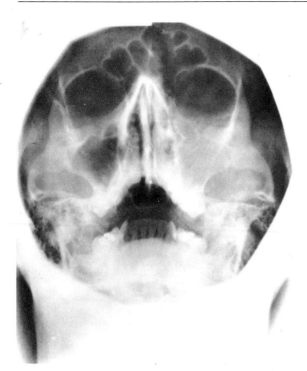

Fig. 3.8 *Occipitomental view of the maxilla. Note the opaque left maxillary sinus; this patient had chronic sinusitis.*

Table 3.1
Occipitomental views

View	Direction of beam	Shows
Basic	Beam is directed through the vertex of the skull towards nasion, perpendicular to the radiographic film	Frontal bones and sinuses, lateral and inferior orbital margins, zygomatic bones and maxillary sinuses
10°	Beam is centred above the occipital protuberance and directed downwards, 10° to the horizontal, towards the lower orbital margin	Superior, inferior and lateral orbital margin, maxillary sinuses
30°	Beam is centred above the occipital protuberance and directed downwards, 30° to the horizontal, towards the upper lip	Anterior aspect of inferior orbital margin, maxillary sinuses, anterior aspect of zygomatic bones

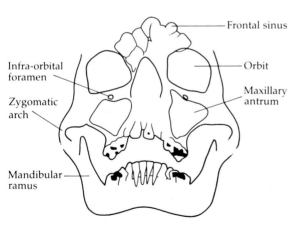

Fig. 3.9 *Anatomical landmarks of an occipitomental view of the maxilla.*

Oblique lateral (sometimes termed lateral oblique)

These radiographic views can be taken in several ways. In general, however, the x-ray beam is directed upwards from below the angle of the mandible towards the opposite side of the jaw (Fig. 3.14). Depending upon the direction of the x-ray beam, oblique lateral views can show the body, angle or ramus of one side of the mandible. They are often the views of choice when orthopantomographic equipment is unavailable but, unlike the latter technique, do not clearly show the maxilla (Fig. 3.15).

Postero-anterior

This view is taken with the radiographic baseline parallel to the horizontal and the x-ray centred in the midline below the occipital protuberance at the level of the angle of the mandible (Fig. 3.16).

Postero-anterior views show the body, angle and ramus of both sides of the mandible and, if the patient's mouth is open, the mandibular condyles may also be seen (Figs. 3.17 and 3.18). Postero-anterior views are especially important for the correct assessment of mandibular fractures, showing displacement in the coronal plane.

Frontal occipital (Townes, half axial)

The radiographic baseline is perpendicular to the film, with the median sagittal plane perpendicular to the horizontal. The x-ray beam is angled downwards 30° to the horizontal and centred 5 cm above the nasion.

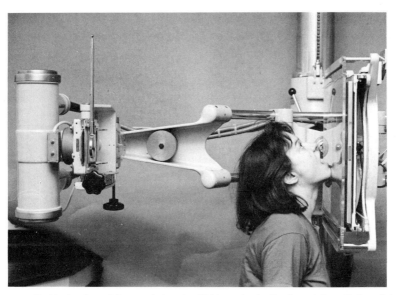

Fig. 3.10 *Positioning for occipitomental views (see Table 3.1 for details of angulation of tube and skull).*

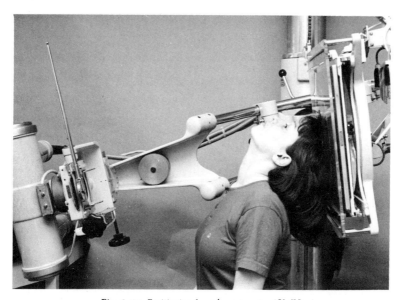

Fig. 3.11 *Positioning for submentovertex (SMV) view.*

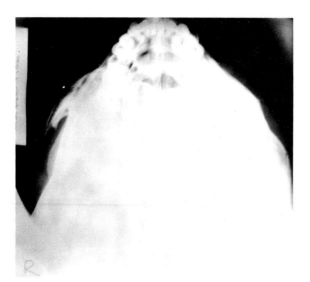

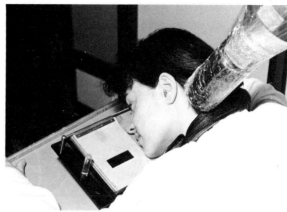

Fig. 3.14 *Positioning for oblique lateral views of the mandible.*

Fig. 3.12 *Submentovertex view of the left and right zygomatic arches. Note the fracture of the left arch.*

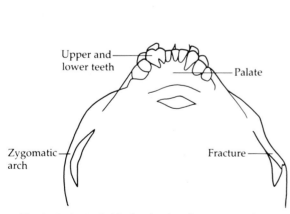

Upper and lower teeth

Palate

Zygomatic arch

Fracture

Fig. 3.13 *Anatomical landmarks of a submentovertex view (see Fig. 3.12).*

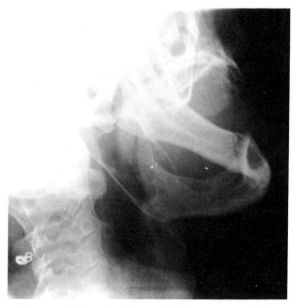

Fig. 3.15 *Oblique lateral view of the left posterior mandible. Note the large radiolucency of the ramus.*

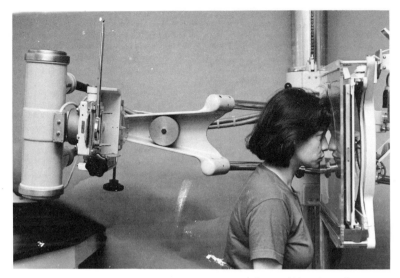

Fig. 3.16 *Positioning for postero-anterior view of the mandible and maxilla.*

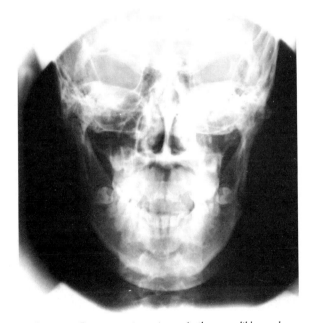

Fig. 3.17 *Postero-anterior view of the mandible and maxilla.*

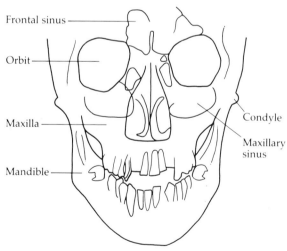

Fig. 3.18 *Anatomical landmarks of a postero-anterior view of the mandible and maxilla (see Fig. 3.17).*

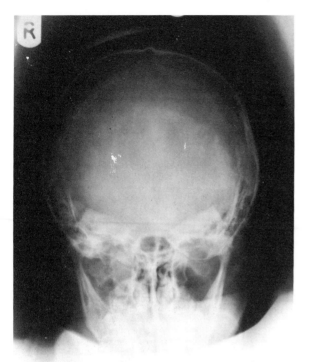

Fig. 3.19 *Fronto-occipital (Townes) view of the mandible.*

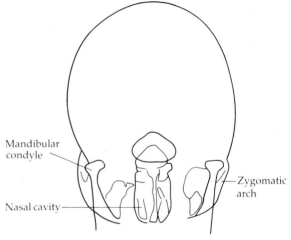

Mandibular
condyle

Nasal cavity

Zygomatic
arch

Fig. 3.20 *Anatomical landmarks of a fronto-occipital view of the mandible.*

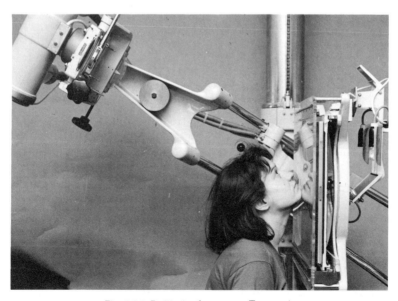

Fig. 3.21 *Positioning for a reverse Townes view.*

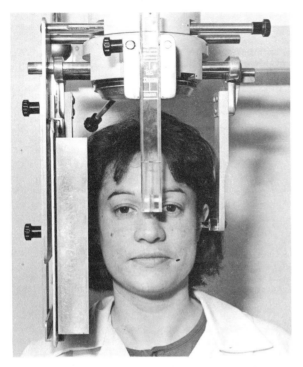

Fig. 3.22 *Positioning for a lateral skull view for cephalometric analysis. The x-ray beam is directed perpendicular to the radiographic film.*

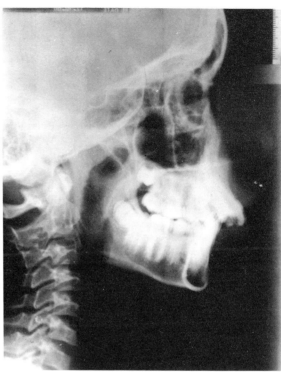

Fig. 3.23 *Lateral skull view for cephalometric analysis.*

Frontal occipital (Towne's) views can demonstrate the neck and the head of both mandibular condyles (Figs. 3.19 and 3.20) but, as outlined earlier, must only be taken when absolutely necessary (due to the radiosensitivity of the lens of the eye). A useful alternative radiographic view is the reverse Townes view in which the x-ray beam is directed in an occipito-frontal direction (Fig. 3.21).

Lateral skull: cephalometric analysis

Using a specifically designed cephalostat (Volume 4), it is possible to obtain standardized lateral radiographs of the skull which allow the anteroposterior and vertical relationships between the cranium, maxilla and mandible to be accurately assessed (Figs. 3.22–3.24). The reference points used in cephalometric analysis are summarized in Table 3.2 and Figure 3.25. Cephalometric analysis is essential in orthodontic assessment and the planning of orthognathic surgery (see Volume 4).

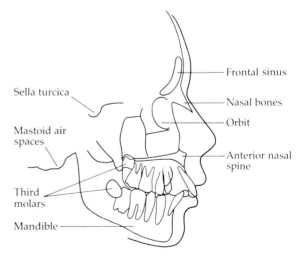

Fig. 3.24 *Anatomical landmarks of a lateral skull view (see Fig. 3.23).*

Table 3.2
Reference points of cephalometric analyses

Point	Definition
N—nasion	The most anterior part of the frontonasal suture
S—sella	Midpoint of the pituitary fossa
A—point A (subspinale)	The most posterior point on the concavity of the anterior surface of the premaxilla below the anterior nasal spine
B—point B (supramentale)	The most posterior point of the concavity on the anterior surface of the mandible
Pog—pogonion	The most anterior point of the bony chin
Gn—gnathion	The point between the most inferior and anterior points on the bony chin
Go—gonion	The most inferior and posterior point at the angle of the mandible, where the bisection of the angle between the tangents of the posterior and inferior borders of the mandible meets the mandibular outline
Me—menton	The most inferior point of the lower border of the mandible
Ar—articulare	The point of intersection of the posterior margin of the ascending ramus and inferior border of the temporal bone
Or—orbitale	The lowest point on the infraorbital margin
ANS—anterior nasal spine	The anterior tip of the anterior nasal spine
PNS—posterior nasal spine	The most posterior extent of the hard palate
Bo—Bolton point	The highest point in the concavity of the fossa behind the occipital condyle
Ba—basion	The lowest point on the anterior margin of the foramen magnum

Angle	Significance	Normal value (degrees)	Normal variation (degrees)
SNA	Anteroposterior relation of the maxilla with the anterior cranium	81	3
SNB	Anteroposterior relation of the mandible with the anterior cranium	78	3
ANB	Anteroposterior relation of the mandible with the maxilla	2	1
MMP	Anterior intermaxillary height	27	4
1/MM	Angulation of the upper incisors to the maxillary plane	108	5
1/MM	Angulation of the lower incisors to the mandibular plane	92	5
1/1	Interincisal angle	133	10

Radiographic views of the temporomandibular joint

There are several methods of obtaining radiographic views of the temporomandibular joint. In one technique (transcranial) the patient is positioned such that the median sagittal plane is parallel to the radiographic film, and the interpupillary plane perpendicular to it. The x-ray beam is directed downwards 25° to the horizontal and centred 5 cm above the temporomandibular joint of the opposite side. Views of each joint can be taken with the mouth open or closed (Figs. 3.26–3.28).

The anteroposterior (Townes) view is often used as an adjunct to the above technique.

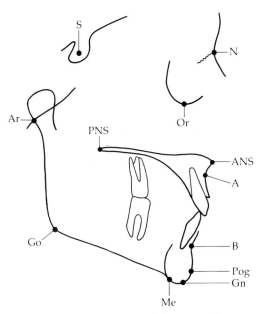

Fig. 3.25 *Reference points for cephalometric analysis (see also Table 3.2).*

Tomography

Tomography is a radiographic technique in which images of slices of the bony skeleton are obtained. The x-ray source moves about an arc around the patient, so blurring the radiographic images of all structures outside the area of clinical interest. Because of this blurring of adjacent structures the definition of tomograms is not as good as that of conventional radiographs; however, tomograms have the great advantage of allowing the investigation of regions not normally accessible by conventional x-ray procedures. Orthopantomography and CT scanning are the main 'dental' applications of tomography (see below); however, tomography is also occasionally used in the assessment of orbital 'blow-out' fractures and in fractures and arthrography of the temporomandibular joint.

Orthopantomography

Orthopantomography is a tomographic technique specifically designed to obtain an image of a curved layer of the mandibular and maxillary arches (Figs. 3.29–3.31). Depending upon the system employed, either the film and x-ray source move about the patient, or vice versa. Orthopantomography demonstrates the entire mandible, and to a certain extent the maxilla, on both sides and is useful, for example, in assessing impacted third molars (wisdom teeth).

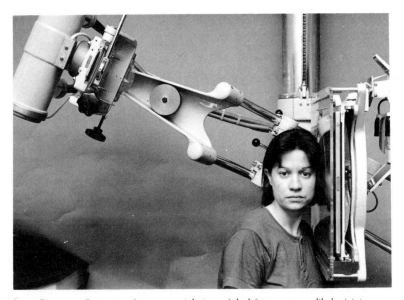

Fig. 3.26 *Positioning for transcranial views of the left temporomandibular joint.*

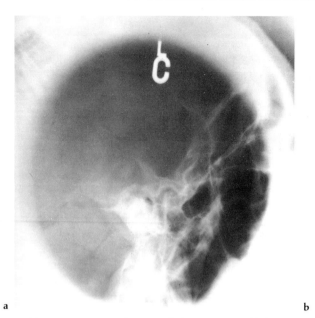

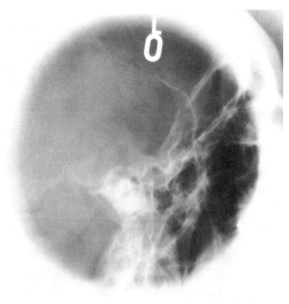

a
b

Fig. 3.27 *Transcranial views of the left temporomandibular joint when (a) closed and (b) open.*

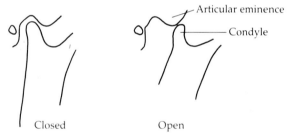

Closed   Open

Fig. 3.28 *Anatomical landmarks of transcranial views of the temporomandibular joint (see Fig. 3.27).*

Orthopantomography is convenient and subjects patients to relatively low levels of radiation. However, it is not without its limitations. Being a tomogram, it shows only a relatively thin 'slice' of tissue. Often the facial contours of patients do not conform to the curvature traced out by the orthopantomograph, and images can be distorted, losing valuable diagnostic information. In addition, the high radiodensity of the cervical vertebrae causes loss of definition due to superimposition in the anterior part of the mandible and maxilla. Intensifying screens and the large object-to-film distance also reduce definition. Therefore, caries and periodontal disease and lesions in the anterior maxilla or mandible cannot be accurately assessed using only this view.

These limitations not withstanding, orthopantomography is a major diagnostic tool in dentistry, since it assists in the localization of teeth (erupted and unerupted), roots, cysts and fractures of the mandible, and, with alteration to a higher horizontal plane, can aid assessment of the maxillary sinuses and condylar heads of the mandible.

Orthopantomography cannot be used with young children since they are unlikely to stand still while the radiograph is being taken. In such circumstances a useful alternative is the bimolar view. This is a modification of the oblique lateral technique which enables images of both sides of the mandible to be obtained on the one extra-oral radiographic film (Fig. 3.32).

Computed tomography

Computed tomography (CT, previously termed computerized *axial* tomography, CAT) is another radiological technique in which images of thin slices of the body are obtained (Fig. 3.33). Unlike conventional tomography which predominantly reveals hard tissues, CT detects both hard and soft tissues.

Each CT scanner has an x-ray source and a series of detectors mounted on a scanning gantry which moves around the supine patient. Slices of 5–13 mm thickness are usually taken in the axial, coronal or sagittal planes.

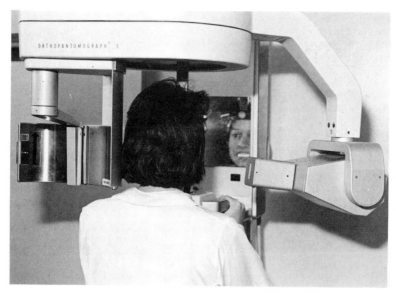

Fig. 3.29 *Positioning for orthopantomography of the mandible.*

CT can detect small variations in tissue radiodensity, and thus allow slices of soft tissue to be visualized.

Since CT can demonstrate inaccessible soft and hard tissue structures, it has become an important diagnostic test for a wide range of clinical problems. In dentistry, it has application especially in the management of patients with severe head injuries and facial fractures (Table 3.3) and can also detail the spread of benign or malignant disorders associated with the orbit, infratemporal fossa, parapharyngeal spaces and paranasal sinuses—areas that are difficult to examine clinically and/or by other radiological techniques.

Table 3.3

Application of computed tomography in orofacial diagnosis

Trauma, e.g.	severe fractures of the maxilla severe head injuries
Neoplasia, e.g.	nasal sinuses salivary glands jaws orbit pharynx larynx
Others, e.g.	soft tissue cysts fibro-osseous lesions

Arthrography of the temporomandibular joint

Arthrography is important in the diagnosis of severe temporomandibular joint dysfunction. However, it is undertaken in only a few specialized centres.

Local anaesthetic is injected around the postero-superior aspect of the mandibular condyle. Iodine-based aqueous contrast medium (provided the patient is not allergic) is then injected into the lower joint space and tomograms of the joint taken as the patient opens and closes his mouth. If tomographic facilities are not available, it is possible to carry out arthrography using an image intensifier (fluoroscope)—an x-ray machine that can provide a radiographic image on a video display unit. The intensifier has the advantage of being able to be linked to a video recorder; thus it is possible to record the movements of each temporomandibular joint (Fig. 3.34).

Xeroradiography

This combines radiography with photocopying (xerography) techniques but though giving clear films with good detail is expensive and has other disadvantages that limit its application in dentistry.

Sialography

Sialography permits the visualization of the duct network of the submandibular or parotid salivary glands. A plain

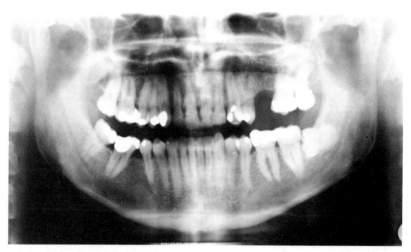

Fig. 3.30 *Orthopantomograph of the mandible and lower part of the maxilla.*

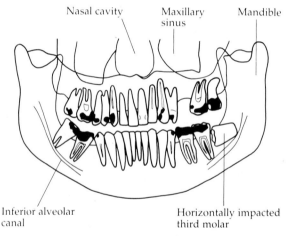

Fig. 3.31 *Anatomical landmarks of an orthopantomograph of the mandible (see Fig. 3.30).*

radiograph is first taken. A radio-opaque contrast medium is injected into the main salivary duct and conventional radiographic views are taken as the gland fills and empties.

The contrast media are iodine based and can be either aqueous (e.g. sodium diatrizoate and sodium metrizoate) or oily (e.g. iodinated unsaturated fatty acids). They can be injected manually, using a hydrostatic technique, or by constant infusion. The latter technique is more useful since it allows medium to accumulate slowly within the gland and eliminates the problem of under-filling (resulting in lack of structural detail) or over-filling (causing pain and loss of definition as the medium overflows into the acini).

Radiographs are taken in two different planes: usually lateral and 15° oblique lateral views for the submandibular gland; and anteroposterior and lateral or 15° oblique lateral views for the parotid gland (Fig. 3.35).

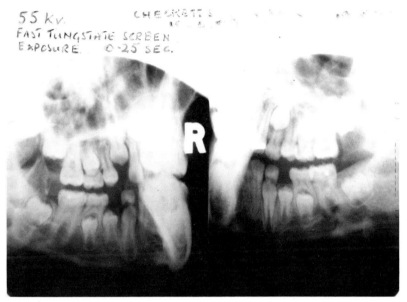

Fig. 3.32 *Bimolar views of the right and left sides of the mandible.*

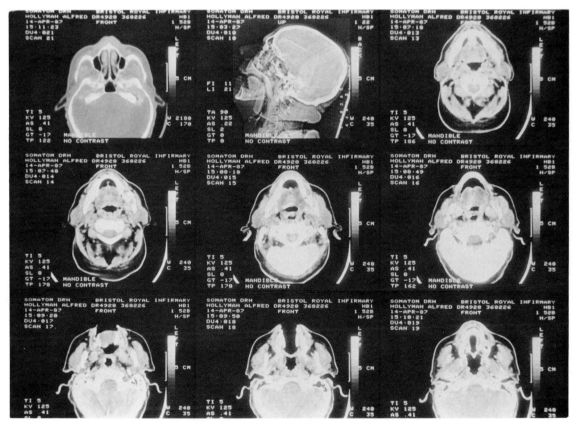

Fig. 3.33 *Axial CT views of the maxillary region.*

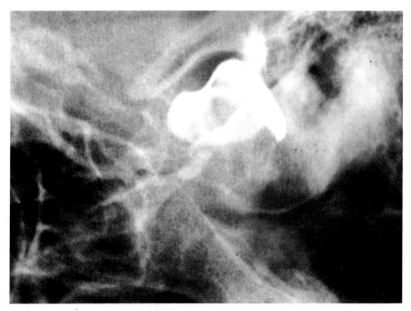

Fig. 3.34 *Arthrography of the temporomandibular joint.*

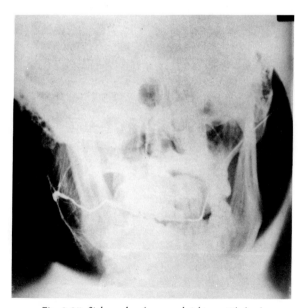

Fig. 3.35 *Sialography of a normal right parotid gland.*

Sialography can be of value in the diagnosis of disorders of the major salivary glands (Table 3.4). However, it must not be undertaken for patients with acute sialadenitis since it is likely to precipitate deeper infection, and it is, of course, contra-indicated in patients who are allergic to iodine.

Radioisotope imaging (radionuclide scanning)

Radioisotope imaging entails the intravenous injection of radioactive isotopes that preferentially concentrate within either specific normal tissues or pathological lesions. The concentrated radioactive material is then detected using either a suitable scanner or a gamma camera. Although the isotopes emit gamma radiation, they are fairly non-toxic since they have a very short half-life and, because scans examine all the tissues of interest, they may do so with a lower radiation dose than would be experienced if multiple x-rays were used. There is a wide range of radioisotope imaging techniques; only those of relevance to the diagnosis of oral disease will be detailed.

Skeletal scanning

Isotopes of technetium (usually technetium diphosphonate) or fluorine are used in skeletal scanning. These radionuclides concentrate in areas of increased bone turnover by exchanging with ions on the surface of hydroxyapatite crystals. The clinical disorders in which bone scanning is often helpful are summarized in Table 3.5, but its widest application is in the detection of metastases, especially when there is clinical suspicion of neoplastic spread yet conventional radiographic views still appear normal (Fig. 3.36).

Table 3.4
Sialographic appearance in disorders of the salivary glands

Disorder	Sialographic appearance
Calculi	Dilatation of ducts. If radiopaque, the calculus will also be detected on the plain film taken before the sialogram
Strictures	Dilatation of ducts; narrowing at stricture
Sjögren's syndrome Recurrent parotitis in adults	Dilatation of ducts and acini. Pooling of contrast medium in the dilated regions gives rise to a 'snowstorm' radiographic appearance, known as *sialectasis*. As disease progresses, so the areas of pooling increase in size and number
Neoplasia (a) Benign	Displacement of the normal ductal network Slight retention of contrast medium within the gland after a sialogogue has been given
(b) Malignant	Destruction of the ductal network Irregular pooling of contrast medium and retention after sialogogue
Extraglandular masses	Displacement of the normal ductal network No retention of contrast medium after a sialogogue

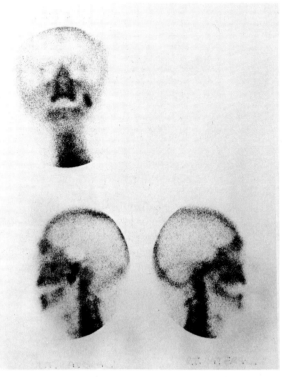

Fig. 3.36 *Skeletal scanning. There is an area of increased radionuclide uptake in the left ramus of the mandible; this was due to a metastasis of breast carcinoma.*

Table 3.5
Clinical applications of isotope scanning in dentistry

	Skeletal disease	Salivary disease	Others
Inflammatory lesions	Osteomyelitis Osteoarthrosis Rheumatoid arthritis Fractures (rarely)	Sjögren's syndrome	Sarcoidosis
Neoplastic lesions	Primary lesions of bone Local invasion or metastases	Salivary neoplasms	Lymphomas
Other lesions	Fibrous dysplasia Paget's disease Cysts	Cysts	

Salivary scintiscanning

Scintiscanning is a test of salivary gland function in which glandular uptake of pertechnetate is measured. Uptake is reduced in chronic inflammatory disorders (e.g. Sjögren's syndrome—Fig. 3.37) and increased in acute salivary gland inflammation. Salivary scintiscanning has the advantage of examining all glands simultaneously.

Thyroid scanning

The site and activity of thyroid tissue can be estimated by thyroid scanning, a technique based upon the ability of thyroid tissue to preferentially trap isotopes (e.g. ^{131}I, ^{125}I, ^{123}I) or analogues (e.g. ^{99}Tc^{m} pertechnetate) of iodine.

The unnecessary removal of lingual thyroid tissue can give rise to hypothyroidism, therefore it is important that thyroid scanning is undertaken before pathological swellings in the posterior dorsum of tongue, which might be ectopic thyroid tissue, are removed.

Other relevant scans

Gallium scans are occasionally used in the diagnosis of sarcoidosis.

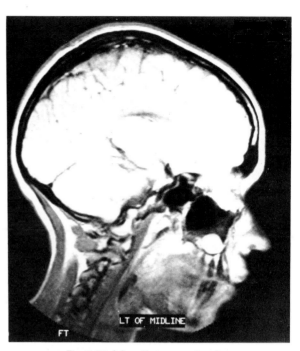

Fig. 3.38 *Magnetic resonance imaging.*

Magnetic resonance imaging (MRI)

This is a newly developed diagnostic technique by which very high-quality cross-sectional images of the body can be obtained (Fig. 3.38). It does not rely upon ionizing radiation; instead it uses high-frequency electric waves and a magnetic field (nuclear magnetic resonance or NMR). To date there have been only a few studies of the application of MRI in dentistry but already it has been found to be of benefit in the diagnosis of temporomandibular joint disease.

HISTOPATHOLOGICAL INVESTIGATIONS

Biopsy

In most instances a biopsy specimen can be obtained following local anaesthesia of the affected tissues. General anaesthesia is required mainly if the patient is very young or uncooperative (e.g. mentally handicapped); where access is poor (e.g. the oropharynx); when the lesion is large and requires detailed surgical investigation; or when it is likely that immediate surgical excision should follow (e.g. for malignancy).

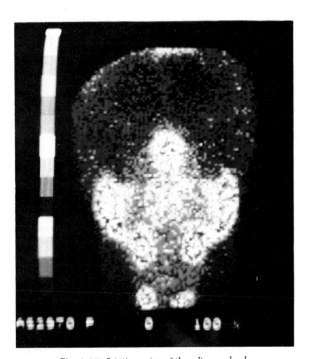

Fig. 3.37 *Scintiscanning of the salivary glands.*

Technique (Fig. 3.39)

When a sample is required for an immediate frozen section or for immunostaining, the receiving laboratory must be given prior warning. This allows time for the liquid nitrogen refrigerant to be sent to the theatre or chairside and for the pathologists to arrange the necessary storage of the sample.

A biopsy must be large enough to include a representative area of pathology plus adjacent normal tissue. Since patients do not normally suffer severe postoperative discomfort, oral mucosal biopsies can be large. However, great care must be taken to avoid cutting important anatomical structures, e.g. major salivary gland ducts, palatine vessels, nerves etc. Whenever possible, to facilitate primary closure of the wound the biopsy should have an elliptical shape (Fig. 3.39).

Biopsies of labial salivary glands may be needed for the diagnosis of, for example, Sjögren's syndrome (Volume 2) and can be taken through a simple incision (Fig. 3.40).

Wounds can be closed with 3/0-diameter gut or silk sutures. Wounds of the hard palate are difficult to close and can either be left open or covered by an acrylic plate or an appropriate antiseptic pack such as Whitehead's varnish soaked in ribbon gauze.

Lesions in bone can sometimes be biopsied with a curette, but a section may need to be removed with chisel or bur. Drill biopsies are sometimes used and lymph nodes and salivary glands are sometimes biopsied by needle biopsy since these methods are less invasive.

For routine histopathological investigations, the biopsy sample is laid with the base upwards on cardboard (to minimize tissue buckling) and is then placed in a small pot containing at least 10 times its volume of 10% formol saline (or formol calcium). The sample is then sent to the laboratory with the request form appropriately completed with at least the patient's name, hospital number, clinical details and provisional diagnosis, and responsible clinician. The pathologist should be warned if the biopsy contains hard tissue such as bone.

Samples for direct immunofluorescence studies are again placed on cardboard, and inserted into small, self-sealing plastic tubes which are dropped into liquid nitrogen.

Samples for routine histopathological investigation are embedded in wax and stained with haematoxylin and eosin (H and E), which demonstrates the general structure of the tissue. Additional staining procedures are occasionally required to demonstrate more specific features such as the presence of micro-organisms or various deposits (Table 3.6).

Table 3.6
Staining of wax-embedded biopsy specimens

Stains	Features denoted
Haematoxylin and eosin	General structure of tissues. This is the standard reference method carried out on all tissues
Periodic acid–Schiff	Mucins, glycogen and some fungi (e.g. *Candida* species)
Gram stains	Bacteria and some fungi
Ziehl–Nielsen	Acid- and alcohol-fast bacteria (mycobacteria)
Haematoxylin and van Gieson	Collagen and fibrous tissue
Alcian blue	Acid mucopolysaccharides
Resorcin–fuchsin elastic stain	Elastic fibres
Congo red or Thioflavin T	Amyloid
Immunostains (including monoclonal antibodies)	Various components depending on antibody used, e.g. immunoglobulin deposits, plasma cells, complement, keratin (see Volume 2)

Autoantibodies to mucosal tissue and other components can be detected by immunostaining. Immunostaining can use probes that fluoresce under ultraviolet light (immunofluorescence) or probes that can be viewed under normal illumination (e.g. immunoperoxidase techniques). Direct immunostaining detects the presence of materials acting as antigens (such as autoantibodies) within lesional tissue, while indirect immunostaining measures levels of autoantibodies in serum.

In direct immunofluorescence, fluorescein-labelled antibodies to human IgG, IgM or IgA are applied to frozen sections of biopsy tissue. If autoantibodies are present, the labelled antibodies bind to them and emit a yellow or green colour when the tissue is examined under a fluorescent microscope (Fig. 3.41). Deposits of complement and fibrin can also be detected by direct immunofluorescence by using fluorescein-labelled antibodies to complement (usually C3) or fibrin. Table 3.7 outlines the typical immunofluorescence patterns of several oral mucosal disorders. Details of the clinical relevance of these findings are discussed in Volume 2).

With indirect immunofluorescence, serum from the

continued on page 88

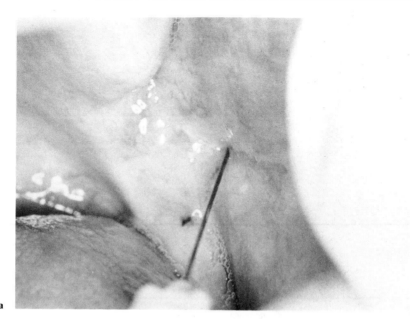

a

Fig. 3.39 *Obtaining a biopsy specimen: (a) local anaesthesia, (b) margin cut—taking both normal and abnormal tissue, (c) tissue is gently pulled up and cut from below, (d) closure of wound with silk sutures. The patient had a squamous cell carcinoma.*

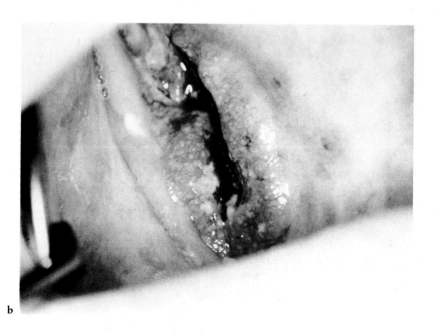

b

(continued)

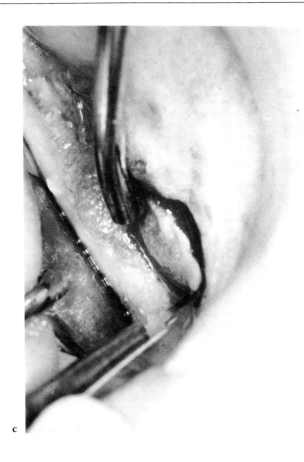

c

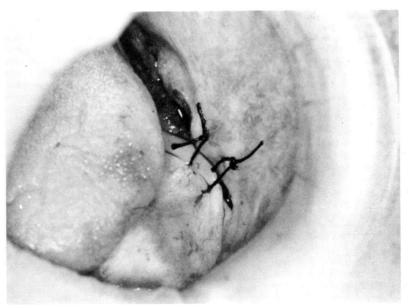

d

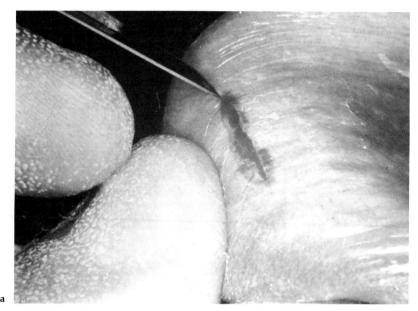

a

Fig. 3.40 *Labial gland biopsy: (a) incision, (b) glands protruding, (c) closure.*

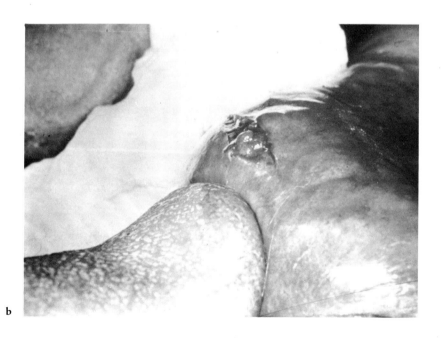

b

(continued)

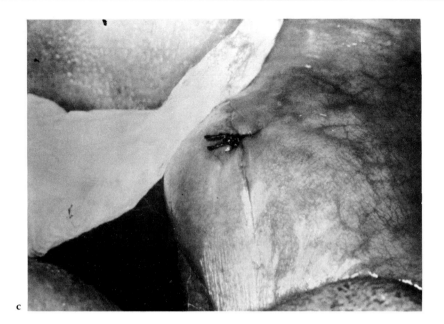

c

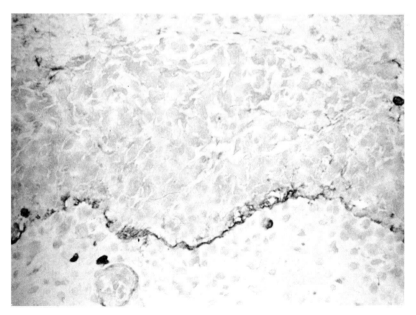

Fig. 3.41 *Direct immunosstaining showing deposits at epithelial basement membrane zone (Courtesy of Dr J. W. Eveson).*

Table 3.7
Typical results of direct immunostaining for oral mucosal disorders (see also Volume 2)

Disorder	Epithelial site of deposits	Deposition	
		Pattern	Typical deposit
Pemphigus	Intraepithelial	Pericellular	IgG, C1, C3
Lichen planus	Basement membrane zone (BMZ)	Linear	Fibrin*, IgG*, IgM*, C3*
Pemphigoid	Basement membrane zone	Linear	IgG, C1, C3
Dermatitis herpetiformis	Basement membrane zone	Granular	IgA, C3
Linear IgA disease	Basement membrane zone	Linear	IgA, C3
Discoid lupus erythematosus (DLE)	Basement membrane zone	Granular	IgG, IgM, IgA, C1, C3
Systemic lupus erythematosus (SLE)†	Basement membrane zone	Granular	IgG, IgM, IgA, C1, C3

* Non-specific deposits.
† In systemic lupus erythematosus there may also be deposition of immunoglobulin and complement in sun-exposed normal skin; this does not occur in discoid lupus erythematosus. In addition, up to 90% of patients with SLE have antinuclear antibodies; only 15% of DLE patients have these autoantibodies.

patient is applied at various dilutions to frozen sections of normal tissue, usually from an animal source. Human autoantibodies to oral mucosa, for example, bind to guinea-pig lip or monkey oesophagus and can be detected by applying the appropriate fluorescein-labelled anti-human antibodies and viewing under a fluorescent microscope.

Cytology

Cytology is a simple, non-invasive technique which examines cells scraped from a lesion, and which at first sight might seem a rather attractive investigative procedure. However, it is rarely employed in the diagnosis of oral mucosal disease except herpetic infection, since results are often unreliable and a biopsy, although more invasive, provides greater and much more reliable information.

Cytology smears are taken using a spatula (wooden or metal) or a dental plastic instrument. The scraped material is evenly spread on a glass slide and a few drops of industrial methylated spirit added. The smear is left to fix for 20 minutes, and then dried and stained.

MICROBIOLOGICAL INVESTIGATIONS
(Table 3.8)

Although some microbial diseases have clinical features that are virtually diagnostic, laboratory confirmation is

often either useful or mandatory. Primary herpetic stomatitis, for example, is usually diagnosed on clinical grounds alone; in contrast, a diagnosis of syphilis must be confirmed by investigations.

Light microscopy, culture, serology or occasionally electron microscopy are the main microbiological investigations available; their application to particular conditions is outlined in the other volumes of this series.

Smears

Examination of stained smears of pus, or microbial samples taken directly from a lesion, facilitates rapid identification of some infecting organisms. This technique can be diagnostic, for example with oral disorders such as acute pseudomembranous candidosis (thrush), acute necrotizing ulcerative gingivitis (ANUG: Fig. 3.42) and tuberculosis. A smear of crushed 'sulphur' granules is an important test supportive of a diagnosis of orofacial actinomycosis.

However, contamination with oral flora means that some infections cannot be diagnosed solely by smear tests. For example, oral smears from patients with possible infection by *Neisseria gonorrhoeae* are of little value, since the smear is likely to be heavily contaminated by commensal oral diplococci. Examination of smears under dark ground or phase contrast microscopy is often helpful in the diagnosis of syphilis. However, oral syphilitic lesions should be washed with saline to remove all com-

Table 3.8
Special tests in the diagnosis of infections

Disorder	Infecting agent	Special tests
Primary herpetic stomatitis	Herpes simplex	Usually clinical diagnosis alone. Viral culture: fourfold rise in levels of specific antibodies between acute and convalescent phases. Electron microscopy or cytology
Herpes labialis	Herpes simplex	Usually clinical diagnosis alone. Viral culture. Patients rarely have a rise in antibody levels
Chickenpox	Varicella zoster	Usually clinical diagnosis alone. Rise in antibody levels
Shingles	Varicella zoster	Usually clinical diagnosis alone
Herpangina	Coxsackie virus A	Usually clinical diagnosis alone. Rise in antibody levels
Hand, foot and mouth disease	Coxsackie virus A	Usually clinical diagnosis alone. Rise in antibody levels
Infectious mononucleosis	Epstein–Barr virus	Abnormal blood film (large number of abnormal lymphocytes). Positive Paul–Bunnell test*
Measles	Measles virus	Usually clinical diagnosis alone
Mumps	Mumps virus	Usually clinical diagnosis alone. S and V antibody titres. Serum amylase and lipase may be raised
Acute necrotizing ulcerative gingivitis (ANUG)	*Fusobacterium nucleatum* and *Borrelia vincentii*	Usually clinical diagnosis alone. Smear (Gram's stain)
Tuberculosis	*Mycobacterium tuberculosis* or atypical mycobacteria	Biopsy or smear (Ziehl–Nielsen stain). Culture*
Syphilis	*Treponema pallidum*	Smear (dark ground microscopy). Serology (see Table 3.10)*
Gonorrhoea	*Neisseria gonorrhoeae*	Culture*
Impetigo	*Staphylococcus aureus* or *Streptococcus pyogenes*	Usually a clinical diagnosis alone. Culture
Diphtheria	*Corynebacterium diphtheriae*	Culture*
Tetanus	*Clostridium tetani*	Diagnosis *must* be based on clinical grounds alone
Angular cheilitis	*Candida albicans* and/or *Staphylococcus aureus*	Usually a clinical diagnosis alone. Culture
Thrush	*Candida albicans* usually	Usually a clinical diagnosis alone. Culture
Chronic atrophic candidosis	*Candida albicans* usually	Usually a clinical diagnosis alone. Culture (from palate and fitting surface of denture)
Chronic hyperplastic candidosis	*Candida albicans* usually	Usually a clinical diagnosis alone. Culture. Biopsy (PAS stain)

* Special tests are not always indicated; only those marked with an asterisk are invariably required.

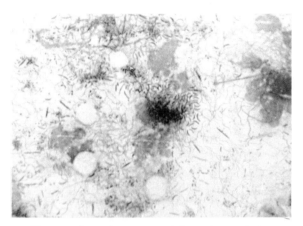

Fig. 3.42 *Smear from an ANUG lesion showing fusiform and spirochaetal bacteria.*

mensal spirochaetes before the smear is taken, and other confirmatory tests such as immunostaining or serology are invariably required.

Culture

Laboratory culture of microbial samples is by far the most common method of identifying an infecting organism. Depending upon the disorder, samples can be taken from one of many sites (Table 3.9).

The length of time required for culture and identification of an infectious agent varies widely, but most bacteria and fungi can be identified within 24–48 hours. Other micro-organisms, such as *Mycobacterium tuberculosis*, require up to 8 weeks before there is adequate growth for identification.

Viruses also vary in their growth characteristics. Herpes simplex can be identified after only 24 hours growth in a suitable cell culture, whereas herpes zoster grows very slowly in vitro.

Serology

Micro-organisms such as *Treponema pallidum* and hepatitis B virus cannot be grown in vitro, and their identification is possible mainly by serological means. Many other micro-organisms are difficult to culture under laboratory conditions, and it may take several weeks before identification is possible.

Serology examines the presence of, or rise in levels (i.e. titre) of, specific antibodies to the infecting organism. A serum specimen taken at the presenting visit is termed the acute serum and at this time levels of specific anti-

body to a new infecting organism are low or not detectable. However, they rise in titre as the body mounts an immune response, and a second sample taken 2–3 weeks later—the convalescent serum—will reveal higher levels of specific antibody. A fourfold rise in antibody titre between acute and convalescent sera indicates infection with the suspected organism.

Bacterial infections

Syphilis is one of the bacterial infections in which serology is diagnostically useful. The serological tests of syphilis can be non-specific or specific.

The non-specific tests (e.g. Venereal Disease Research Laboratory test (VDRL), and the reagin test) detect an antibody that appears in treponemal diseases and is not specific to syphilis. False positive results can arise following acute viral infections (e.g. infectious mononucleosis, mumps, measles, chickenpox, herpes simplex), chronic bacterial infections (e.g. tuberculosis), immunization against typhoid or yellow fever, or autoimmune diseases (e.g. lupus erythematosus, haemolytic anaemia).

The specific tests all detect a treponemal antigen and include the fluorescent treponemal antibody test (FTA), treponemal haemagglutination test (TPHA) and treponemal immobilization test (TPI). The specific tests are less prone to false positive or negative results than the non-specific tests but are still not specific enough to differentiate syphilis from other treponemal disorders (e.g. from yaws or pinta).

The expected serological results of the different stages of syphilis are outlined in Table 3.10. Syphilis is discussed further in Volume 2.

Fungal infections

Anti-candidal antibodies can be detected in patients with oral candidal infection, but these are rarely needed for diagnosis since most forms of candidosis can be diagnosed on clinical grounds, supplemented if necessary by a Gram-stained smear, or culture (Volume 2).

Viral infections

Many viral infections of the mouth can be diagnosed clinically. Diagnosis can, if necessary, be confirmed by detecting a fourfold rise in titre of specific antibodies between the acute and convalescent phases, but this approach is, of course, retrospective.

Acute infection by Epstein–Barr virus (EBV) can be confirmed by a positive Paul–Bunnel test which detects high levels of heterophil antibodies to different com-

Table 3.9
Microbiological sampling

Specimen	Comments
Pus	Specimens are taken using a swab or sterile syringe and needle. A swab should be immediately placed in its accompanying transport medium; while pus should be placed in a sterile bottle. Whenever possible, bottled pus rather than a swab should be sent to a microbiology laboratory, since organisms such as mycobacteria and actinomyces are scarce and may only be detected in large amounts of pus. All samples must be rapidly sent to the relevant laboratory. Samples collected out of normal working hours can be stored overnight, at 4–8°C in a conventional refrigerator.
Blood	Blood for culturing must be collected carefully. To avoid contamination, the overlying skin should be thoroughly cleaned with an alcohol-based swab such as isopropanol (water-based antiseptics are often contaminated) after changing the needle of the syringe. Blood is collected in the conventional manner and injected into inoculation bottles. The inoculation bottles should be sent to the laboratory as soon as possible. Out of hours they should be stored at 35–37°C.
Urine	A midstream sample (MSU) is the more common urine specimen. However, samples may also be collected by catheterization or suprapubic aspiration. To avoid growth of contaminants, samples must be sent to the laboratory within 1 hour of collection. The dip-inoculation method of collecting urine avoids the need to rush samples to the laboratory. With this technique, a dip-slide containing culture medium is dipped in newly collected urine and placed in a sterile container. Bacteria will remain viable for 5 days; however, cell counts cannot be made unless a fresh urine sample is sent separately.
Nasal secretions	Swabs should first be moistened by dipping into peptone water (saline kills some organisms). If a nasal lesion is being investigated, only the appropriate nostril is swabbed; however, if the patient is being investigated for carriage of micro-organisms, the same swab should be used for both nostrils.
Conjunctival fluid/discharge	Discharge can be swabbed, taken from the space between the conjunctivae of the lower eyelid. Care must be taken to avoid contamination with skin organisms.

Table 3.10
Serological tests for diagnosis of syphilis

	Before treatment		After treatment	
	VDRL	TPHA/FTA	VDRL	TPHA/FTA
Primary	−/+	+	−	−/+
Secondary	+	+	−	+
Early latent	+	+	−	+
Late latent	+	+	+	+
Tertiary	+	+	+	+
Quaternary	+	+	+	+
Quaternary (late)	−/+	−/+	−/+	−/+

Latent	= period between secondary and tertiary stages, when there are no clinical symptoms.
Tertiary	= gumma formation.
Quaternary	= CVS + CNS problems.
VDRL	= Venereal Disease Research Laboratory test.
TPHA	= *Treponema pallidum* haemagglutination test.
FTA	= Fluorescent treponemal antibody test.

ponents of EBV (Volume 2). Serology is thus helpful in differentiating EBV-associated 'glandular fever' (infectious mononucleosis) from other types of 'glandular fever' which are Paul–Bunnel negative (e.g. CMV or HIV infection).

The serological markers of hepatitis B virus and human immunodeficiency virus (HIV) are discussed in Chapter 2.

Electron microscopy

Rapid diagnosis of viral infections (e.g. herpes simplex and herpes zoster) is possible by electron microscopic examination of vesicular fluid or biopsy tissue. This technique is costly and only readily available in a few clinical centres and is therefore not in common usage.

HAEMATOLOGICAL AND BIOCHEMICAL INVESTIGATIONS

Haematological investigations may be indicated preoperatively (for example to exclude anaemia if GA is indicated), and are often essential for the accurate diagnosis of oral lesions, such as those of leukaemia. Tables 3.11 and 3.12 provide a summary of the haematological, biochemical and immunological features of many systemic and oral disorders. Further details may be found in Volume 2, but it should be noted that since there is some interlaboratory variation in values, results should be interpreted only in relation to local normal values.

Taking a blood sample

Blood and serum are potentially infectious and therefore great care must be taken to avoid needlestick injury or the contact of these fluids with skin or mucosa (Chapter 2). Resheathing the needle is dangerous (Table 3.13).

Blood samples are usually taken from the veins of the antecubital fossa, which are large, superficial and easily

Table 3.11
Interpretation of haematological results

	Normal range	Raised	Lowered
Haemoglobin	Male 13–18 g/dl Female 11.5–16.5 g/dl	Polycythaemia; Myeloproliferative disease	Anaemia; fluid overload
Red cell count (RBC)	Male 4.2–6.1×10^{12}/l Female 4.2–5.4×10^{12}/l	Polycythaemia	Anaemia; Fluid overload
Packed cell volume (PCV)	Male 40–54% Female 37–47%	Polycythaemia; Dehydration	Anaemia; fluid overload
Mean cell volume (MCV)	78–99 fl	Vitamin B_{12} or Folate deficiency; Liver disease; Alcoholism; Hypothyroidism	Iron deficiency; Thalassaemia
Mean cell haemoglobin (MCH)	27–31 pg	Pernicious anaemia	Iron deficiency; Thalassaemia; Sideroblastic anaemia
Mean cell haemoglobin concentration (MCHC)	32–36 g/dl		Iron deficiency; Thalassaemia; Sideroblastic anaemia; Anaemia in chronic disease
White cell count	4–10×10^9/l	Pregnancy; Exercise; Infection; Trauma; Leukaemia; Malignancy	Early leukaemia; Some infections; Bone marrow disease; Drugs; AIDS; Idiopathic
Neutrophils	3×10^9/l	Pregnancy; Exercise; Infection; Bleeding	Endocrinopathies; Bone marrow disease; Idiopathic
Lymphocytes	2.5×10^9/l	Physiological; Some infections; Leukaemia; Bone disease	Some infections; AIDS
Eosinophils	0.15×10^9/l	Allergic disease; Parasitic infection; Skin disease; Lymphoma	Immunodeficiency
Platelets	140–440×10^9/l	Thrombocytosis in myeloproliferative disease	Thrombocytopenia related to leukaemia, drugs, infections; Autoimmune; Idiopathic
Reticulocytes	150–400×10^9/l	Haemolytic states; During treatment of anaemia	
Erythrocyte sedimentation rate (ESR)	0–15 ml/h ⎫	Pregnancy; Infections; Anaemia; Connective tissue disease;	
Plasma viscosity	1.4–1.8 cp ⎬	Myelomatosis; Temporal arteritis; Malignancy	

Table 3.12

Interpretation of biochemical and immunological blood tests

	Normal range	Raised	Lowered
Alkaline phosphatase	30–110 i.u./ml 3–13 KA units*	Puberty; Pregnancy; Paget's disease; Liver disease; Malignancy in bone	Hypothyroidism
Aspartate transaminase	3–40 i.u./l	Liver disease; Biliary disease; Trauma	—
Bilirubin	1–17 mol/l	Liver disease; Biliary disease; Haemolysis	—
Calcium (total)	2–2.6 mmol/l	Hyperparathyroidism; Malignancy in bone; Sarcoidosis; Thiazide diuretics	Hypoparathyroidism; Rickets; Renal failure
C1-esterase inhibitor	0.1–0.3 g/l	—	Hereditary angioedema
Ferritin: adult male adult female child	25–190 ng/ml 15–99 ng/ml 21 ng/ml	Liver disease; Haemachromatosis; Leukaemia; Lymphoma; Thalassaemia	Iron deficiency
Folate (red cell)	120–650 μg/l	Folic acid therapy	Alcoholism; Diet deficiency anaemias; Malabsorption; Phenytoin
Free thyroxine index (FTI)	1.3–5.1 i.u.	Hyperthyroidism	Hypothyroidism
Glucose (fasting)	2.8–5.0 mmol/l	Diabetes mellitus; Hyperthyroidism; Cushing's disease; Liver disease	Hypoglycaemia; Addison's disease; Hypopituitarism; Hyperinsulinism
Total immunoglobulins	7–22 g/l	Liver disease; Infection; Sarcoidosis; Connective tissue disease; AIDS	Immunodeficiency
IgG	5–16 g/l	Myelomatosis; Connective tissue disease	Immunodeficiency
IgA	1.25–4.25 g/l	Alcoholic cirrhosis	Immunodeficiency
IgM	0.5–1.75 g/l	Primary biliary cirrhosis; Nephrotic syndrome; Parasitic infection; Infections	Immunodeficiency
Phosphate	0.8–1.5 mmol/l	Renal failure; Hypoparathyroidism;	Hyperparathyroidism; Rickets; Malabsorption; Insulin
Potassium	3.5–5.0 mmol/l	Renal failure; Addison's disease	Vomiting; Diarrhoea; Diabetics; Diuretics; Cushing's disease; Malabsorption
Sodium	130–145 mmol/l	Dehydration; Cushing's disease	Oedema; Renal failure; Addison's disease
Steroids	110–525 nmol/l	Cushing's disease	Addison's disease; Hypopituitarism
Thyroxine	50–138 nmol/l	Hyperthyroidism; Pregnancy; Contraceptive pill	Hypothyroidism; Nephrotic syndrome; Phenytoin
Urea	3.3–6.7 mmol/l	Renal failure; Dehydration	Liver disease; Nephrotic syndrome; Pregnancy

*KA units = King–Armstrong units.

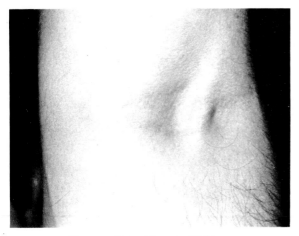

Fig. 3.43 *Veins of the antecubital fossa.*

visualized (Fig. 3.43). In addition, puncturing in this site causes less pain than in other sites such as the veins of the forearm and dorsum of the hand. Only when it proves impossible to take a sample from the above sites are the femoral or jugular veins used.

The only occasion when arterial blood is likely to be needed from oral surgery patients is when blood-gas analysis is required for a patient in intensive therapy. The artery used is usually the femoral artery in the groin; a physician should be asked to take this specimen.

Table 3.13 and Figure 3.44 summarize how blood samples may be obtained. Until recently, this was by simple venepuncture using a disposable syringe and needle, but now many use a vacuum system in which samples are rapidly and automatically 'sucked' into a pre-evacuated sample bottle (Vacutainer—Fig. 3.45). Figure 3.46 illustrates how blood is obtained using the Vacutainer system.

IMMUNOLOGICAL INVESTIGATIONS

Investigations of the immune system (other than assay of antibody levels as discussed above) can examine the *cellular* or the *humoral* components. Both may need to be examined in patients with suspected immune defects but, in others, investigations are in general limited to the humoral response since investigations of cellular responses are difficult, expensive, and not always especially helpful. A total white cell count and a differential count are, however, useful screening procedures.

Table 3.13
Obtaining a blood sample

1. Place a tourniquet around the arm* and, as this is tightened, gently palpate to find a suitable vein.
2. Clean overlying skin with an isopropyl alcohol swab.
3. Insert a 21-gauge (green) needle attached to a disposable syringe through the skin overlying the vein. The needle should be pointed towards the heart at an angle of 45° to the skin. As the needle crosses the blood vessel wall, there is an increase in resistance which then decreases as the lumen is reached.
4. Loosen the tourniquet.
5. Slowly withdraw an aliquot of blood (too rapid withdrawal of blood will cause haemolysis). Any air in the syringe indicates that the needle is not completely in the vein and therefore it should be gently pushed forward or pulled backward slightly.
6. Once an adequate amount of blood has been obtained, slowly withdraw the needle and press a cotton swab over the sample site.
7. Carefully remove the needle and place it in the sharp's box (e.g. Burnbin)—do not recap the needle, this is how many needlestick injuries occur. The blood should be carefully placed in the appropriate sample bottles. Bottles containing EDTA, citrate or lithium heparin should be gently rolled to ensure the sample does not clot.
8. The blood bottles should be labelled with patient's details and the time and date of collection.
9. A request form should be filled in and sent to the laboratory with the appropriate blood sample.
10. Patients who belong to hepatitis B or HIV high-risk groups must be treated carefully. The clinician must wear gloves, mask, goggles and disposable apron (see p. 36).
11. All splashing of blood must be avoided and any contaminated surfaces immediately cleaned with sodium hypochlorite or glutaraldehyde solutions.
12. The high-risk status of any blood sample must be clearly indicated on both the bottle and request form.

* The tourniquet must not be overly tight, since this causes patient discomfort and, perhaps more importantly, can decrease local arterial supply and venous return, both of which affect the platelet count and calcium levels.

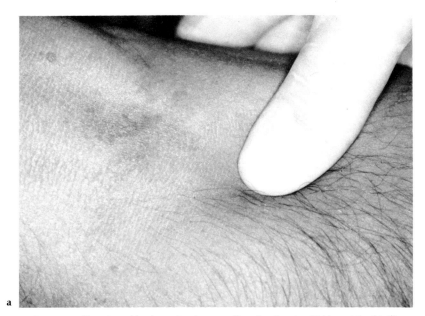

a

Fig. 3.44 *Obtaining a blood sample using a needle and syringe (see Table 3.13 for details).*

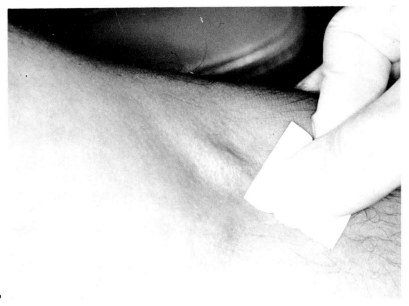

b

(continued)

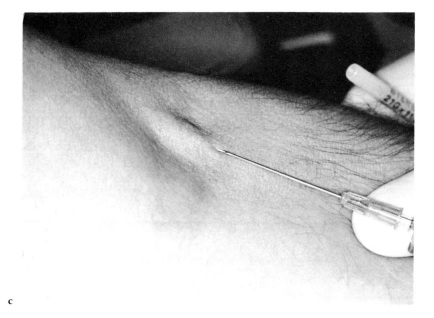

c

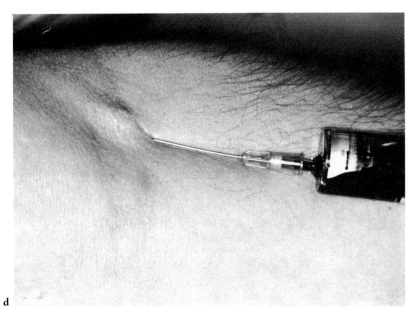

Fig. 3.44 *continued*   **d**   *(continued)*

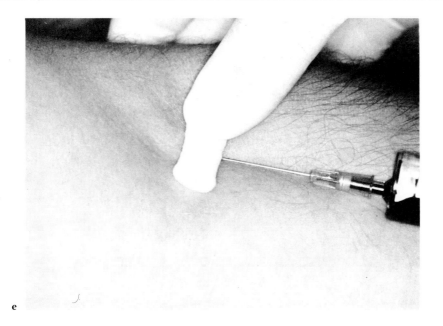

e

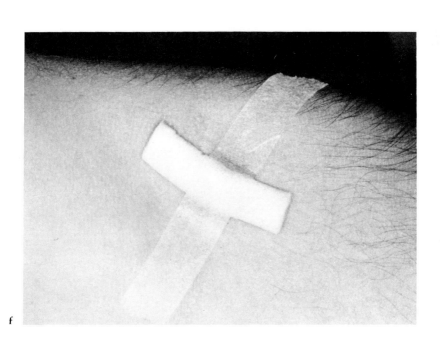

f

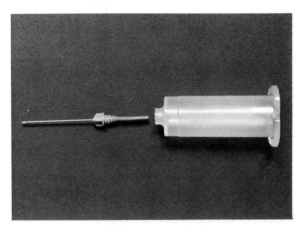

Fig. 3.45 *The Vacutainer system.*

Serum immunoglobulins

Quantitative changes in serum immunoglobulins occur in a number of systemic disorders, some of which have oral manifestations (see Table 3.12). For example, an increase in IgG is found in rheumatoid arthritis and some other autoimmune diseases. Qualitative alterations in serum immunoglobulins arise in plasma-cell disorders where there is excess production of defective immunoglobulin or of immunoglobulin light or heavy chains (Fig. 3.47). These additional proteins are known as paraproteins. In multiple myeloma, not only is there hypergamma-globulinaemia, but light-chain paraproteins are present in urine. These were originally discovered in urine as proteins that deposited on heating urine but then dissolved on further heating (Bence–Jones protein).

Decreases in serum immunoglobulins are found in, for example, humoral immune defects such as hypogamma-globulinaemia and IgA deficiency (Volume 2).

Immune complexes

Immune complexes are usually complexes of antigen with antibody and may be associated with disorders such as lupus erythematosus. There are several methods by which serum immune complexes can be detected, but the results of different methods do not always correlate. Precipitation by polyethylene glycol (PEG) is the most simple technique but is non-specific since complexes involving any of the three major immunoglobulin classes will produce a positive result. More specific techniques include C1q binding (which detects IgM and IgG complexes) and platelet aggregation (which detects IgG-containing complexes). Blood samples for measurement of serum immune complexes should be sent to the appropriate laboratory as soon as possible, since sample storage may give rise to false positive results. Samples may need to be collected and stored at 37°C since some complexes precipitate at lower temperatures (cryoglobulins).

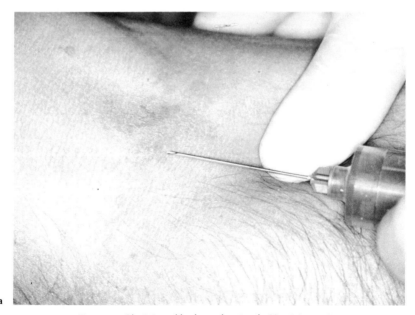

a

Fig. 3.46 *Obtaining a blood sample using the Vacutainer system.*

(continued)

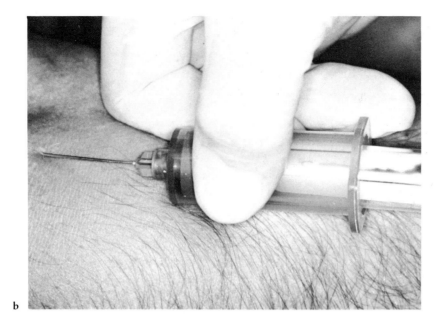

b

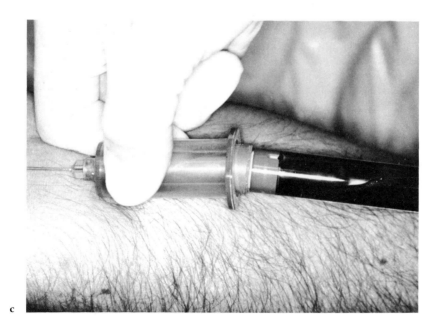

c

(continued)

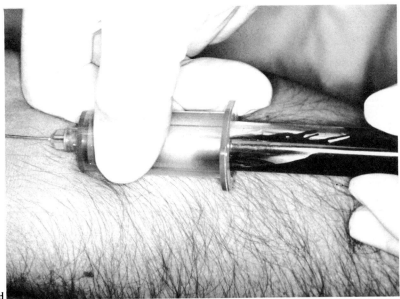

Fig. 3.46 *continued* **d**

Autoantibodies

Autoantibodies are, in the main, measured by specific, indirect immunofluorescence assays. Pemphigus is the most typical autoimmune disease of relevance (Volume 2). The more well-characterized autoantibodies and the disease associations are listed in Table 3.14, but it must be remembered that the mere presence of an autoantibody is *not* indicative of concurrent or even inevitable disease, since autoantibodies may occur (usually in low titre) in healthy patients and relatives of affected subjects—in general, autoantibodies are more common in the elderly and females. The clinical significance of an autoantibody usually depends upon its titre.

Complement

Complement assays are rarely required in dentistry except in suspected hereditary angioedema where C1 esterase inhibitor levels are reduced and the patient may have angioedema and airway obstruction after dental treatment (p. 61).

Cellular studies

Investigations of leucocyte numbers and function are indicated in suspected immune defects. In HIV infection, for example, there are reduced lymphocyte counts (lym-

Table 3.14
The clinical association of autoantibodies

Autoantibody specificity	Main clinical associations
Antinuclear, e.g. double stranded DNA, Ribonucleoprotein	Systemic lupus erythematosus Sjögren's syndrome Mixed connective tissue disease
IgG	Rheumatoid arthritis
Smooth muscle	Chronic active hepatitis
Mitochondria	Primary biliary cirrhosis
Reticulin	Coeliac disease Dermatitis herpetiformis
Gastric parietal cell	Pernicious anaemia
Thyroid microsome	Autoimmune thyroid disease
Adrenal tissue	Idiopathic Addison's disease
Salivary duct; Ro/La*	Sjögren's syndrome
Skeletal muscle	Myasthenia gravis
Stratified squamous epithelium	Pemphigus Pemphigoid

*Extractable nuclear antibodies also known as SSA and SSB antibodies.

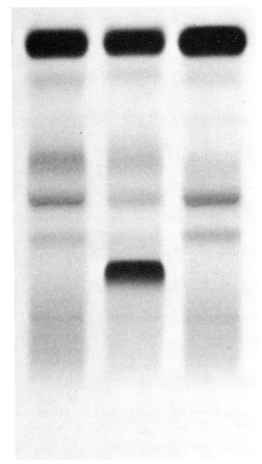

Fig. 3.47 *Electrophoresis of serum immunoglobulins. Note the middle sample comes from a patient with multiple myeloma: the lower dense band is due to IgG paraproteins. The other samples are of normal serum.*

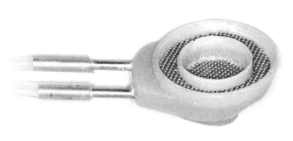

Fig. 3.48 *Cup for the collection of parotid saliva.*

phopenia) and depression of one particular type of T lymphocyte (T4 or CD4 cell).

OTHER INVESTIGATIONS

Sialometry

Sialometry is the measurement of salivary flow rates. It most commonly involves the parotid glands, since the parotid duct orifice can be easily identified and isolated and the parotid gland is more prone than the others to disease apart from duct obstruction. Sialometry of the submandibular and sublingual glands is rarely undertaken and, without specialized equipment, it is difficult to distinguish between the specific secretions of each gland.

Technique

Parotid saliva is collected using a suitable plastic collection cup such as a Carlsson–Crittenden cup (Fig. 3.48) which has an inner chamber that sits over the duct opening and from which the saliva is collected, and an outer chamber which connects to a dental suction unit and ensures close contact between the cup and the buccal mucosa. Care must be taken to ensure the suction is not so strong as to occlude the duct opening or cause the patient pain. Whenever possible, both parotid glands should be tested at the same time.

One millilitre of 5–10% (w/v) citric acid is applied to the dorsum of the tongue to stimulate salivation and saliva is collected in a calibrated sterile glass or plastic bottle such as a measuring cylinder. The flow rate is estimated by dividing the total sample volume by the time of collection (in minutes). The mean salivary flow rate of the parotid gland following stimulation with 10% citric acid is at least 1.5–2.0 ml/minute per gland. A stimulated parotid salivary gland flow rate of under 1 ml/minute usually indicates salivary hypofunction.

Aspiration of a suspected cystic lesion

The cystic nature of a lesion may be confirmed by inserting a large sterile needle (gauge 19 or 21) directly into the lesion and withdrawing a sample of fluid into a sterile disposable syringe. This is a useful clinical investigation, especially if a haemangioma or vascular lesion is suspected, and can avoid some unpleasant operative complications. The fluid can also be sent for analysis either in the syringe (with needle removed and a cap fitted) or in a sterile glass or plastic container.

At present it is not possible to distinguish with absolute reliability between the fluid content of specific cyst types. The presence of cholesterol crystals (detectable by polarized light microscopy) can be useful in identifying dentigerous and radicular cysts. There are, however, no laboratory tests to differentiate between the fluids from these two cystic disorders.

Levels of soluble protein in cyst fluid can, however, distinguish keratocysts from other odontogenic cysts: keratocysts have a lower protein concentration (2–3 g/ 100 ml) compared with the fluid of radicular, residual or dentigerous cysts which have a protein concentration of approximately 7 g/100 ml. However, since *infected* keratocysts can have this latter higher concentration of

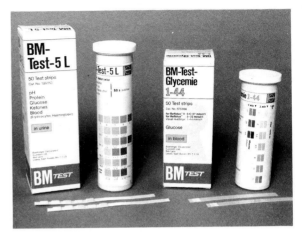

Fig. 3.49 *Urinalysis sticks (BM-Test-5L) and blood analysis sticks.*

soluble protein, measurement of the protein concentration of cyst fluid is not an absolutely satisfactory diagnos-

Table 3.15
*Urinalysis: interpretation of results**

	Protein	Glucose†	Ketones	Bilirubin‡	Urobilinogen‡	Blood§
Health						
Usually	None	None	None	None	Present	None
Occasionally	Trace can be normal in young people	Trace can be normal in 'renal glycosuria' and pregnancy	Ketonuria may occur in vomiting, fasting or starved patients			
Disease						
Raised levels usually indicate	Renal diseases	Diabetes mellitus	Diabetes mellitus	Jaundice	Jaundice	Genitourinary diseases
Occasionally	Cardiac failure, diabetes, myeloma, amyloid, some drugs, some chemicals	Pancreatitis, hyperthyroidism, Fanconi syndrome, sometimes after a head injury, other endocrinopathies	Febrile or traumatized patients on low carbohydrate diets	Hepatocellular and obstructive liver disease	Hepatocellular and obstructive liver disease	Bleeding tendency, some drugs

* Using test strips, e.g. Ames reagent strips or BM-Test-5L. Normal or non-fresh urine may be alkaline; normal urine may be acid.
† Dopa, ascorbate or salicylates may give false negative.
‡ May be false negative if urine not fresh.
§ Ascorbic acid may give false negative.

tic test. Biopsy of the lining is the only absolutely reliable diagnostic method.

Urinalysis

Analysis of urine at the bedside or chairside is a quick, simple, relatively cheap investigation capable of detecting some relevant conditions such as diabetes mellitus.

Urine levels of blood, bilirubin, ketones, urobilinogen, and glucose can be measured using a suitable test kit (Fig. 3.49). Raised levels of these in urine may indicate disease (Table 3.15). However, false positives can arise due to contamination of the container or due to concurrent drug therapy. In addition, test kits are unsuitable for detailed urinalysis such as microbial investigation or the measurement of specific proteins.

FURTHER READING

Beeching B. (1981). *Interpreting dental radiographs.* Update.

Cirbus M. T., Smiback M. S., Beltram J., Simon D. C. (1987). Magnetic resonance imaging in confirming internal derangement of the temporomandibular joint. *J. prosthet. Dent.,* **57**: 488–494.

Falace D. A. (1978). An evaluation of the clinical laboratory as an adjunct to dental practice. *JADA,* **96**: 261–265.

Fraser C. G. (1985). Urine analysis. *Br. med. J.,* **291**: 321–325.

Gold B. D., Wolfersberger W. H. (1980). Findings from routine urinalysis and hematocrit on ambulatory oral and maxillofacial surgery patients. *J. oral Surg.,* **38**: 677–678.

Leading Article (1988). 'Is routine urinalysis worthwhile?'. *Lancet,* **i**: 747.

Mason R. A. (1982). *A guide to dental radiography,* 2nd edn. Bristol: Wright.

Porter S. R., Scully C. (1988). *Radiographic interpretation in dentistry.* Oxford: Oxford University Press (in press).

Scully C. (1985). *The hospital dental surgeons guide.* London: British Dental Association.

Scully C., Cawson R. A. (1987). *Medical problems in dentistry,* 2nd edn. Bristol: Wright.

Smith N. J. D. (1980). *Dental radiography.* Oxford: Blackwell Scientific.

Sutton D. (1987). *A textbook of radiology and imaging,* 4th edn. Edinburgh: Churchill Livingstone.

Wilson N. H. F. (1987). Dental xeroradiography. In *Dental annual* (Derrick D. ed) pp. 261–271. Bristol: Wright.

Chapter
4
Management of emergencies

✓Emergencies should be prevented whenever possible—by careful assessment of the patient, especially by taking a reliable medical history, and care in treatment, particularly when general anaesthesia is used.

Only a few emergencies can or should be treated definitively in the dental surgery, but all dentists should know how to clear and maintain the airway, and how to carry out cardiopulmonary resuscitation (CPR).

Confidence and satisfactory management of emergencies can be increased by always having readily available:

(a) the telephone numbers of the local hospital and of the patient's general medical practitioner (or another helpful local medical practitioner);

(b) ancillary staff trained in emergency procedures;

(c) an emergency kit that is frequently checked and working (Table 4.1; Fig. 4.1).

Essential items include an efficient aspirator so that the airway can be sucked clean, oxygen, adrenaline solution 1 in 1000 for intramuscular injection, and a corticosteroid such as 200 mg hydrocortisone hemisuccinate for intravenous injection.

The following are the most common emergencies in dental surgery.

1. Sudden loss of consciousness, including: fainting, collapse in a diabetic patient, cardiac arrest, collapse in a patient with a history of systemic corticosteroid therapy, and stroke.

2. Adverse reactions after injections.

3. Fits.

4. Disturbed or unusual behaviour.

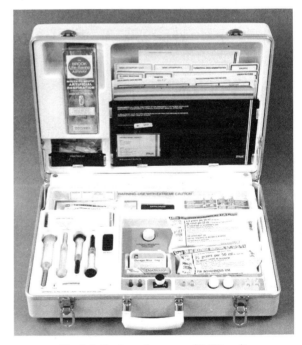

Fig. 4.1 *One type of emergency kit (Zita pak).*

✓ **Table 4.1**
Suggested emergency kit

Portable apparatus for administering oxygen, e.g. Pneu PAC
    Ventilator
Oral airway
Aspirator
Tourniquet
Disposable syringes and needles
Adrenaline injection BP (0.5 ml ampoules of 1 in 1000 solution)
Hydrocortisone sodium succinate injection BP (100 mg)
Diazepam for injection (10 mg vials)
Sugar, such as Lucozade, or Dextrosol tablets, for oral use, and
    dextrose injection BPC (50% solution)
Nitrous oxide/oxygen (anaesthetic machine, relative analgesia
    machine or Entonox)

---

5. Postoperative bleeding.
6. Inhaled foreign body.
7. Acute chest pain.
8. Asthmatic attack.
9. Severe maxillofacial injuries.
10. Emergencies in general anaesthesia and sedation (see Chapter 6).

SUDDEN LOSS OF CONSCIOUSNESS

Sudden loss of consciousness may be caused by fainting, myocardial infarction (heart attack), stroke, corticosteroid insufficiency, epilepsy, drug reactions, hypoglycaemia, bradycardia or heart block.

The cause of sudden loss of consciousness may be suggested by the patient's history. Collapse of a diabetic at lunchtime, for example, is most likely to be caused by hypoglycaemia. Collapse at the sight of a needle or during an injection is likely to be a simple faint, but if it follows some minutes after an injection of penicillin, is most likely to be anaphylaxis—an acute allergic reaction characterized by hypotension, sometimes with bronchospasm and urticaria. The simple precaution of laying patients flat *before* giving injections will prevent fainting (and a great deal of anxiety on the part of the operator!).

The clinical features of an episode of collapse may also aid the diagnosis. For example, severe chest pain suggests a heart attack. Collapse in a patient with angina or previous myocardial infarction may clearly be caused by a myocardial infarct.

Fainting

Fainting (vasovagal attack or syncope) is the most common cause of sudden loss of consciousness. It seems to be due to an initial emotionally induced, sympathetically mediated tachycardia and rise in blood pressure which induce a parasympathetic (vagal) response with skeletal blood vessel dilatation, bradycardia and a fall in blood pressure which reduces the blood flow to the brain.

Predisposing factors include:

(a) anxiety
(b) pain
(c) fatigue
(d) fasting
(e) high temperature and relative humidity.

About 1 in every 50 patients having tooth extraction under local anaesthesia faint and this is especially common in young adult males. Prevention is better than

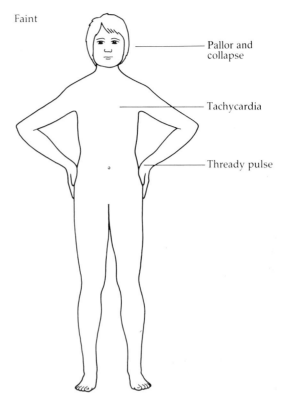

Faint

— Pallor and collapse

— Tachycardia

— Thready pulse

Fig. 4.2 *Features of a faint.*

cure: if injections are always given with the patient prone, he *cannot* faint!

Signs and symptoms of fainting include dizziness, weakness or nausea, pallor, cold moist skin, and a pulse initially slow and weak, then rapid and full. The patient loses consciousness (Fig. 4.2).

Management

1. Lower the head—preferably by laying the patient flat (Fig. 4.3), with the legs higher than the head, or putting his head between his knees. If the patient is not laid flat he may start to convulse because of cerebral hypoxia.
2. Loosen clothing if tight.
3. Smelling salts may help but are unpleasant.

Recovery is usually rapid and the patient should be reassured. If the patient is not recovering, consider other causes of collapse—especially anaphylaxis, myocardial infarction, and hypoglycaemia (diabetic). Further treatment should be deferred where possible.

If there is not immediate recovery, the following steps should be taken.

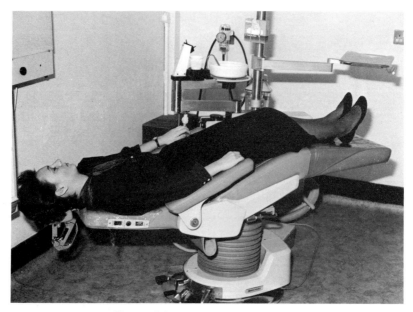

Fig. 4.3 *Management of a fainting patient.*

1. Give glucose, orally (four sugar lumps) if the patient has not completely lost consciousness; or 50 ml of 50% sterile glucose intravenously if unconscious; or 1 mg glucagon intramuscularly. A hypoglycaemic patient will rapidly improve with this regimen. If there is still no improvement, medical assistance should be summoned, and in the meantime:

2. maintain the airway and give oxygen;

3. give hydrocortisone sodium succinate (hemisuccinate) 200 mg intravenously.

Collapse of a diabetic patient

Collapse may be caused by fainting or, for example, myocardial infarction, since ischaemic heart disease is a common complication of longstanding diabetes, as well as by hypo- or hyperglycaemia.

Increasing drowsiness, disorientation, excitability or aggressiveness in a diabetic, especially if a meal is known to have been missed, suggests hypoglycaemia (Fig. 4.4). Try to carry out dental treatment on diabetics early in the morning to avoid this problem.

Management

Hypoglycaemia is the most dangerous complication of diabetes since the brain is starved of glucose. Glucose *but*

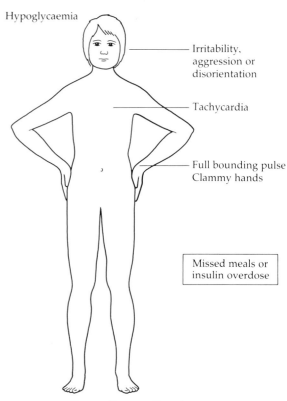

Hypoglycaemia

Irritability, aggression or disorientation

Tachycardia

Full bounding pulse
Clammy hands

Missed meals or insulin overdose

Fig. 4.4 *Features of hypoglycaemia.*

Table 4.2
Hypoglycaemia compared with hyperglycaemia

	Hypoglycaemia	Hyperglycaemia
Onset	Rapid	Slow
Mood	Irritability or aggressiveness	Drowsiness or disorientation
Pulse	Full and rapid	Weak
Skin	Moist	Dry
Blood sugar	Low	High
Urine sugar	Negative	Usually positive

not insulin should therefore be given to the diabetic who collapses, unless it is *certain* that the cause is hyperglycaemia.

1. Lay the patient flat and clear the airway.
2. If conscious give glucose orally (Lucozade, Dextrosol or at least four sugar lumps). If unconscious, give sterile glucose intravenously (50 ml of 50% solution).
3. Call an ambulance.

The differences between hypo- and hyperglycaemic coma are summarized in Table 4.2.

Cardiac arrest

Sudden cessation of effective cardiac beating leads to cerebral hypoxia which, after 3–4 minutes, produces irreversible brain damage. The heart may cease beating altogether (asystole) or, more commonly, beats rapidly, irregularly, and ineffectually (ventricular fibrillation).

Causes

Cardiac arrest may be caused by myocardial infarction, hypoxia, anaesthetic overdose, anaphylaxis, or severe hypotension.

Diagnosis

Suggestive features are sudden pallor and respiratory depression (Fig. 4.5) in a patient who collapses with:

(a) sudden loss of consciousness, and
(b) absence of arterial pulses—palpate the carotid artery in the neck anterior to the sternomastoid (Fig. 4.6).

During general anaesthesia, cessation of bleeding, darkening of the blood, absent pulses, irregular or cessation of respiration may signify cardiac arrest.

Other signs too late to be of use include:

(c) cyanosis,
(d) pupil dilatation, absence of light reaction,
(e) no measurable blood pressure.

Management

The main aim is to restore a flow of oxygenated blood to the brain by cardiopulmonary resuscitation

1. Summon assistance and note the time.
2. Lay the patient on the floor and clear the airway.
3. Give two firm sharp blows to the midsternum with the side of the closed fist; this occasionally restarts the heart in normal rhythm.
4. Give external cardiac compression at 60/minute. (Depress the sternum at the junction of the upper two-thirds with the lower third, 5 cm (2 inches) at each compression.)
5. Artificially ventilate once every five or six cardiac compressions. (Use face mask and oxygen, or mouth-to-mouth or mouth-to-nose or, if experienced, endotracheal intubation.)
6. Electrical defibrillation if the heart is fibrillating; drugs may also be required but these procedures are the province of the physician. However, the dentist can usefully put up an intravenous line to facilitate their administration.
7. Persist until there is restoration of a good spontaneous pulse, of blood pressure, purposeful movements (not twitches), reflex activity or of consciousness.

If the patient recovers, he should be admitted to hospital. If the patient is not resuscitated by 15 minutes, recovery is unlikely.

Collapse in a patient with history of systemic corticosteroid therapy

Fainting and other causes of collapse are possible, but adrenal insufficiency in general anaesthesia, trauma, infections or other stress must be excluded.

Diagnosis

1. Pallor.
2. Pulse rapid, weak or impalpable.
3. Loss of consciousness.
4. Rapidly falling blood pressure.

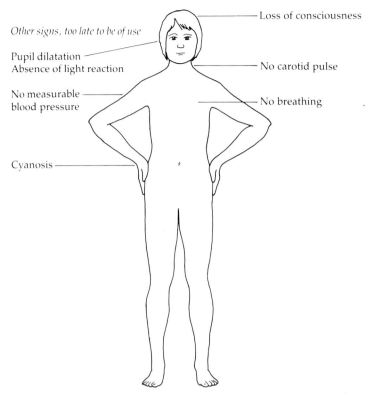

Other signs, too late to be of use

Loss of consciousness

Pupil dilatation
Absence of light reaction

No carotid pulse

No measurable
blood pressure

No breathing

Cyanosis

Fig. 4.5 *Features of cardiac arrest.*

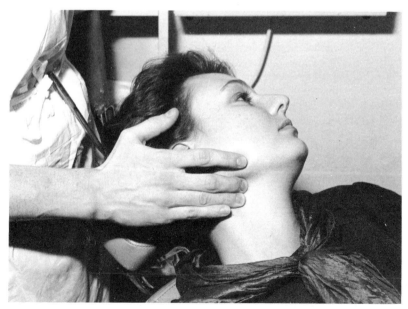

Fig. 4.6 *Palpation of carotid pulse—much more value than taking the radial pulse in suspected cardiac arrest.*

Management

Even if the cause of the collapse is unclear, it is safest to give corticosteroids immediately.

1. Lay patient flat, raise legs, and clear airway.
2. Give at least 200 mg hydrocortisone sodium succinate intravenously.
3. Call an ambulance.
4. Give oxygen.
5. Consider cause and other possible reasons for collapse.

Strokes

Patients are usually hypertensive and middle-aged or elderly.

Diagnosis

1. Loss of consciousness.
2. Weakness of arm and sometimes leg on one side.
3. Side of face may droop.

Management

1. Maintain a clear airway.
2. Call an ambulance.

ADVERSE REACTIONS AFTER INJECTION OF A LOCAL ANAESTHETIC OR OTHER DRUG (see also Chapter 6)

Most reactions are simple faints, though, rarely, other causes of collapse are involved. Some other reactions are very rare and no specific treatment is needed.

Anaphylactic shock

Causes

This is usually caused by penicillin, but also by methohexitone.

Diagnosis

Anaphylactic shock occurs within a few minutes usually, but may be delayed 30 minutes or so. Its features are listed below (Fig. 4.7).

1. Facial flushing, itching, paraesthesia or peripheral coldness.
2. Wheezing, abdominal pain, nausea.
3. Loss of consciousness.

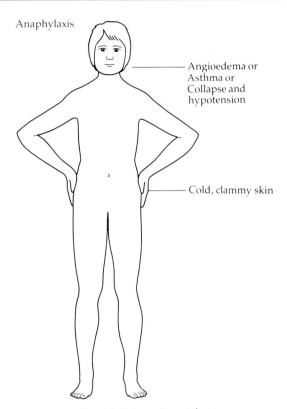

Anaphylaxis

— Angioedema or Asthma or Collapse and hypotension

— Cold, clammy skin

Fig. 4.7 *Features of anaphylaxis.*

4. Pallor going on to cyanosis.
5. Cold clammy skin.
6. Rapid, weak or impalpable pulse.
7. Facial oedema, or sometimes urticaria (Fig. 4.8).

Management

1. Lay patient flat with legs raised.
2. Give 1 ml of 1 in 1000 adrenaline intramuscularly (adult), and
3. give 200 mg of hydrocortisone sodium succinate intravenously.
4. Give oxygen.
5. Call an ambulance.

Reactions to intravascular injection of local anaesthetic

Causes

1. Failure to use aspirating syringe.
2. Rapid injection.

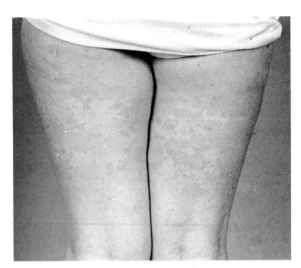

Fig. 4.8 Urticaria from penicillin allergy.

Diagnosis

Possible effects may include agitation, confusion, drowsiness, fits or loss of consciousness.

Management

1. Lay patient flat.
2. Give reassurance.
3. Maintain the airway.

Most patients recover spontaneously within half an hour.

Local anaesthetic allergy

Allergy to local anaesthesia is *very* rare but is managed as for anaphylaxis.

Cardiovascular reactions

Following local anaesthesia these are usually only palpitations caused mainly by the vasoconstrictor. The patient should be reassured while the symptoms subside naturally. If the reaction is severe, such as myocardial infarction (whether coincidental or not), treat as above.

Overdosage of local anaesthetics

Overdosage with local anaesthetics is uncommon and reactions vary from convulsion to drowsiness, respiratory failure or even cardiac arrest. The patient should be reassured, the airway kept patent and oxygen given.

Temporary facial palsy, diplopia (double vision) or localized facial pallor following local anaesthetic

This can occasionally result when the local anaesthetic tracks towards the facial nerve or orbital contents. The eyelids should be closed and a protective dressing worn until the anaesthetic abates.

Needle fracture

Fracture of a needle is rare unless the needle is re-used or repeatedly bent and then straightened. However, needles should never be re-used or bent. If the protruding end of a broken needle cannot easily be grasped with mosquito forceps, the patient should be immediately referred to a surgeon for its removal (Chapter 6 and Fig. 10.3).

General anaesthetic overdose or hypotension

Maintain the airway, give oxygen and consider giving corticosteroids.

PATIENTS WHO HAVE FITS

Most fits are related to epilepsy and in known epileptics, but a not uncommon cause is also the failure to lay a fainting patient flat when there may be cerebral hypoxia which can precipitate a fit.

Epilepsy (see also Chapter 2)

Causes of a fit in a known epileptic include starvation, menstruation and some drugs such as methohexitone, tricyclics or alcohol.

Diagnosis of grand mal attack (Fig. 4.9)

1. Loss of consciousness with rigid, extended body. Sometimes preceded by a brief cry.
2. Widespread jerking movements.
3. Incontinence sometimes.
4. Slow recovery.

Management

1. Put the patient prone in the head-injury (see Fig. 6.49, p. 168) position. All that is needed is to keep the airway clear and to stop the patient damaging himself.
2. If the convulsions do not stop within 5 minutes, or if another attack starts:

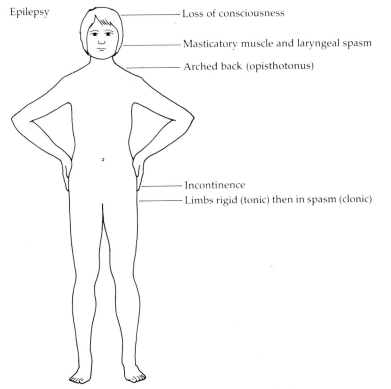

Epilepsy

Loss of consciousness

Masticatory muscle and laryngeal spasm

Arched back (opisthotonus)

Incontinence

Limbs rigid (tonic) then in spasm (clonic)

Fig. 4.9 *Features of a major convulsion (grand mal fit).*

(a) give 0.1 mg/kg diazepam intravenously (or intramuscularly),

(b) call an ambulance,

(c) repeat diazepam if there is no recovery within 5 minutes.

DISTURBED OR UNUSUAL BEHAVIOUR IN THE DENTAL SURGERY

Patients can be disturbed or show abnormal behaviour because of intoxication with alcohol or other drugs, organic disease such as diabetes or head injury, or psychiatric disease (Chapter 2). For example, many patients attending casualty services are intoxicated with alcohol and some patients attempt to relieve dental pain or get courage to attend the dentist by taking alcohol or other drugs.

Patients with head injuries may show disturbed behaviour because of brain damage. Diabetic patients who become hypoglycaemic may become irritable and aggressive.

Psychogenic disorders ranging from simple aggressive personality disorders to severe psychoses are important causes of abnormal behaviour.

Many complaining or aggressive dental patients are otherwise normal individuals who act in that way because of acute anxiety or panic, sometimes aggravated by chronic discomfort or pain (Chapter 1).

Psychiatric emergencies

Management

1. Summon psychiatric assistance or call an ambulance.

2. Do not sedate the patient since this may confuse the diagnosis and may occasionally be fatal. Diazepam 20 mg intravenously or intramuscularly may, however, be needed in an emergency.

Emergency admission procedures are shown in Table 4.3.

Table 4.3
*Compulsory procedures for management of patients with psychiatric disease**

Section	Purpose	Duration	Persons making application	Medical recommendations
Mental Health Act, 1983				
2	Hospital admission for observation	28 days	Nearest relative or authorized social worker	Both: 1. Registered medical practitioner, and 2. recognized psychiatrist
3	Hospital admission for treatment	1 year; may be renewed if appropriate. Patient may appeal to a Mental Health Tribunal in the first 6 months	Nearest relative or authorized social worker (the latter must, where practicable, first consult the nearest relative)	Both: 1. registered medical practitioner who knows patient, and 2. recognized psychiatrist
4	Hospital admission for observation in emergency (when only one doctor is available and the degree of urgency does not permit delay to obtain a second medical opinion)	72 hours	Any relative or authorized social worker	Registered medical practitioner
5	Emergency detention of an informal patient already in hospital	3 days, beginning on the day on which report furnished		The responsible consultant psychiatrist in charge of the case; his deputy may act on his direct instructions
136	Removal by police to a place of safety. Persons who appear to be mentally disordered in a place to which public have access, if in immediate need of care or control, may be taken by police to a place of safety to await examination by doctor or authorized social worker	72 hours	Police officer	—
Mental Health Act Scotland, 1960				
24	Hospital admission for observation	28 days	Nearest relative or authorized social worker	Both: 1. registered medical practitioner and 2. medical practitioner recognized under Section 27
31	Hospital admission for observation in emergency (where Section 24 is not applicable) or emergency detention of an informal patient already in hospital	7 days	Any relative or authorized social worker	Registered medical practitioner who has examined the patient on that day
104	Removal by police to a place of safety	72 hours	Police officer	—

* Call the Duty Psychiatrist or Medical Practitioner.

Hyperventilation syndrome

Overbreathing may induce collapse. Usually the patient is an anxious or hysterical young woman who over-breathes until carbon dioxide washout results in alkalosis producing tetany and paraesthesia and cerebral vaso-constriction that may cause collapse. In contrast to a faint, the hyperventilation syndrome causes a flushed appear-ance and rapid pulse rate.

Organic causes include pain and cardiovascular or ner-vous system disease. Hyperventilation is also a response to acidosis (either metabolic or drug associated) and to poor respiratory exchange, but in these cases is a com-pensatory physiological response.

The common denominator underlying the hyperventi-lation syndrome is usually anxiety.

Management

Patients should be reassured. Otherwise, the most im-portant aspect of treatment, if reassurance is ineffective, is to get the patient to rebreathe exhaled carbon dioxide by placing her cupped hands or a paper bag over her nose and mouth (Fig. 4.10), or using sedation, usually with diazepam. If, however, there is obvious sympathetic overactivity, as shown particularly by tachycardia or arrhythmias, a cardiologist's opinion should be obtained as treatment with a beta blocker may be necessary. In patients with hysterical personalities, however, the re-sponse to treatment may be poor.

POSTOPERATIVE BLEEDING

Post-extraction bleeding usually has a local cause, par-ticularly traumatic extractions with soft tissue damage. It is uncommonly caused by haemorrhagic disease, but this must always be considered (Chapter 2).

Management

Because a little blood makes a great mess, especially when diluted with saliva, post-extraction bleeding often worries the patient excessively.

1. Reassure the patient.
2. Ask relatives to leave unless the patient is a very young child.
3. Clean the mouth with a saline-soaked swab.
4. Locate the source of bleeding.
5. Inquire into history, especially family and previous operative history, to exclude a systemic cause.
6. Give local anaesthesia.
7. Suture the socket.
8. Keep the patient rested until bleeding stops.
9. If bleeding is persistent or severe and there has been loss of more than about 500 ml, or if the patient is severely anaemic or debilitated, then admit to hospital. Tranexamic acid (5 ml containing 500 mg by injection intravenously) may be effective in the interim.
10. Call an ambulance if bleeding is uncontrollable.

INHALED FOREIGN BODY

The best treatment is prevention. The use of rubber dam will prevent all but the most bizarre incidents. In the ab-sence of rubber dam, a parachute chain (Fig. 4.11) should

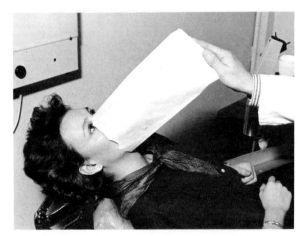

Fig. 4.10 *Management of hysterical hyperventilation.*

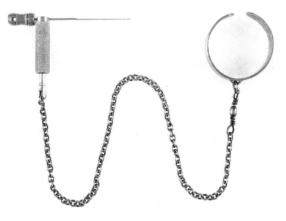

Fig. 4.11 *A parachute chain.*

always be attached when endodontic hand instruments are used.

An inhaled foreign body such as an inlay or crown causes, at the very least, anxiety and embarrassment, and can cause serious illness such as a lung abscess or worse.

Management

1. Ask the patient to cough deliberately. If this fails, take a chest radiograph (two views at right-angles, i.e. posterior-anterior and lateral chest views) to locate the object (Figs. 4.12 and 4.13).
2. Use the Heimlich manoeuvre (Fig. 4.14).
3. Refer for endoscopy (and inform your Medical Defence Society!). Even thoracotomy might become necessary. Record the details of the incident.

Ingested foreign bodies are less dangerous and usually pass uneventfully (Fig. 4.15).

ACUTE CHEST PAIN

Acute, severe chest pain is often caused by angina or myocardial infarction.

Diagnosis of angina/myocardial infarction

1. Severe crushing retrosternal pain.
2. Breathlessness, vomiting and loss of consciousness if there is an infarct.
3. Pulse may be weak or irregular if there is an infarct.

Management

1. If the patient has a history of angina, give anti-anginal drugs if he has them (glyceryl trinitrate 0.5 mg sublingually). If there is no relief of pain in 3 minutes, the cause is probably an infarct.
2. Summon assistance.
3. Do not lay the patient flat if this increases breathlessness.
4. Give nitrous oxide and oxygen (50/50) to relieve pain and anxiety.
5. Reassure the patient.

ASTHMATIC ATTACK

Anxiety, infection or exposure to an allergen can precipitate an attack of asthma.

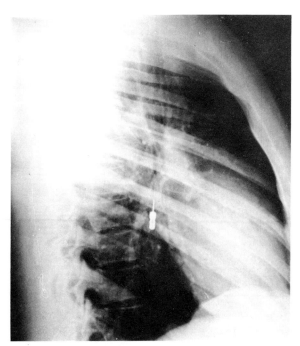

Fig. 4.12 *Lateral chest radiograph showing an inhaled endodontic instrument (rubber dam was not used: Volume 3).*

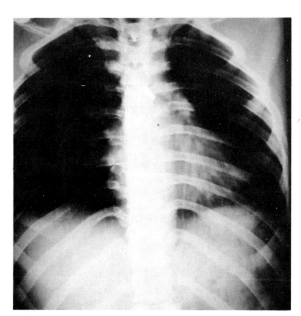

Fig. 4.13 *Postero-anterior chest radiograph showing an inhaled endodontic instrument.*

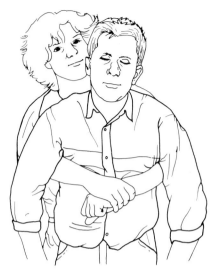

Fig. 4.14 *Heimlich manoeuvre.*

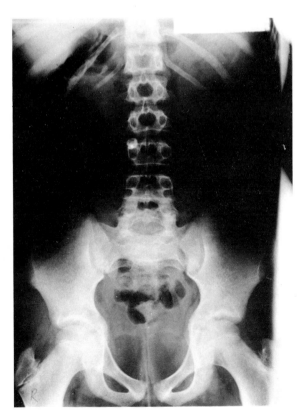

Fig. 4.15 *Ingested tooth crown (rubber dam was not used: Volume).*

Diagnosis

1. Breathlessness.
2. Expiratory wheezing.
3. Accessory muscles of respiration in action.

Management

1. Give the anti-asthmatic drugs normally used (such as salbutamol).
2. Give oxygen.
3. If there is no response within 2–3 minutes, give 0.5 to 1 ml of 1 in 1000 adrenaline intramuscularly (adult).
4. Do not lay the patient flat.
5. Reassure the patient.
6. Call an ambulance.
7. Give hydrocortisone sodium succinate 200 mg intravenously if there is no response to adrenaline.

SEVERE MAXILLOFACIAL INJURIES (Volume 2)

Management

1. Lay the patient in the head-injury (see p. 168) position.
2. Establish and maintain a clear airway.
3. Check for head injury.
4. Check for chest injury or damage to cervical spine, liver, spleen or kidneys.
5. Check for ocular injuries.
6. Call an ambulance.

EMERGENCIES IN GENERAL ANAESTHESIA OR SEDATION (see also Chapter 6: p. 70)

Respiratory complications

Respiratory obstruction produces see-saw breathing and a sense of vibrations around the neck, often with noisy inspiration (stridor).

Commonly, obstruction is caused by the tongue falling back against the posterior pharyngeal wall, and is readily corrected by pushing the mandible forwards by exerting anterior pressure against both angles. Fragments of teeth, fillings, blood or vomit should not be allowed to enter the airway. The most dangerous times are during induction of anaesthesia, dental treatment, and postoperatively. No food or drink should be taken for at least 4 hours before a GA. Care should therefore be taken during intubation not to damage teeth or fillings, to ensure dentures have been removed, and to make sure that the patient has had no food or drink for 4–6 hours before a GA.

A pack should be used to protect the airway during treatment, and endotracheal intubation increases the safety. Care must be taken to segregate debris such as extracted teeth, etc. from clean swabs to be used in the mouth, lest debris be carried back into the mouth on a swab. The mouth and pharynx should carefully be aspirated before extubation after removal of throat packs.

Postoperatively, the mouth and pharynx should be cleared carefully and the patient laid in the tonsillar position (see Fig. 6.49, p. 168). *This is a very dangerous period and the patient should not be left unsupervised or inadequately supervised.* (See Chapter 7.)

Should obstruction occur because of foreign material, the mouth and throat must be aspirated with the patient in the tonsillar position, and oxygen given until he or she can be transferred to hospital.

Laryngeal spasm may be caused by hypoxia, irritant anaesthetic agents, or foreign material. The pharynx should be cleared and oxygen given.

Respiratory depression is usually caused by an anaesthetic overdose, when the anaesthetic should be stopped and oxygen given. Hypoxia and cardiac arrest are other causes—again oxygen should be given.

Convulsions

Epilepsy is rare under GA: treat by giving oxygen and intravenous diazepam.

Allergy to anaesthetic (see page 109)

Cardiovascular complications

Cardiac arrest is discussed on page 107.

Hypotension may also result from anaesthetic overdose, drug interactions, or autonomic blockade during anaesthesia. Treatment consists of placing the patient head down (Trendelburg position) and giving oxygen. Intravenous atropine 0.6–1.2 mg may correct bradycardia; vasopressors (such as metaraminol, methoxamine or ephedrine) may also prove useful.

Sedation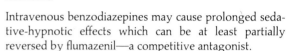

Intravenous benzodiazepines may cause prolonged sedative-hypnotic effects which can be at least partially reversed by flumazenil—a competitive antagonist.

FURTHER READING

Editorial (1981). Inhaled foreign bodies. *Br. med. J.*, **282**: 1649–1651.

Edmondson H. D., Frame J. W. (1986). Medical emergencies in general practice. *Dent. Update*, **11**: 263–273.

Lowenstein S. R. *et al.* (1981). Cardiopulmonary resuscitation by medical and surgical house-officers. *Lancet*, **ii**: 679–681.

The Dental Clinics of North America (1982). *Medical emergencies in the dental office.* Philadelphia: Saunders.

Tinker J. (1981). How to manage a cardiac arrest. *Br. J. hosp. Med.*, **25**: 83–84.

Scully C. (1985). *The hospital dental surgeon's guide.* London: British Dental Association.

Scully C., Cawson R. A. (1987). *Medical problems in dentistry*, 2nd edn. Bristol: Wright.

Shirlaw P. J., Scully C., Griffiths M. J. *et al.* (1986). General anaesthesia, parenteral sedation and emergency drugs and equipment in general dental practice. *J. Dent.*, **14**: 247–250.

Chapter

✓ 5   *Principles of prescribing*

This chapter deals with the basics of prescribing but not the fundamentals of pharmacology, which are covered in specialist texts (see Further reading). The therapy of specific disorders is discussed elsewhere in this and other volumes of the series under relevant sections.

The legislation governing the supply, administration, marketing and sale of medicines includes mainly the Medicines Act (1968) and the Misuse of Drugs Act (1971) and Regulations (1985).

THE MEDICINES ACT 1968

The Medicines Act 1968 resulted in description of medicines as:

(i) prescription-only medicines (POM)—those available only on prescription,

(ii) general sale list (GSL)—those for general sale,

(iii) pharmacy medicine (P)—those available only through a pharmacy.

The Act also resulted in the Medicines Commission, an advisory body with subsidiary bodies including the Committee on Dental and Surgical Materials and the Committee on Safety of Medicines (CSM).

Prescription-only medicines

Prescription-only medicines are those medicinal products described as such in The Medicines (Products Other than Veterinary Drugs (Prescription-only)) Order 1983 as amended. Such medicines are marked POM and may only be supplied or sold by a pharmacy in accordance with a prescription given by an appropriate practitioner—a dentist, doctor or veterinary surgeon. In addition, a pharmacist may provide a limited supply of prescription-only medicines without prescription under strictly defined circumstances.

Prescription writing for drugs that are *not* controlled drugs

A prescription must meet requirements set out in the legislation in order to be valid. It must:

1. be signed in ink with the name of the practitioner giving it;

2. be written in indelible ink (this includes typewriting) unless it is a National Health Service (NHS) prescription which is not for a controlled drug, in which case it may be written by means of carbon paper or similar material but must be signed in indelible ink by the practitioner giving it;

3. contain the following particulars:

    (a) the address of the practitioner giving it,

    (b) the appropriate date,

    (c) particulars to indicate that the practitioner giving it is a dentist (or doctor),

    (d) Where the practitioner giving it is a dentist (or doctor), the name and address and the age, if under 12, of the person for whom the treatment is given.

The prescription should also contain (Fig. 5.1):

1. the full name of the drug,

2. the dose and dose frequency, preferably stated in English without abbreviation,

3. the quantity to be supplied *or* length of treatment required,

4. the symbol *NP* if the medicine is to be labelled with the name of the preparation (NHS forms already have this printed on them).

Great care should be taken with dosage, particularly where decimal points are involved. The rules given at the front of the *British National Formulary* or *Dental Practitioner's Formulary* should be adhered to: quantities less than 1 g should be written as milligrams (for example, 500 mg *not* 0.5 g) and those less than 1 mg should always

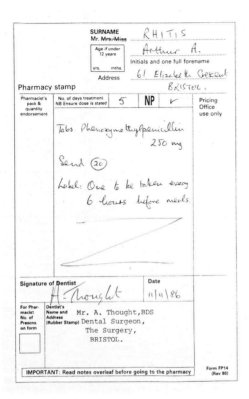

Fig. 5.1 *Sample prescription for course of penicillin V.*

Drugs (Prescription-only)) Order 1983, as amended, provides an exemption for such POM products for parenteral administration to humans. Section 58 (2)b of the Medicines Act, however, prohibits the administration of such products (other than to oneself) by anyone who is not a practitioner (dentist or doctor) or who is not acting in accordance with a practitioner's directions (such as a dental student in a hospital setting or a state registered nurse). The only other exemption is if a drug is being administered in an emergency for a life-saving purpose.

General Sale List and pharmacy medicine

The Medicines (General Sale List) Order 1980 details medicinal products which can be sold or supplied with reasonable safety other than by a pharmacist. The GSL includes small packs of drugs such as aspirin or paracetamol and products such as chlorhexidine. Section 52 of the

be written in full (for example, 100 microgrammes *not* 0.1 mg). If decimals are used, a zero should be inserted before the decimal point if no other figure is indicated (Fig. 5.1).

A prescription must not be dispensed more than 6 months later than the 'appropriate date' unless it is a 'repeatable prescription' (see below), in which case it will not be dispensed for the first time after the end of this period or other than in accordance with directions contained in the repeat prescription. An NHS prescription cannot be repeated. These terms are defined as follows:

The appropriate date. In the case of NHS prescriptions, this is the date on which it was signed by the practitioner or a date indicated by him or her as being the date before which it will not be dispensed; in every other case, it is the date on which the prescription was signed.

A repeatable prescription is one which contains a direction that it may be dispensed more than once (see above).

The Medicines (Products Other Than Veterinary

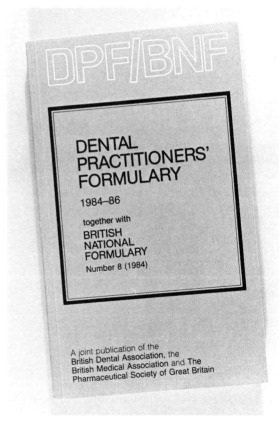

Fig. 5.2 *The* Dental Practitioners' Formulary *(DPF). New editions are available at frequent regular intervals.*

Medicines Act permits a dentist to sell or supply such medicinal products to a patient or to a person caring for a patient.

Labelling of medicines

Pharmacists are now recommended by the Pharmaceutical Society to label medicines with typed or mechanically printed instructions. As well as the patient's name, date and the directions for use, the label should bear the name of the drug and quantity dispensed, since this information can be invaluable in emergencies.

Storage of medicines

Drugs are potentially dangerous, especially to children, and are therefore best stored in 'childproof' containers, preferably in a locked cabinet. They should be kept at the surgery, not at home, and in general terms are best kept cool, out of the light and protected from ambient moisture.

Controlled drugs *must* be stored as outlined below (page 124).

Drug information

The *British National Formulary* (BNF) gives a useful and practical guide to therapeutics. The *Dental Practitioners' Formulary* (DPF) outlines the dental preparations approved by the Secretary of State which can be prescribed by dental practitioners on form FP14 (Figs. 5.2 and 5.3). The list includes titles in the British Pharmacopoeia 1980 (BP) and British Pharmaceutical Codex 1973 (BPC) which comply with the Medicines Act (Section 65) as well as some preparations not included in BP or BPC. Information can also be obtained from Drug Information Centres (Table 5.1). *Monthly Index of Medical Specialities* (MIMS) gives a useful generic index and other information.

General principles of therapeutics

Drugs can be valuable in the treatment of many different conditions but should only be given if no more suitable treatment is available or effective, since *all* drugs may produce unwanted, or adverse, effects ranging from the trivial to severe and even life-threatening complications (such as anaphylaxis). It is the duty of the practitioner to be aware of these possibilities and to weigh the pros and

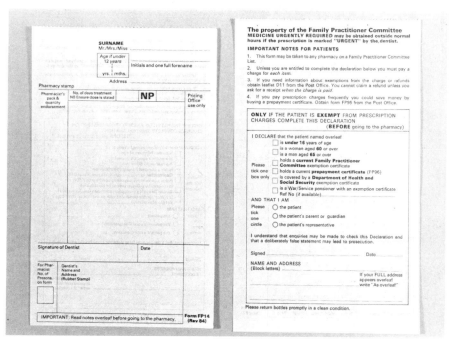

Fig. 5.3 *National Health Service form FP14 for dental prescriptions (showing both sides of form).*

Table 5.1
Drug information centres

Belfast	0232 248095
Birmingham	021 471 3884
Bristol	0272 298632/260256
Edinburgh	031 229 3901
Glasgow	041 552 3535
Leeds	0532 432799 or 0532 430715
London	01 407 760
Newcastle	091 232 1525

cons before prescribing or not prescribing. Drugs are not always the most appropriate treatment. For example, the most appropriate treatment of an oral pyogenic infection such as an apical abscess is, in most cases, drainage of pus rather than antibiotic treatment.

Drugs can be extremely valuable, however. For example, because systemic corticosteroids are life-saving in the treatment of pemphigus; then the side-effects such as hypertension are 'acceptable' hazards. In contrast, systemic corticosteroids are not acceptable as treatment in less serious conditions such as minor aphthae. Furthermore, the safest of the group of drugs indicated should always be used where possible. For example, the dangers of using full general anaesthesia clearly exceed those of relative analgesia or local analgesia.

Drug interactions are sometimes very important in dental practice, where the main interactions are with general anaesthetic agents (see below).

The age of the patient influences the drugs that can be prescribed (Chapter 2). Children should not be given aspirin (because of the danger of inducing Reye's syndrome) or tetracyclines (which cause tooth discoloration: Fig. 5.4). Doses of most drugs should be reduced in the elderly.

The medical history of the patient also influences the drugs that can be prescribed. Aspirin, for example, because it interferes with haemostasis, should not be given to patients with a bleeding tendency. In general terms, however, it is again the general anaesthetic agents that are the greatest risk to the medically compromised patient.

In summary:

1. use drugs only if they are the best treatment available;
2. ensure that the advantages of drug treatment outweigh the disadvantages of withholding treatment;

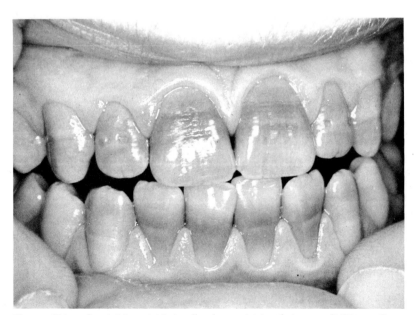

Fig. 5.4 *Tetracycline staining—intrinsic yellow-brown staining that can result if tetracyclines are given to children. The fetus can be affected if the mother is given tetracyclines.*

3. use the safest effective drug and consider age, medical history and drug interactions;

4. use general anaesthesia only where there are very good indications;

5. restrict the number of drugs given to an absolute minimum.

6. warn the patient about any possible adverse effects.

Route of administration

In general terms, oral administration is preferred since it is painless and thus more acceptable to the patient, and is simpler for the practitioner to administer. Incidentally, anaphylaxis is probably less likely to occur with oral drugs than with those given by injection (parenterally). The main disadvantages of the oral route are that absorption can be unpredictable, especially if the patient vomits, and that, unless the anaesthetist directs otherwise, oral drugs should not be given when the stomach needs to be empty, such as within 4–6 hours before GA (Chapter 6).

Topical application

Lignocaine, antifungal agents, and corticosteroids are the most commonly used topical preparations in dentistry. All are effective preparations.

Sublingual drugs

Lorazepam, buprenorphine, and glyceryl trinitrate can be absorbed sublingually.

Oral drugs

Despite the unpredictability of absorption, improvements in drugs and their formulation result in this being the favoured route. Some drugs such as amoxycillin are so well absorbed orally that they give high blood levels comparable with those reached by injection.

Absorption may be impaired by food, milk, and antacids and therefore drugs such as penicillin, erythromycin, tetracycline, and paracetamol should be given at least 30 minutes before food. Drugs that are gastric irritants (such as aspirin) are best given with food.

Parenteral administration

The parenteral route is a prerequisite when a rapid onset of effect is required as, for example, in intravenous seda-

tion or intravenous induction of anaesthesia. It is also a useful route to ensure that drugs reach the therapeutic level in, for example:

(a) patients of poor compliance (e.g. mentally handicapped),
(b) persistent vomiting,
(c) general anaesthesia.

Another big advantage of (intramuscular) injections is that long-acting preparations (depot injections) can be given, though these injections can be painful. For example, depot penicillins (e.g. procaine penicillin and benethamine penicillin) give sustained effective blood levels for several hours or days, depending on the preparation used.

Antimicrobials and, in certain circumstances, various other drugs (e.g. corticosteroids, diazepam) may be given intramuscularly (i.m.). The indications for i.m. antimicrobials in dentistry have been reduced somewhat since the advent of oral amoxycillin which gives acceptably high blood levels within 1–2 hours, persisting 9–10 hours, and obviously increased compliance. Diazepam is poorly absorbed if given i.m. and, therefore, the rectal route is preferred if for some reason the intravenous route is inappropriate.

For any i.m. (or any other) injection, it is wise to have the patient lying down beforehand, since he then cannot fall down if he faints. If he collapses while having an injection when standing, he not only may damage himself, but you may have a few moments of anxiety trying to differentiate a simple faint from anaphylaxis.

If an i.m. injection *is* indicated, check that:

(a) the patient is not allergic to the drug or that the drug is not otherwise contraindicated;
(b) the expiry date of the drug has not passed;
(c) the correct drug (and solvent) is used: this is especially important if another person (e.g. a nurse) makes up the drug;
(d) adrenaline 1 in 1000 is available for i.m. injection if anaphylaxis occurs (see Chapter 4).

Method

1. With the patient lying down, rub the site with an isopropyl alcohol swab. The anterolateral aspect of the thigh is the preferred site for i.m. injections since injections may be given into the vastus lateralis muscle on the anterolateral aspect of the thigh where there is a mass of muscle free from important vessels or nerves.

The anterior part of the upper and outer quadrant of

the buttock can be used but is a less safe site than the thigh because of the proximity of the sciatic nerve. To find the safest place for an i.m. injection, place the tip of the left index finger on the anterior superior iliac spine and the tip of the middle finger, abducted as shown in Figure 5.5, just below the iliac crest. The injection site is then into the gluteal muscles within the triangle formed by the fingers and the iliac crest. *Do not inject* into the 'bottom' or there is then danger of damage to the sciatic nerve with possible paralysis of the leg.

Small injections can be given into the deltoid muscle on the outer aspect of the shoulder, but the shirt or blouse must be removed so that you will not inject too low, since there is danger of damage to the radial nerve. Damage to nerves may cause pain, paraesthesia or even paralysis.

2. Leave the alcohol to dry before injecting.
3. Check again that you are about to inject the correct drug.
4. Rapidly pierce the skin and muscle with the needle (size 19 or 20 for large volumes of fluid; size 21 or 23 for small volumes).
5. Aspirate to ensure the needle is not in a blood vessel.
6. Inject slowly.
7. Withdraw the needle; swab the area.
8. Observe for adverse reactions (30 minutes in the case of antimicrobials): especially watch for difficulty in breathing, rashes or collapse.

Drug doses

Drug doses are given in appropriate publications such as the *British National Formulary* (BNF) and *Dental Practitioners' Formulary* (DPF) and should be checked before prescribing. Doses must be reduced in:

(a) children (Chapter 2);
(b) the elderly (Chapter 2);
(c) medically compromised patients: particularly relevant are liver or kidney disorders (Chapter 2);
(d) patients taking drugs with synergistic effects: sedative drugs, for example, should be given in lower doses if the patient is taking drugs such as tranquillizers or alcohol that have a CNS depressive effect.

Timing of administration

The timing of administration of drugs can be critical, especially in the following situations.

1. Prophylaxis for endocarditis, when the antibiotic cover should only be given 1–2 hours preoperatively. This gives maximum blood levels at the time of operation and, if given sooner, resistant micro-organisms may appear (Chapter 2).
2. Premedication, when the patient should arrive in the anaesthetic room suitably premedicated (Chapters 6 and 9).
3. Corticosteroid cover, when a high level of corticosteroids is required at and after operation (Chapter 2).

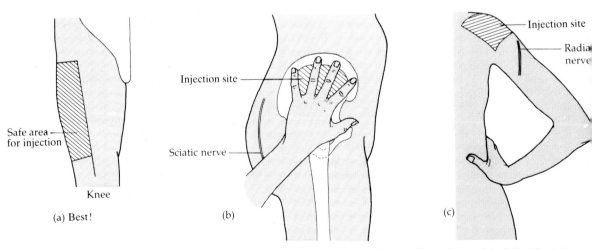

Fig. 5.5 *Sites for intramuscular injection: the lateral aspect of the thigh is the safest. Oral amoxycillin produces such high blood levels that it is often preferred to an injection. (a) Anterolateral aspect of the thigh. (b) Anterior part of the upper and outer quadrant of the buttock. (c) Outer aspect of the shoulder.*

4. Diabetics, when drugs should be administered at appropriate timing in relation to other factors that alter blood sugar levels (especially meals) such that hypoglycaemia does not occur (Chapter 2).

Duration of administration

Medicines may need to be given long term, e.g. antihypertensive therapy, or short term, e.g. analgesia and antibiotics. In either case adverse reactions to the medicine may need a reduction in dosage or alternative medicines being tried.

Where drugs are given for long periods, problems associated with adverse effects can be significant and the patient may need to be monitored clinically, sometimes with estimation of drug levels in serum or saliva (e.g. anti-epileptic drugs) or investigations for adverse reactions such as with a blood count (e.g. with carbamazepine, which may cause leukopenia).

Patient compliance

Patients do not always comply with prescribed treatment. Nearly 1 in 5 prescriptions given are not collected from the pharmacist and even those that are collected may never be used or may be used incorrectly. Even in accident and emergency departments, up to 1 in 10 patients given a prescription fail to collect it from pharmacy.

The following are the main reasons for non-compliance.

1. The failure to understand the reason for the medication and the dosage requirements, especially when many medicines are being taken by the patient.
2. The patient sees his own clinical improvement and so stops taking the medication.
3. There is no apparent improvement after many months of taking medication and therefore it is seen to be pointless to continue.
4. The patient suffers an adverse reaction.

The only practical way to increase compliance is to counsel the patient with regard to the need for the prescription, when and how to take the drug and for how long, and the possible adverse effects and drug interactions (Chapter 2).

Drug interactions

Drug interactions are important but uncommon in routine dental practice unless GA is used. The major

likely interactions are discussed in Chapter 2 and summarized below.

Metronidazole gives an unpleasant Antabuse type of reaction with facial flushing, headaches and hypotension if the patient takes alcohol. This is the same type of reaction experienced by a patient taking Antabuse (disulfiram) if he drinks alcohol (see p. 26).

Aspirin can potentiate anticoagulants and increases the likelihood of peptic ulceration in alcoholic patients or those on corticosteroids. Paracetamol does not have these disadvantages.

General anaesthetic agents potentiate antihypertensive agents, and CNS depressants. With monoamine oxidase inhibitors (MAOI) there is the danger of precipitating a hypertensive crisis with GA agents, codeine, pethidine and opiates as well as from sympathomimetics such as ephedrine. This danger persists for up to 2 weeks after stopping MAOI treatment. Sympathomimetics may cause cardiac dysrhythmias in patients anaesthetized with halothane or cyclopropane (Chapter 6).

There can be reduced efficacy of the *contraceptive pill* in patients on oral antibiotics—but it is a small possibility.

Adverse drug effects

Most drugs have some adverse effects, sometimes trivial and, only in a minority of patients, serious. The more common adverse effects of drugs used in dentistry are discussed in Chapter 2. The greatest risks are from general anaesthetic agents: for example, because of the risk of halothane hepatitis, repeated halothane anaesthetics are contraindicated.

The detection and recording of adverse reactions, particularly those related to new drugs, are important, and any suspected reactions should be reported in writing to the Committee on Safety of Medicines (Figs. 5.6 and 5.7).

Adverse drug reactions are reduced by:

(a) only using drugs when there are good indications;
(b) avoiding the drug or reducing the dose if there have been previous untoward reactions or there is a drug history or relevant medical history;
(c) using only those drugs with which you are familiar;
(d) warning the patient of any possible adverse reaction and asking him to stop the drug if he has untoward symptoms or signs.

The possibility of adverse drug effects on the fetus means that, wherever possible, drugs should be avoided in pregnancy (Chapter 2).

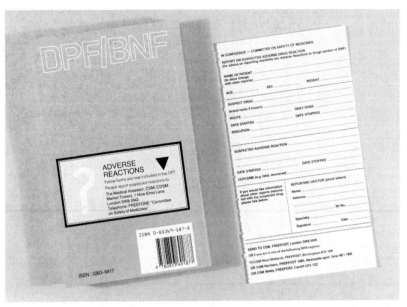

Fig. 5.6 *Reporting adverse drug reactions—pull-out form from DPF for forwarding to the Committee on Safety of Medicine (CSM).*

MISUSE OF DRUGS ACT 1971

This act has two associated regulations: the Misuse of Drugs Regulations and Misuse of Drugs (Safe Custody) Regulations.

Misuse of Drugs Regulations 1973 (amended 1974, 1975, 1985)

These regulations define classes of persons authorized to supply and possess controlled drugs, and enable dentists to possess, produce, supply, prescribe or administer controlled drugs (CD—formerly termed dangerous drugs) in the practice of their profession. They also apply selective control to groups of drugs which are defined in the schedules to the regulations.

Schedule 1 specifies the most strictly controlled drugs such as cannabis resin and LSD. Their use and possession require a special licence.

Schedule 2 is in practical terms the most important, although of the hundred or so drugs listed, only a few are in regular use (for instance, pentazocine, pethidine, morphine and papaveretum). Dentists have authority to possess, supply and produce drugs in Schedule 2. Dentists

may also administer or direct any person other than a doctor or dentist to administer such drugs to a patient. Dentists may only supply or offer to supply such drugs to those who may lawfully possess them—that is, patients under their care.

Schedule 3 contains only five drugs and some of their derivatives, none of which is in wide clinical use in the UK.

Schedule 4 contains 33 benzodiazepines, including those such as diazepam and temazepam used in dentistry. Midazolam is not included. These drugs require no statutory safe custody requirements, no special prescription requirements, and no record-keeping requirements.

Schedule 5 includes preparations which because of their strength are exempt from most CD requirements.

Drugs in these schedules must be supplied on prescription. Under the NHS, this currently limits prescribing by dentists under Schedules 2 and 3 to pethidine and pentazocine. Privately, any drugs in Schedules 2 and 3 may be prescribed providing this is solely for the purpose of meeting the strictly dental needs of the patient. When supplied in this way, the drug becomes the property of the patient (and strictly speaking is no longer a controlled drug).

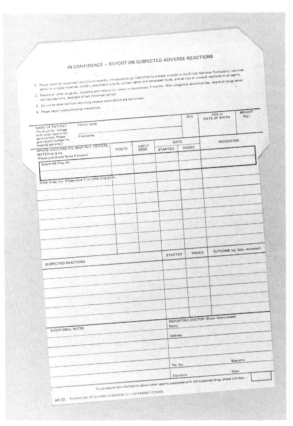

Fig. 5.7 *Reporting adverse drug reactions—CSM yellow form.*

Prescription writing for controlled drugs

A prescription issued for controlled drugs in Schedules 2 and 3 must comply with the following.

A. Except for the prescriber's address, the whole prescription must be in the prescriber's handwriting and be written in ink or some other indelible material and contain the following details.

1. The name and address of the patient.
2. The dose to be taken.
3. Where the controlled drug is prescribed in the form of a preparation (for example, tablets), then the form must be stated. If the preparation exists in more than one strength, the appropriate strength must be stated. If only one strength exists, this detail may be omitted since it is implicit in the name of the preparation.
4. The total quantity (in both words and figures) or

the number of dosage units (in both words and figures) of the preparation.

5. Where the prescription is not a preparation, the total quantity (in both words and figures) of the drugs to be supplied must be stated.

6. The prescription must be endorsed with the words 'for dental treatment only'.

7. The signature and date must both be written by the prescriber.

B. A prescription for controlled drugs in Schedules 2 and 3 can only be dispensed if:

1. The prescription complies with the above requirements;
2. The address of the prescriber is one within the UK;
3. The dispenser is acquainted with the signature of the prescriber or has no reason to doubt it is genuine.

Prescriptions will not be filled prior to the date specified or more than 13 weeks after this date.

It is not a legal requirement that the age of the patient (if under 12) be specified.

Misuse of Drugs (Safe Custody) Regulations 1973 (amended 1985)

These regulations mean that all controlled drugs must be kept in a locked receptacle which can only be opened by the dentist or somebody authorized by him. This receptacle must be securely fastened to a wall. Details of structural requirements for cabinets, safes and rooms suitable for keeping such drugs are given in Schedule 2 of these regulations. A locked car is not considered a locked receptacle.

Storage of controlled drugs

Dentists may personally obtain controlled drugs specified in Schedules 2, 3 and 4 of the Misuse of Drugs Regulations 1973 for use in dental practice. This needs a written requisition to a pharmacist which must state the dentist's name, address, profession or occupation, the purpose for which the drug is supplied and the total quantity, and be signed. A person delegated by a practitioner to collect such a drug will only be supplied with it if the requisition is accompanied by a statement signed by the practitioner that he or she has empowered the recipient to receive it on his or her behalf. The supplier must be satisfied that the request is bona fide.

Registers must be kept for recording the receipt of controlled drugs for use in practice. A register must be a bound book, suitably ruled and with headed columns. Entries must be in chronological order in ink or indelible material and give particulars of every quantity of drug obtained or supplied whether by way of administration or otherwise.

A separate register or part of a register must be used for each class of drug, the name of which must be given at the top of the page. Entries must be made on the day of receipt or supply or, if this is unreasonable, no later than the next day. No entry may be cancelled, obliterated or altered but corrections may be made by dated marginal comments or footnotes.

Separate registers are required for each set of premises and must be preserved for 2 years from the date of the last entry. A dentist must—on demand by the appropriate Secretary of State or other authorized person—give, as requested, particulars of any drug in Schedule 2 or 4 obtained, supplied or stocked by him.

Destruction of controlled drugs

No person who is required by the Misuse of Drugs Regulations 1973 to keep a register of transactions on controlled drugs (Schedules 2 and 4) may destroy such a drug except in the presence of an authorized person (such as a police officer or regional pharamaceutical officer). These provisions do not apply to patients, and if they have unwanted controlled drugs in their possession, these should be destroyed (by, for instance, flushing small quantities down the toilet). This avoids them falling into the wrong hands and complications over record-keeping obligations.

FURTHER READING

British Dental Association/British Medical Association/ Pharmaceutical Society of Great Britain (1986). *Dental practitioners' formulary*. London: Pharmaceutical Press.

Cawson R. A., Spector R. G. (1982). *Clinical pharmacology in dentistry*, 3rd edn. Edinburgh: Churchill Livingstone.

Chapter
6   *Pain and pain control*

Pain is perhaps Nature's earliest sign of disease and is a common feature of many oral diseases. The mouth is an especially sensitive part of the body. An organic basis can be identified in most cases of pain and most respond to local treatment and/or mild analgesia. Pain can also accompany and follow dental treatment. In contrast, a few patients develop orofacial pain which appears to have no organic basis and for which a psychogenic cause is probable, and these patients not infrequently also have other psychogenic aches and pains such as abdominal pain (irritable bowel syndrome). In all patients who have pain, psychological reactions are important. Severe chronic pain, such as in occasional patients with neuralgia after shingles, may even lead to attempts at suicide (Volume 2).

PHYSIOLOGY OF PAIN PERCEPTION

Pain receptors are densely distributed in oral mucosa, facial skin and deeper orofacial tissues. From these regions they relay centrally, mainly via trigeminal neurones (see Volume 2). Painful stimuli induce a change in polarity of the cell membrane of the receptor, which results in a sodium ion influx, and nerve depolarization and subsequent repolarization, with the production of an action potential. The action potential passes along the nerve axon centrally. Large A-delta fibres transmit pain sensation rapidly; C fibres transmit more slowly. Sensory neurones synapse with neurones running in the trigeminothalamic tracts to the thalamus, there to relay with tertiary neurones whose axons extend to the cerebral cortex of the parietal and frontal lobes of the brain as well as to the sensory cortex. There are thus three neurones in a sensory pathway (whereas motor paths involve two neurones only).

Pain results mainly from stimuli that injure the tissue (i.e. pricking, cutting, pinching, burning or freezing) but,

in muscle, pain also results from prolonged contraction and ischaemia (lack of blood supply and oxygenation). Such muscle pain appears to underlie, for example, tension headaches and mandibular pain-dysfunction syndrome (Volume 2). Masticatory muscles also go into spasm, with pain and trismus, if irritated by local infection (e.g. pericoronitis).

Peripheral mediators of pain include a range of chemicals such as 5-hydroxytryptamine, histamine, bradykinin, prostaglandins, and interleukins, as well as other polypeptides and low pH metabolites released by tissue injury, ischaemia, complement activation, etc. Some analgesics block these peripherally released mediators: aspirin, for example, inhibits prostaglandin synthesis.

Centrally, pain may be provoked by natural CNS transmitters or modulators such as gamma-amino butyric acid (GABA) and glycine, and may be suppressed by natural peptides with opiate-like analgesic actions—the enkephalins and endorphins. The activity of these peptides may provide an explanation for the obvious effects of psychological and other factors on pain perceptors and response, usually regarded as 'the attitude of the mind', and for the analgesic effects of placebos, acupuncture and other techniques. Opiates themselves, such as morphine, appear to cause analgesia by a central effect on the receptors for these natural peptides.

The threshold for pain perception is actually about the same in most patients, but the response varies widely depending largely on psychological make-up, emotional state and other influences. Anxious and neurotic patients tend to react excessively or abnormally. Emotions such as rage or fear or distractions such as sound (audioanalgesia) tend to reduce awareness or response to pain. Interestingly, pain threshold and tolerance are increased by improving the information given to the patient before any operative intervention. Drugs can, by peripheral (e.g. aspirin) or central action (e.g. morphine), raise the pain threshold. Local anaesthetics or nerve sectioning can block pain transmission; general anaesthetics and sedatives act centrally.

Theories of pain perception include a *specificity theory* that postulates a specific pain pathway from receptor to a brain pain centre and predicts that the intensity of pain is proportional to the degree of tissue damage. Melzack and Wall have proposed the *gate control* theory that postulates a spinal cord 'gate' that controls the flow of pain impulses to the brain under the influence of peripheral and central modulatory signals. Pain is then regarded as a state of perception in which the organism as a whole reacts to apparent injury only if the gate is appropriately set.

PAIN CONTROL

Reduce tissue damage

Avoidance of damage is the best way to avoid pain (Chapter 8).

Remove causes of pain

Oral pain is best treated by removing the cause. This can be immediately effective. For example, drainage of an acute dental abscess by incision of the fluctuant abscess or opening the tooth pulp chamber to drain can provide immediate pain relief. Removing an opposing tooth that is biting on the operculum can readily reduce the pain of pericoronitis.

Reassurance

The psychological benefit received from calm, confident reassurance can produce surprising benefit in many patients, particularly in those who have pain with a psychogenic basis.

Improve general health

Depression, malaise associated with infection, lack of sleep, and fatigue, may all impair the resilience of a patient suffering pain.

Analgesic drugs

Most pain responds to analgesic drugs but, for perioperative pain, and occasionally other pain, local anaesthetic injections, cryoanalgesia (see p. 129), relative or general anaesthesia, or sedation techniques may be required.

Intractable pain may respond only to sensory nerve

blockade by long-acting local anaesthetics such as bupivicaine, or destruction peripherally (e.g. using cryosurgery—cryoanalgesia), or centrally by various neurosurgical techniques.

Most oral pain responds to paracetamol or aspirin. Codeine or more potent analgesics are only occasionally required.

Some of the more useful analgesic drugs are discussed below. Sedation and local and general analgesia (anaesthesia) are discussed later.

Aspirin is a useful mild analgesic but may cause gastric irritation and interfere with haemostasis. It is therefore contraindicated for patients with peptic ulcers and bleeding disorders. Aspirin is also contraindicated for children (in which it may precipitate Reye's syndrome), and some asthmatics (who may be allergic).

Mefenamic acid is a mild analgesic. It may be contraindicated in asthma, gastrointestinal and liver disease, and pregnancy, and may cause diarrhoea or haemolytic anaemia.

Paracetamol is a useful mild analgesic, though it is hepatotoxic in overdose or prolonged use, and is contraindicated in liver or renal disease.

Diflusinal is an analgesic with long duration of action, useful for the control of mild to moderate pain and particularly effective against pain from bone and joints. It is contraindicated in pregnancy, peptic ulcer, allergies, renal and liver disease.

Codeine phosphate, an analgesic for moderate pain, is contraindicated in late pregnancy and liver disease and may cause sedation and constipation.

Dihydrocodeine tartrate, an analgesic for moderate pain, may cause drowsiness, dizziness and constipation and is contraindicated in children, hypothyroidism, asthma and renal disease.

Buprenorphine is a potent analgesic, effective when given as a sublingual drug, more potent than pentazocine and of longer action than morphine. Unlike pentazocine, it causes no hallucinations but it may cause salivation, sweating, dizziness and vomiting. There may be respiratory depression in overdose, and buprenorphine can cause dependence. It is contraindicated in children, pregnancy, liver disease or respiratory disease.

Meptazinol is another potent analgesic. Side-effects are as for buprenorphine but it is claimed to have a lower incidence of respiratory depression.

Pentazocine is a potent analgesic which may produce dependence and hallucinations, and may cause withdrawal symptoms in narcotic addicts. It is contraindicated in pregnancy, children, hypertension, respiratory depression, head injuries or raised intracranial pressure. There is a risk of dependence.

Pethidine is less potent and causes less respiratory depression than morphine. Pethidine and morphine are used mainly in premedication and postoperative analgesia. Both drugs can cause dependence.

Morphine is a useful, potent analgesic. Morphine (and the related papaveretum: Omnopon) is useful in premedication and analgesia for in-patients but should not be used for patients with head injuries since it causes respiratory depression and nausea or vomiting, and also pupillary constriction (which interferes with neurological observations) (see Volume 2 and Chapter 7).

Methods of pain control other than analgesics

Hypnosis and acupuncture may be of value in inducing analgesia but are usually too time consuming and unpredictable to find favour with most patients and practitioners. Acupuncture may be more effective in situations of cultural conditioning, but even in the laboratory can induce analgesia comparable to that produced by 33% nitrous oxide inhalation.

Electroanalgesia—passing a 40–50 µA current through the dental handpiece—may be of some value but is still in its infancy.

CRYOANALGESIA

Cryoanalgesia is the application of low temperature to nerves to produce anaesthesia or analgesia.

Nitrous oxide, or carbon dioxide, is pressurized and pumped through a small aperture at the end of a tube in a closed system, and recirculated. When the gas passes through the aperture rapid expansion occurs with pronounced cooling (the Joule–Thompson effect). It is possible to achieve temperatures of $-70°C$ using nitrous oxide.

The basic machinery is modified to include thermocouples to measure accurately and regulate the tip temperature, and the system has been made small enough to be fashioned into a needle so that areas deep in the body can be frozen without recourse to open surgery (percutaneous cryotherapy). To assist accurate localization, nerve stimulators in the tip can also be used.

With this system working at maximal efficiency, frozen tissues, termed an 'ice-ball', of a diameter of up to 2 cm can be achieved. The size of the cryolesion depends on factors such as probe tip temperature, and the thermal conductance and vascularity of the tissue. It must be realized that although the 'ice-ball' may be large, the temperature of the periphery may be only just sub-zero, whereas for cell necrosis to occur, temperatures below $-20°C$ must be achieved.

Using liquid nitrogen (at a temperature of $-196°C$) rather than nitrous oxide, much lower temperatures can be reached, and with these much more powerful machines the thermocouple needle can be placed distant from the probe tip for accurate control of the 'ice-ball' size.

Mechanism of action

Although nerve conduction can be completely blocked at temperatures well above freezing point, prolonged conduction block can only be achieved by freezing below $-20°C$.

The cryoprobe has allowed us to freeze neural tissue accurately to these very low temperatures and produce degenerative neural changes with anaesthesia that may last for many months.

Animal studies have shown that this type of cryolesion produces a combination of intra- and extra-axonal ice crystal formation, fluid and electrolyte fluxes, with disruption of the cellular membrane, and vascular changes leading to local ischaemia. Wallerian and retrograde degeneration follow. The epi-, peri- and endoneurium are preserved and there is a minimal inflammatory reaction and little scarring on healing. Preservation of the structural framework of the nerve bundle facilitates regeneration from the viable proximal nerve stump, and recovery rate is similar to that for crush injury of a nerve, but more complete.

Small (C) fibres seem to be more resistant to freezing than the more heavily myelinated large (A) fibres. To ensure maximum effect, liquid nitrogen should be used with fast-freeze, slow-thaw cycles.

In most series of open human nerve freezing (i.e. where nerves are surgically identified and exposed before freezing), subjective and objective sensation return within 3 months.

There appears to be a very low incidence of neuroma formation, or neuritis, which is not so for neurolytic injections (absolute alcohol, phenol in glycerine) or neurectomy.

Uses of cryoanalgesia

Cryoanalgesia is indicated in painful conditions where a long-term anaesthetic or analgesia is desirable. The duration of even the most long-acting local analgesics (such as bupivicaine) is only 12 hours.

There may be some limitations to the treatment if the area of interest is supplied by a mixed nerve, since the cryolesion is not selective and motor paralysis may be unacceptable.

There are four broad indications for the use of cryo-analgesia.

1. The treatment of neuralgias, particularly where medical treatment has failed.
2. To facilitate postoperative pain control.
3. The relief of chronic pain such as in the palliative treatment of malignancy.
4. Local treatment of painful lesions.

The response in post-herpetic neuralgia is disappointing, as with all other treatment modalities. Although in one series treatment resulted in pain relief of more than 6 weeks for 50% of patients, essentially all had relapsed by 6 months.

Personal experience suggests that cryosurgery to the affected nerves may precipitate pain projected to the cutaneous distribution of that nerve, despite anaesthesia of that area of skin or mucosa, analogous to anaesthesia dolorosa, seen uncommonly after neurosurgery for PTN. Further, recrudescence of the pain with sensory recovery may be particularly severe and difficult to control.

In the treatment of trigeminal neuralgia (PTN) many series have shown that pain control outlasts the period of sensory return, although the results for the treatment of a typical facial pain are less encouraging.

Cryoanalgesia has a place in the management of PTN. Long-term follow-up of open nerve freezes shows that PTN refractory to maximum dose medication can be controlled for between 1 and 2 years following cryosurgical application.

LOCAL ANALGESIA

The history of local analgesia is interesting, but only one or two events will be mentioned to highlight the nature of this relatively recent, common form of medication. In the second part of the 19th century, cocaine was extracted and exploited—first for topical anaesthesia and later for injection. Procaine was introduced in 1904 and was superseded by lignocaine, first synthesized in 1943 and introduced over the next few years. Since then many other local analgesics have been developed, but lignocaine remains the most commonly used drug in dentistry.

Further details of the anatomy of the jaws and, in particular, the trigeminal nerve, the physiology of nerve conduction and pain, and the pharmacology of local analgesics should be sought in the relevant specialist texts.

The drugs

Local analgesics

Local analgesics are used to prevent impulse transmission in nerves. This action is reversible. The drug acts at the sodium channels in the axon membranes, preventing the influx of sodium ions necessary for depolarization.

The useful local analgesics belong to two series, the esters and the amides. These are characterized by their chemical structures. The esters are often used in topical preparations, but a typical example of an injectable drug in this group is procaine (Fig. 6.1). Lignocaine is a representative member of the amides (Fig. 6.2).

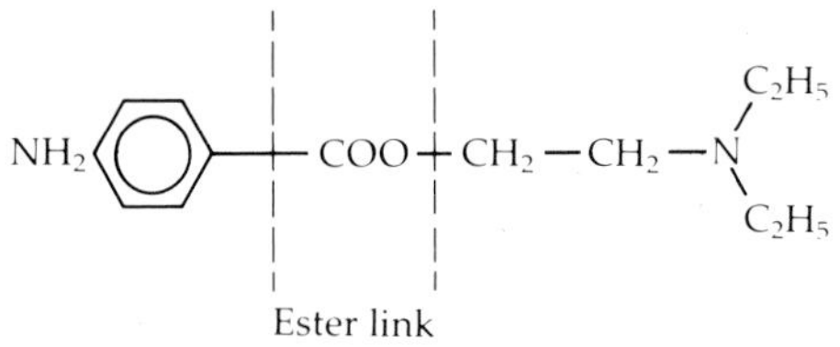

Fig. 6.1 *Procaine—showing ester link.*

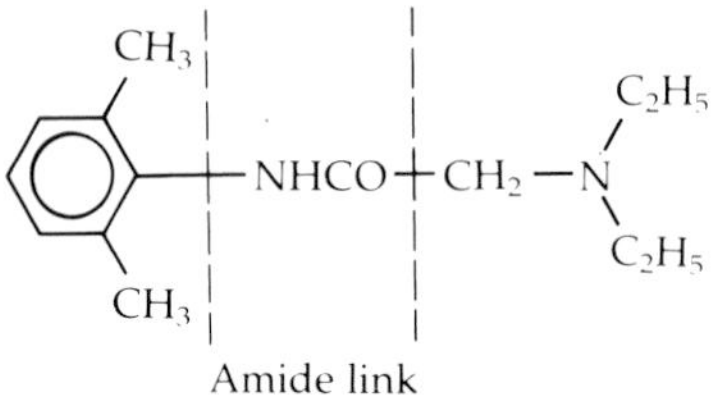

Fig. 6.2 *Lignocaine—showing amide link.*

There are several useful amide local analgesics, three in particular being employed in dentistry—these are lignocaine, prilocaine and mepivacaine. Two further agents, bupivacaine (similar to mepivacaine) and etidocaine (similar to lignocaine) are long-acting analgesics with no particular use in general dentistry, although they are used in other clinical situations.

Lignocaine

First synthesized in 1943 by Lofgren in Sweden, lignocaine was extensively tested before being marketed about 5 years later. It is produced in solution as the hydrochloride salt, and a 2% concentration has been shown to be satisfactory in general dental use, although other strengths have been employed in special circumstances.

Early investigations were carried out by Swedish workers using a method of electrical pulp testing. In these tests it was clearly demonstrated that, for infiltration analgesia of a maxillary lateral incisor, 2% lignocaine containing adrenaline was completely successful.

The most common preparation used in the UK for dental local analgesia is 2% lignocaine with 1 in 80 000 adrenaline—there are many commercial products. Plain solutions of 2% lignocaine are available, but, despite early comments about the success of this preparation, later studies have shown that it is inefficient.

Lignocaine has a swift onset of action, and infiltration analgesia is often satisfactory in less than a minute after injection. There is, however, a delay in the onset of block (regional) anaesthesia (see later) and it may take 3 or 4 minutes for a successful inferior alveolar block to become established.

It is important to appreciate that soft tissue anaesthesia is not always an indication of dental (pulpal) anaesthesia. Lignocaine with adrenaline probably gives about 30 minutes pulpal anaesthesia, but the soft tissue (lip) numbness from a block may last for about 4 hours.

Prilocaine

This amide is used as a 3% solution containing a vasoconstrictor (in the UK this vasoconstrictor is felypressin), but it is also available as a 4% plain solution which is sometimes used for inferior alveolar nerve blocks.

Prilocaine (marketed as Citanest by Astra) is slightly less toxic than lignocaine and may induce less vasodilatation. It found favour mainly when it was considered unwise to use solutions containing adrenaline (see section on vasoconstrictors). Prilocaine can, however, induce the formation of methaemoglobinaemia so it must be used with some care in patients with anaemia and cardiac failure; infants may also be at greater risk. The amounts administered for dental treatment are unlikely to be troublesome. Prilocaine crosses the placenta more easily than lignocaine, so is not the drug of choice for use during pregnancy.

Pulpal anaesthesia is less profound when prilocaine is used. Unfortunately the duration of unwanted soft tissue anaesthesia may be prolonged, even more than with the use of lignocaine with adrenaline.

Mepivacaine

Although less frequently employed in the UK now, mepivacaine is a useful local analgesic. As a 3% plain solution it produces pulpal anaesthesia for short procedures (about 15 minutes) and also shorter soft tissue symptoms.

Vasoconstrictors

The mouth is a very vascular region and drugs are rapidly absorbed across the mucosa or after injection. The effectiveness of a local analgesic depends on there being an adequate concentration of the drug within the sensory nerves (Fig. 6.3). In the vascular oral tissues, concentrations fall rapidly due to uptake of the analgesic into circulation (Fig. 6.4).

When a vasoconstrictor is added to the local analgesic solution, the local blood flow is considerably reduced. The immediate effect is to increase the rate at which nerve blockade occurs and the resultant depth of anaesthesia is improved. The continued vasoconstriction prolongs this state as the pool of analgesic is maintained around the nerve. The analgesic 'wears off' once the local blood flow returns to normal and the reservoir of drug is depleted, allowing the concentration within the nerve to fall.

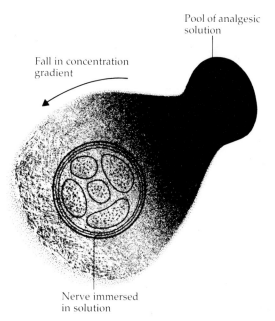

Pool of analgesic solution

Fall in concentration gradient

Nerve immersed in solution

Fig. 6.3 *Analgesia depends on an effective concentration of drug throughout the fasciculi.*

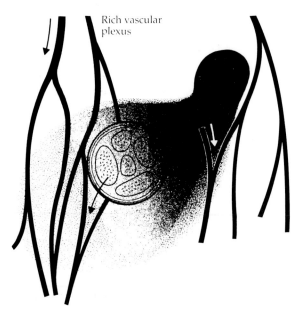

Rich vascular plexus

Fig. 6.4 *The concentration of local analgesia falls rapidly due to uptake into the vascular network.*

An additional factor is that local analgesics themselves influence blood flow. At clinically used concentrations, all of these drugs cause some degree of vasodilatation and therefore in plain solution (i.e. without a vasoconstrictor) have a very short duration of action.

Adrenaline and noradrenaline

Adrenaline causes intense vasoconstriction, mainly on the arterial side of the microcirculation, and is added to local analgesics to improve the rate, depth and the duration of anaesthesia. Lignocaine benefits most from the addition of adrenaline, then prilocaine, and mepivacaine least of all; this is said to be related to the inherent vasodilatation from these agents, which is greatest from lignocaine and least from mepivacaine.

An additional benefit from the presence of adrenaline is the improved visibility during surgery due to reduced bleeding. This is so useful that injections of preparations containing adrenaline may be given when oral surgery is carried out under general anaesthesia.

It was thought that the addition of adrenaline reduced the systemic uptake of local analgesics to such an extent that greater doses could be given safely—but there is increasing evidence that this is not true of oral injections.

Some dental surgeons are reluctant to administer local analgesics which contain adrenaline to patients who suffer from cardiovascular disorders. The amounts of adrenaline infiltrated during dental injections are small and are slowly absorbed. There is no evidence that such preparations present a risk to any patients, provided that an intravascular bolus is avoided by the use of an aspirating technique.

Other sympathomimetic amines have been added to local analgesics, and of these only noradrenaline is commonly used. This agent is less powerful than adrenaline, but, when used in local analgesics, it is effective. High doses may well be harmful, so that there seems little advantage in its use.

Felypressin

This is one of the synthetic vasopressins similar to the natural pituitary hormone. These agents, of which there are many, have two principal actions. The first is vasoconstriction, which is most effective on the venous side of the vasculature, and the second is antidiuresis via the renal tubular system. Although several vasopressins are useful in local analgesics, felypressin is one which has a satisfactory combination of effects, being a reasonable constrictor, but causing less water retention than some other analogues. Water retention can be potentially harmful, particularly in patients with heart failure.

Felypressin is available with prilocaine as Citanest with Octapressin (Astra) and this preparation *may* be selected if a patient has reported unpleasant reactions to solutions containing adrenaline (a rare but recognized problem) or if a patient has poorly controlled hypertension or disorders of cardiac rhythm (although there is no evidence that solutions containing adrenaline cause harm). Care must be greater when felypressin is used, as it causes coronary arterial constriction.

Although felypressin does cause a reduction in blood flow, it does not give the same bloodless field for surgery as adrenaline. Its predominant effect on the venous vessels sometimes appears to increase bleeding during oral surgery.

Systemic effects of local analgesics

Local analgesics are toxic agents, but only produce undesirable systemic effects when present in the blood in sufficient concentration. Lignocaine has been studied more than other agents and serves as a good example.

As soon as lignocaine has been injected into the submucosal connective tissues, its absorption begins. The rate at which it is taken up into the bloodstream depends very much on the vascularity of the tissues and also on the way in which it is injected. A rapid rate of injection and multiple injection sites both spread the solution over a large vascular bed and enhance uptake.

The absolute levels of drug in the circulation depend on the dose administered. For any particular dose, a large volume of solution will increase absorption as it will be exposed to a large vascular bed, whereas a smaller volume of a more concentrated solution produces lower blood levels (despite theoretical concentration gradient effects).

Once lignocaine has been absorbed it is redistributed; the very vascular tissues such as the liver, heart and brain attaining the highest levels first. In the liver, lignocaine (like all of the amides) is rapidly metabolized. The blood level of lignocaine represents the balance between con-

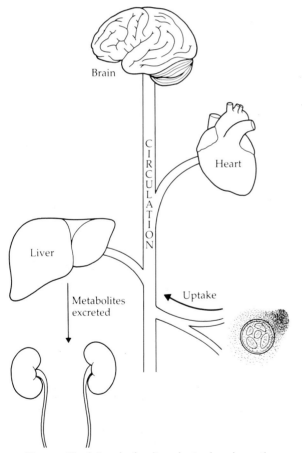

Fig. 6.5 *Circulating levels of analgesic depend on the balance between rate of uptake and distribution.*

tinuous absorption from the injection site and the rate of metabolism (Fig. 6.5).

Patients who have impaired liver function or who have cardiac failure (where perfusion of the liver is reduced) therefore metabolize local analgesics more slowly and the dose they receive should be carefully controlled.

Dental local analgesia has an excellent record of safety, but many of the short-lived unpleasant effects experienced by patients after an injection, often attributed to 'psychological' disturbance or 'fainting', are due to transient significant plasma levels of local analgesic affecting the brain. This can occur within seconds of an injection and is then probably due to an accidental intravascular injection; or it can occur 10–15 minutes after injection, when peak levels of lignocaine appear in the blood from absorption from the injection site. Tachycardia and similar cardiovascular changes may well be due to the vasoconstrictor (see Chapter 4).

The features of systemic responses to circulating lignocaine include headache, drowsiness, dizziness and nausea. Slightly higher blood levels cause stimulation which may be seen as restlessness, talkativeness, nystagmus (involuntary jerking eye movements), and fine fibrillation in small muscles, for example in the hand. Very high levels (which could only be expected following multiple or intravascular injections) may lead to convulsions and death.

Contraindications

There are very few absolute contraindications to the use of local analgesics. However, there are situations in which additional factors may make the operator select general anaesthesia, i.e.:

1. If the extent of treatment would cause the patient emotional distress, even if pain control is adequate.
2. If several minor surgical procedures are planned, it may prove sensible to complete these under one general anaesthetic rather than having repeated visits for local analgesia. This is of particular relevance if a patient requires antibiotic prophylaxis for surgery.
3. Indications discussed on p. 156.

Precautions (see also Chapter 2)

Where there is a significant systemic disorder, additional consideration may be required.

1. *Ischaemic heart disease.* Angina, or a history of myocardial infarction, should alert the dental surgeon to the need for careful management and painless treatment.

Emotional disturbance (fear) and pain are more likely to provoke cardiovascular disturbance, and coronary ischaemia, than injected local analgesic agents. It is, however, mandatory to use an aspirating system. Lignocaine (2%) with adrenaline (1 in 80 000) is the most reliable local analgesic and should be the agent of choice.

Some specialists believe that sedation offers improved management in these situations. Intravenous benzodiazepines should be used cautiously for patients with cardiovascular or respiratory impairment, particularly the elderly.

2. *Diabetes.* Although diabetics do not represent a particular difficulty with local analgesia, they can constitute a management problem. It is essential to ensure that those patients controlled by drugs (oral hypoglycaemics and more particularly, insulin injections) have their normal diet and medication before treatment. (It is thought possible that adrenaline may promote slightly raised blood sugar levels—but this would be advantageous.)

Some diabetic patients have impaired healing. There is a theoretical problem, if profound vasoconstriction results from an injection, that surgical wounds (extraction sockets) may be more prone to breakdown and infection. It is perhaps wise to use a preparation such as Citanest (prilocaine with felypressin) as the vasoconstrictor is less intense—even though the depth of analgesia may be reduced. It would be wise to prescribe antibiotics postoperatively.

3. *Irradiated bone.* Similar considerations are necessary when operating on bone in a site of direct radiotherapy (e.g. after treatment of an oral malignant lesion).

4. *Epilepsy.* Uncontrolled epileptics may be difficult to manage, and prolonged procedures are best performed under intravenous sedation with benzodiazepines (with local analgesia) or under general anaesthesia.

Well-controlled patients can be treated under local analgesia. Although high levels of circulating local analgesics can cause cerebral irritation (and fits), the mechanism is different from that of classical epilepsy and there is no evidence that the administration of local analgesics for dental surgery is harmful (but it is necessary to use an aspirating syringe and avoid accidental intravascular bolus injections).

5. *Severe hepatic or renal failure.* It is highly unlikely that a patient with significant liver or kidney failure will present to a general dental practitioner for treatment. However, it may happen in hospital practice.

The amide local analgesics are metabolized almost exclusively in the liver (Chapter 2), and if administered to patients with significant hepatic damage, can accumulate in the circulation. It is therefore necessary to perform only limited treatment at each visit to reduce the amount of analgesic administered. There are no guidelines as to the amounts recommended in degrees of liver failure. However, as prilocaine is metabolized to an extent in other tissues (e.g. lungs) and is inherently less toxic than lignocaine or mepivacaine, it would be the drug of choice in these circumstances.

The products of (hepatic) metabolism of local analgesics are excreted via the kidneys. In severe renal failure, these metabolites can be cleared slowly and repeated injections would lead to their accumulation. The metabolites are themselves toxic. Similar precautions, therefore, should be taken as for patients in liver failure.

An additional consideration for patients with liver failure exists if a disturbance of haemostasis is evident (see below).

6. *Mental handicap.* In such cases, treatment under local analgesia may prove difficult or impossible. Where co-operation can be gained, it is sensible to do the minimum at each visit. If the treatment is short, mepivacaine should be used so that there is the shortest postoperative soft tissue anaesthesia.

7. *Allergy.* Allergy to the amide local analgesics is *extremely* rare. Many patients will say that they 'are allergic' if they remember an adverse experience which they attribute to the local analgesic, e.g. a faint. However, the patient's history should not be ignored, and every effort should be made to dispel or substantiate the 'allergy' before treatment commences. It is quite wrong to label the patients 'allergic to local analgesics' on a doubtful history. However, if a patient had a definite allergic reaction, the local analgesic used (and similar drugs) should be avoided.

It must be remembered that some patients will declare an 'allergy' in an attempt to secure treatment under general anaesthesia. If their cooperation is in doubt, a general anaesthetic may be preferable for lengthy or particularly uncomfortable aspects of treatment, but the 'allergic' state should be disproved.

8. *Haematological disorders.* Patients who have a bleeding tendency (for example haemophiliacs, anticoagulated patients, those in significant hepatic failure etc.) should not be given 'block' injections. Nerve block injections are normally given where there is a neurovascular bundle (e.g. the inferior alveolar nerve block) or a venous plexus (e.g. the posterior superior alveolar nerve block) so that there is a risk of uncontrolled haemorrhage deep inside the tissues which may cause swelling and obstruct the airway. Superficial infiltration injections are safer, but these also lead to quite extensive bruising—although this is not life-threatening. Intraligamentary injections have been shown to be valuable in this clinical situation.

9. *Local pathology.* It is unsafe to infiltrate directly into a haemangioma or other local pathological lesion. Nerve block injections are indicated, and if these cannot be given successfully, general anaesthetics will be necessary.

10. *Sepsis.* Where there is cellulitis or an abscess, local infiltration is contraindicated and block injections should be given. In either case infection may spread, and in the former the injection is unlikely to work (see section on failures) and in the latter, injection into an abscess cavity is futile.

Where there is sepsis in a patient with a systemic disorder which predisposes to infection (and its spread) such as or immunological suppression, it may be preferable to employ general anaesthesia.

Techniques of local analgesia

Patient management

A caring, sympathetic attitude will improve the apparent success of local analgesia, for no matter how powerful the drug, if the patient is apprehensive, reactions to treatment will be evident and denials of the adequacy of the analgesic will be frequent. The extremely nervous patient may not respond initially to this approach, and premedication or sedation will prove invaluable (Chapter 1).

Patient co-operation is important, not only for a successful outcome but also for safety. A controlled technique is important to prevent needle injuries for, although the dental surgeon will be wearing rubber gloves, these offer almost no significant protection against an accidental needlestick which may occur if a patient is agitated or struggling.

General

The patient will be in a supine position, or at least well reclined—and a good light is essential. Sterile instruments are prepared out of the patient's vision.

The site for injection is inspected to exclude local contraindications, such as an abscess or other pathology (e.g. haemangioma), and then dried. Drying cleans the surface and improves vision. It is not necessary to apply an antiseptic in a healthy patient as needle track infections are almost unheard of. In the days of re-usable needles this was a more common problem, not from surface bacteria being inoculated, but from the injection of material within the lumen of the needle. For patients compromised immunologically by disease or treatment, it is sensible to take the precaution of applying antiseptic, such as chlorhexidine, prior to injecting.

Topical analgesics, such as lignocaine gel, applied beforehand remove any discomfort from the penetration, and their application assists in gaining patient confidence, particularly with children.

The mucosa is drawn taut so that the surface and the 'target' can be seen more clearly—the needle will pass through the stretched mucosa swiftly and painlessly.

Equipment

Disposable needles *must* be used and never reused on another patient. Their introduction has effectively eliminated a major source of cross-infection and also needle fractures. Traditionally, short needles were used for infiltrations and long needles for nerve block injections. It is now common practice to use long needles throughout. The long needle is used so that if a needle does break, then it is more likely that sufficient shaft will be left protruding to enable the dentist to retrieve it immediately. Needle fracture is *extremely rare.*

The cartridge syringe system is very convenient and simplifies the administration of local analgesics; several designs of syringe are available. The non-aspirating syringe is commonly used, but intravascular accidents can occur as a result. These accidents rarely have serious consequences—leading some authorities to question the value of aspiration. However, aspiration is recommended.

Aspiration can be achieved using a positive draw-back syringe, where some form of claw-grip is engaged into the rubber bung and the plunger is retracted using a thumb ring (Fig. 6.6). The system is effective, but is not generally adopted as it tends to be clumsy.

Passive or 'automatic' systems exploit the recoil in the diaphragm or rubber bung of the cartridge. The power is less but usually adequate to display blood in the cartridge if a vessel is penetrated. The most popular system is the 'self-aspirating' bung (Fig. 6.7), but this is not entirely reliable. Other passive systems are under investigation.

Cartridges of local analgesics are of two sizes, containing either 1.8 ml or 2.2 ml of solution. The contents are

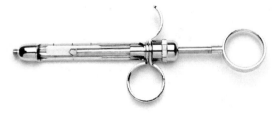

Fig. 6.6 *An aspirating syringe with a positive claw-grip action (Bayer).*

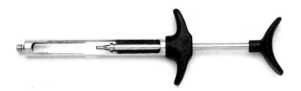

Fig. 6.7 *A 'semi-automatic' passive aspirating system (Astra).*

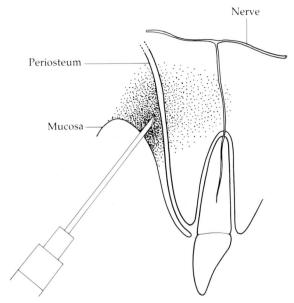

Fig. 6.8 *Diagrammatic representation of a dental infiltration injection.*

sterile and contain the appropriate concentration of local analgesic (e.g. 2% lignocaine) and vasoconstrictor (e.g. 1 in 80 000 adrenaline). An anti-oxidant is included to extend the shelf-life of the adrenaline and often an antiseptic to secure the sterility of the solution. 'Parabens', used for the latter purpose, were the cause of many of the allergic reactions and manufacturers are gradually withdrawing these from their products.

Partially used cartridges must *never* be used on a second patient since they may contain blood or tissue fluid, or be infected.

Procedures

Dental injections are of two basic types—infiltrations and blocks. Infiltration injections are those given directly into, or very close to, the tissues or tooth to be operated upon (Fig. 6.8). The solution diffuses into the tissues and affects the fine branches of the nerve. Typically, the analgesic is infiltrated slowly into soft tissues, or placed directly adjacent to the apex of a tooth. Rapid injection of solution may cause significant discomfort at the time and afterwards.

The onset of analgesia after an infiltration is very rapid; in the soft tissues it is almost immediate. When an infiltration injection is given for treatment of a tooth, for example a maxillary premolar, there is about a 1-minute delay before pulpal analgesia is adequate. The duration of effect depends on two factors—the binding ability of the analgesic (i.e. its relative potency) and the vascularity of the tissue. Lignocaine with adrenaline will give about 30 minutes of pulpal analgesia, after which time the concentration of the solution in the nerves becomes significantly reduced. The local circulation begins to return to normal after about 15 minutes and then the analgesic is taken up into the bloodstream at a greater rate; but the depletion in the tissue is not effective in removing analgesic from nerve (due to its being bound to the connective tissues and nerve membranes) until the levels are extremely low.

A nerve block injection refers to an injection of solution around a nerve trunk, and a large peripheral area of tissue is then anaesthetized (Fig. 6.9). The benefits of a block technique are that an extensive region can be anaesthetized with a relatively small volume of solution and a single injection and that if local disease elsewhere precludes the use of infiltration injections, then a block can often be employed safely.

Once the solution is deposited, there is a short period during which no effects are apparent. The pool of analgesic is close to the neurovascular bundle (sometimes it surrounds the nerve trunk) and must diffuse through the sheath to the nerve bundles and penetrate the connective tissues around the fasciculi to be taken up by the individual axons (Fig. 6.10). This 'latency' of onset varies depending on the analgesic used, but, for the three commonly employed in dentistry, little difference can be detected. Once through the sheath, the analgesic diffuses throughout the bundles until a sufficient concentration is present to block conduction in the axons. In a composite nerve with several fasciculi (like the inferior alveolar nerve), some bundles of fibres may be affected first and some axons are blocked before others (typically the unmyelinated and smaller fibres block first—but this is not always the case). There is, therefore, a further delay from the onset of symptoms—the patient first declaring

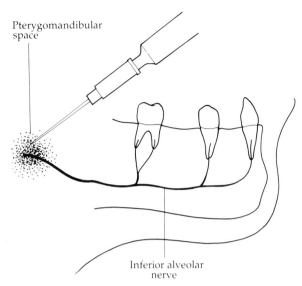

Fig. 6.9 *Diagrammatic representation of a dental nerve block injection.*

some patchy 'tingling' in the lip—to the whole region becoming completely anaesthetized—'numb' or 'dead'. As time progresses, the blood flow again reduces the amount of analgesic in the tissues until the concentration gradients allow analgesic to leave the nerve. However, because the analgesic is bound to the lipids and proteins in the membranes and connective tissues in the nerve, this recovery process is slower than the onset of analgesia.

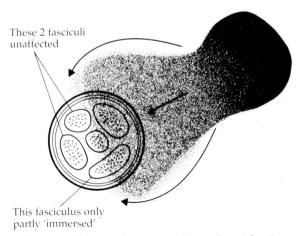

Fig. 6.10 *The connective tissue barriers to the uptake of analgesic into a nerve trunk.*

Injections for the maxillary teeth

1. Buccal/labial infiltration procedures.
2. Palatal injections (anterior and posterior).
3. Nerve block (infraorbital and posterior-superior-alveolar).

The pulps of most upper teeth can be anaesthetized successfully using infiltration injections on their outer aspects, i.e. into the submucosa of the labial (or buccal) sulcus. If 2% lignocaine with 1 in 80 000 adrenaline in the solution is used, about 0.5 ml will anaesthetize a tooth with a single root (incisor or canine), although 1.0 ml is usually required for a premolar or molar tooth. When several teeth are being treated, the number of injections can be reduced due to the 'spread' of the analgesic solution by carefully selecting suitable sites between adjacent teeth.

Infiltration techniques

It is important to visualize clearly the tissue into which the injection is to be delivered. The lip or cheek is retracted and the reflected mucosa is drawn taut (Fig. 6.11); the sulcus is then inspected (see earlier) and dried. A topical analgesic can be applied. The needle is inserted through the tense mucosa—this is virtually painless—just adjacent to the alveolus (Fig. 6.12). The syringe should be held so that the needle is inclined towards the apex of the tooth. For anterior teeth the syringe should be aligned with their long axes to prevent inaccuracy. To approach posterior teeth, however, the syringe is tilted to gain access through the mouth, so care must be taken to ensure that the needle point is positioned adjacent to the tooth being treated and not inadvertently advanced distally (Fig. 6.13).

In the incisor region, the needle point is held just beneath the surface of the mucosa, but for some other teeth it may be necessary for the needle to be a few millimetres deeper, to be positioned opposite the estimated position of the root apex.

Once the needle is positioned, aspiration is performed and then, if a negative result is obtained (i.e. no backflow of blood), the solution is slowly injected. A slow injection allows the solution to pool precisely where the needle tip has been carefully sited; a fast injection is painful due to distension and disruption of the tissues and also spreads the solution over a wider area. Although 1.0 ml may be comfortably delivered in about 15 seconds in the posterior region, a much slower rate of injection is required for incisors and canines. Soft tissue anaesthesia (a numb lip) may be apparent almost immediately, but it is desirable to

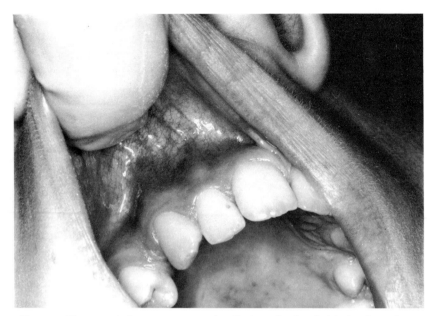

Fig. 6.11 *The mucosa is drawn taut to expose the reflection and so that the injection site can be seen clearly.*

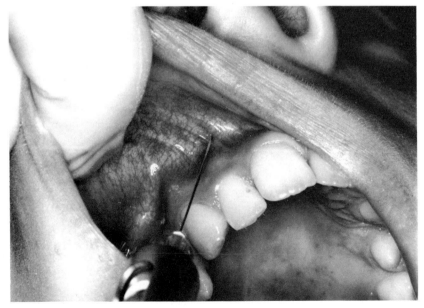

Fig. 6.12 *Needle position for infiltration analgesia of maxillary lateral incisor.*

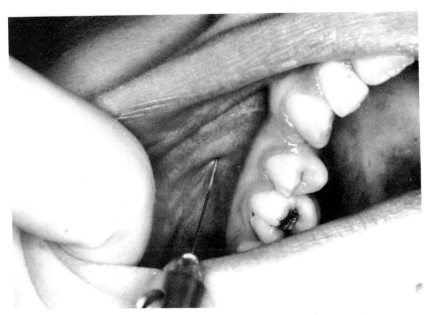

Fig. 6.13 *Needle position for infiltration analgesia of a maxillary first molar.*

wait for at least a minute or two to allow a sufficient depth of pulpal anaesthesia to develop.

Palatal injections

It is necessary to provide analgesia of the palatal tissues if an extraction or other surgical treatment is to be performed. Sometimes a deep cavity preparation or endodontic manipulation of a palatal root will require palatal analgesia.

Anterior palatal injection. Injection of the terminal branches of the long sphenopalatine nerve at the incisive canal will provide analgesia of an area of palatal mucosa adjacent to the incisor, and usually canine, teeth. The syringe is positioned so that the mucosa is penetrated by the needle at right-angles to the surface adjacent to the estimated position of the foramen (Fig. 6.14). (Injecting directly into the foramen can be very painful for the patient.)

The tissues are bound firmly to the palatal bone, so only 0.25–0.5 ml of solution is deposited, under pressure. This is usually painful (a 'burning' or 'stinging' sensation) and the tissues usually blanch.

Posterior palatal injection. An injection around the greater palatine nerve provides analgesia of the palatal tissues at the injection site and more anteriorly, perhaps as far forward as the canine tooth.

The injection site is selected corresponding to the tooth being treated, or a little distal to it, and is approached from the opposite side of the mouth; and the tissues penetrated at right-angles to the surface (Fig. 6.15). The gingiva and the midline raphe are incapable of accepting much analgesic solution—the most comfortable and successful site is midway between the two.

When treatment is being provided at the distal aspect of the arch, e.g. the extraction of an upper third molar, the injection is best given towards the anterior of the tooth, because as the solution diffuses distally it can affect the soft palate, causing some patients considerable distress.

Nerve block injections

These are rarely indicated in the maxilla, but can be used if a tooth cannot be anaesthetized adequately by an infiltration injection, perhaps due to thick cortical bone—this may occur with first molars and canines. Nerve blocks may also be useful if local inflammation renders an infiltration relatively ineffective.

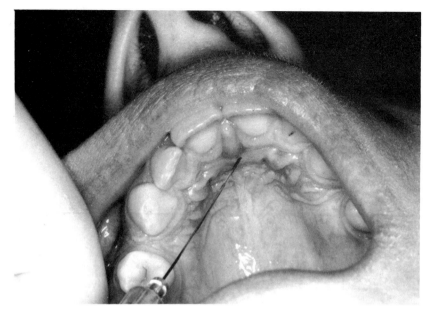

Fig. 6.14 *Injecting adjacent to the incisive foramen for analgesia of the premaxilla.*

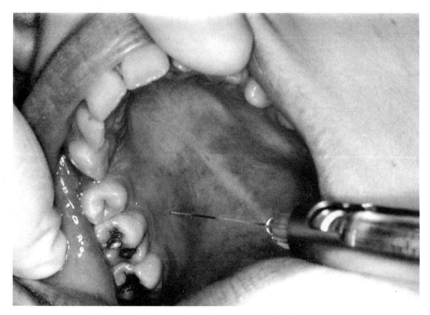

Fig. 6.15 *The approach for the posterior palatal injection.*

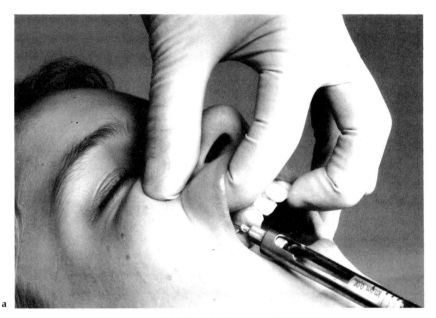

a

Fig. 6.16a and b The infraorbital nerve block injection.

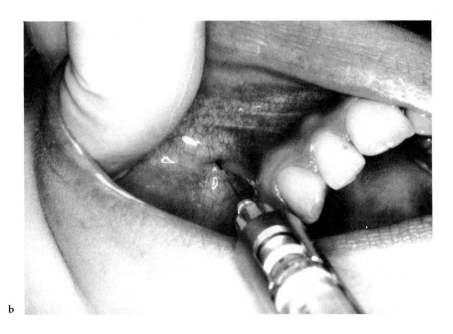

b

The following nerve blocks are sometimes used in dentistry:

1. *Infraorbital block.* The infraorbital nerve is approached via the labial sulcus above the canine. The lip is grasped firmly using the thumb and first finger and then is pulled upwards towards the orbit (Fig. 6.16a). The full height of the sulcus is then revealed. A finger is placed on the face on the lower aspect of the orbital rim. The syringe is held parallel to the canine tooth and the tense mucosa is penetrated (Fig. 6.16b). The needle is then advanced to the estimated position of the foramen (previously palpated) and about 1.0 ml of solution is slowly deposited. Firm pressure by the finger on the orbital rim discourages solution from diffusing upwards.

The solution blocks conduction in the infraorbital nerve and in the anterior alveolar nerves arising close to the foramen.

2. *Posterior-superior-alveolar (PSA) block.* The PSA nerve is approached via the buccal sulcus opposite the third (or second) molar (Fig. 6.17). The tissues are retracted and inspected (as described for an infiltration) but the syringe is held inclined away from the maxilla, so that the needle is directed towards the alveolus. The syringe is also inclined so that the needle is pointing backwards. The mucosa is penetrated opposite the apex of the third molar and the needle is advanced for about a further 1.5 cm and must be kept close to bone.

Aspiration is carried out and, if negative, 1.0 ml of solution is deposited slowly, taking no less than 15 seconds. If there is a positive aspiration of blood, then the needle may have entered the pterygoid plexus of veins and should be withdrawn for about 0.5 cm—it is likely that a bruise will appear in the sulcus due to a small venous ooze within the lax tissues. Injecting into the plexus, particularly quickly, will disrupt the vessels to a greater extent.

Injections for the mandibular teeth

1. Inferior-alveolar nerve block.
2. Mental foramen injections.
3. Buccal (long buccal) injections.
4. Infiltration injections.

The nerve supply of mandibular teeth is mainly derived from the inferior alveolar nerve. Due to relatively thick and dense cortical bone, infiltration injections are rarely successful (there are exceptions), so that 'block' of the inferior alveolar nerve is usually needed. This is carried out where the nerve leaves the bony mandible at the foramen on the medial aspect of the ramus within the pterygomandibular space: it also anaesthetises the lingual nerve.

Analgesia of the first premolar, canine and incisors may be obtained sometimes by injecting at the mental

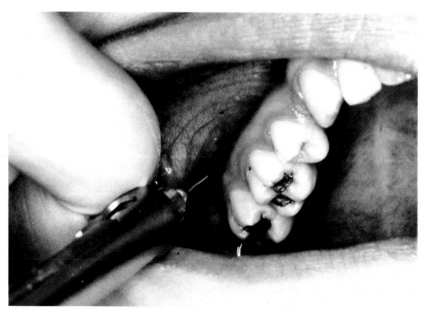

Fig. 6.17 *The posterior-superior-alveolar nerve block injection.*

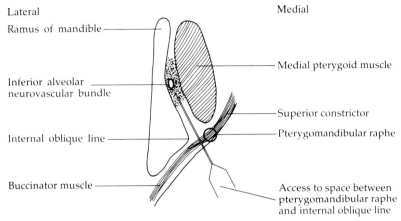

Lateral

Ramus of mandible

Inferior alveolar
neurovascular bundle

Internal oblique line

Buccinator muscle

Medial

Medial pterygoid muscle

Superior constrictor

Pterygomandibular raphe

Access to space between
pterygomandibular raphe
and internal oblique line

Fig. 6.18 *The pterygomandibular space: horizontal section above the lingula.*

foramen, and incisors may be anaesthetized by infiltration injections. For surgery of molar teeth including their extraction, it is also necessary to infiltrate the buccal tissues separately (see p. 146).

Inferior alveolar nerve block

The accessible part of the nerve traverses the pterygomandibular space from the mandibular foramen to the base of the skull. The pterygomandibular space is a narrow slit between the ramus and the medial pterygoid muscle (Fig. 6.18). Its anterior (oral) aspect is limited laterally by the internal oblique line of the mandible and medially by the pterygomandibular raphe: the raphe lies just anterior to the medial pterygoid muscle. (The 'roof' of the space is the lateral pterygoid muscle, and the posterior 'wall' is the parotid gland with its fascia.)

The approach to the pterygomandibular space is made anteriorly through the mouth. The injection site can only be revealed and inspected when the patient's mouth is widely open; this is vital to the procedure and assists in the identification of the landmarks which are (laterally) the bony internal oblique line and (medially) the soft tissue pterygomandibular raphe (Fig. 6.19). The raphe runs from the pterygoid hamulus to the posterior of the mylohyoid line and it becomes tense when the mouth is stretched widely open and is therefore frequently seen clearly. If it is obscured by overlying mucosal folds, it can be palpated. The internal oblique line is identified by palpation, using the index finger of the left hand (right-handed operator).

To anaesthetize the right side of the patient's lower jaw, the surgeon approaches from in front and places the tip of the left index finger on the anterior aspect of the ramus in the retromolar region, and firmly compresses the

soft tissues against the bone, so that bony ridges may be felt. The finger is moved gently medially until the internal oblique line is appreciated and then the finger is *retained in that position* so that the tip indicates the bony landmark.

It is essential to the technique that the needle passes through the pterygomandibular space, i.e. between the mandible and medial pterygoid muscle; the syringe is held with the barrel over the opposite (i.e. patient's left) canine and first premolar teeth (Fig. 6.20). The needle is inserted through the tense mucosa in the narrow interval between the pterygomandibular raphe and the left fingertip (indicating the internal oblique line of the mandible). The height of the puncture is best gauged from the insertion of the raphe into the mandible, being 1.0–1.5 cm above this (Fig. 6.21). As the entrance to the space is an 'inverted triangle', this allows a little more freedom of access than an injection at a lower level. In the dentate this height will allow the syringe to pass above the teeth—but the occlusal plane is a poor reference, due to the frequent loss or tilting of teeth.

The syringe is advanced for about 1.0 cm—the inferior bundle is situated approximately 1.0 cm from the internal oblique line of the mandible despite the very great variation in the shape and size of lower jaws. (This depth of injection can only be recommended if the technique is followed precisely so that the left index finger is firmly pressed against the internal oblique line, thus eliminating soft tissue inaccuracies.) It is likely that the medial aspect of the ramus will be contacted—but this is not essential. (Beginners find this a reassuring aspect of the procedure, but, if bony contact does occur, then the needle must be withdrawn slightly to prevent painful subperiosteal injection.) Errors may occur if the surgeon attempts to 'find' the inner aspects of the ramus, because the angle of the

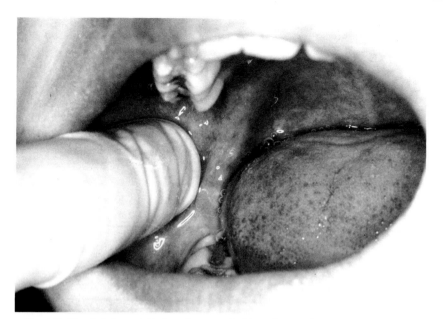

Fig. 6.19 *The first finger indicating the internal oblique line of the mandible. The pterygo-mandibular raphe is clearly seen.*

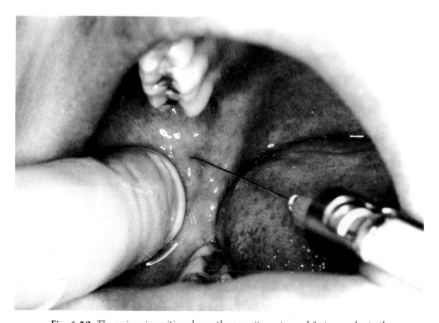

Fig. 6.20 *The syringe is positioned over the opposite canine and first premolar teeth.*

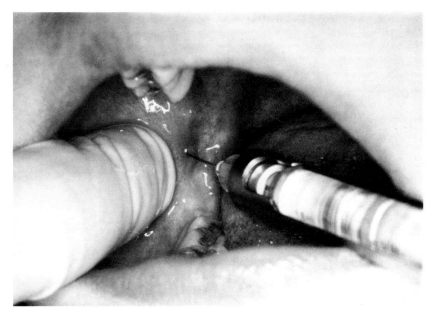

Fig. 6.21 *The needle is inserted about 1.0–1.5 cm above the insertion of the raphe into the mandible. (The entrance to the space is an inverted triangle.)*

ramus to the body of the mandible (often referred to as the flare) may be pronounced. The needle may therefore pass parallel to the jaw and be inserted far too deeply (Fig. 6.22).

When the needle has been positioned, aspiration *must* be performed. As the technique depends on injecting at the neurovascular bundle, intravascular involvement is relatively common—aspiration is even more important when the mandible has been contacted, due to the pos-

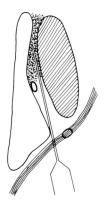

Fig. 6.22 *The needle is inserted too deeply in an attempt to touch the mandible.*

sibility of 'transfixing' the vessels. Then 1.5 ml of solution is slowly injected, taking no less than 30 seconds in order to reduce discomfort and to allow the solution to 'pool' accurately where it has been deposited.

The lingual nerve is very close to the inferior alveolar nerve and is invariably anaesthetized. Occasionally, fascial sheets separate the two nerves, so it is usual to deposit a small amount of solution as the needle is withdrawn in order to disperse the solution around the lingual nerve.

Throughout the procedure and until the needle is finally withdrawn from the tissues, it is important to ensure that the patient's mouth is kept widely open.

There is a short latency of onset before the patient reveals the first symptoms of 'tingling' in the lower lip, which indicates that the analgesic is taking effect. Often the patient is more aware of the onset of symptoms in the lingual nerve and positive enquiry is necessary to confirm the beginning of labial anaesthesia. These first signs of success should occur between about 30 seconds and 1 minute; if they are delayed, the final outcome may be suspect—the procedure was probably inaccurate. Once the onset of analgesia is established, the surgeon should wait for several minutes to allow the depth to improve as the concentration of analgesic increases within the fasciculi and the nerve fibres. It is frequently possible to commence operating after about 3 minutes, provided that the patient has confirmed a densely numb lip. Depth of analgesia will improve for at least a further 10 minutes.

The teeth which are usually anaesthetized fully by this injection are the molars, premolars and canines. The incisors are sometimes completely anaesthetized, but more often are inadequately anaesthetized, requiring additional infiltration injections (see below). This is due to overlap of nerve supply from the opposite inferior alveolar nerve at the midline. The molar area can retain sensitivity from a nerve supply other than the inferior alveolar nerve and, if this is discovered, buccal and infiltration injections will block the other nerves (lingual, mylohyoid, buccal and sometimes cervical).

The extraction of posterior teeth or other surgical procedures always require additional buccal analgesia (see below).

Mental foramen injection

At the level of the premolar teeth (usually the second premolar), the inferior alveolar nerve divides into its two peripheral branches: the incisive nerve which runs forward within the mandible to supply the canine and incisor teeth, and the larger mental nerve which leaves the mandible via the mental foramen to supply the skin of the lower lip to the midline, the intraoral mucosa over the corresponding area and the labial gingiva. Terminal filaments of the mental nerve often re-enter the dental plexus via the labial plate and this gives partial innervation to the incisor teeth (Fig. 6.23).

Injections at the mental foramen are delivered for two reasons: (i) to affect the incisive nerve when treatment is to be carried out on canine or incisor teeth; and (ii) to affect the mental nerve when operations are to be carried out on the soft tissues labial to the lower canine incisor region.

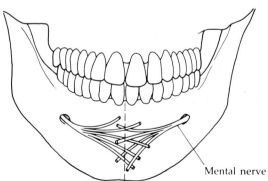

Fig. 6.23 *The mandibular midline. The overlap of sensation is due partly to the mental nerves entering the dental plexus.*

The lip is retracted and the mucosa inspected. If possible, the foramen is located by palpation. The operator is seated behind the patient's head and the lip is now firmly retracted, using the thumb and forefinger of the left hand, so that the mucosa is taut and the syringe is directed downwards and forwards, so that the needle enters the foramen (Fig. 6.24). Then 1.0 ml of solution is slowly injected, taking at least 20 seconds over the delivery; if analgesia of the incisive nerve is required, it is customary to 'massage' the area to encourage the solution to enter the canal.

The lower lip will become numb quite rapidly and, although this usually implies that the incisive nerve is anaesthetized, it may not be the case.

The inferior alveolar nerve block is more reliable and is preferred.

Buccal (long buccal) injections

The long buccal nerve supplies the mucosa on the buccal aspect of molar teeth and gives sensitivity to the periosteum and buccal bone; it may contribute to the nerve supply of one or more molar teeth. Analgesia of this nerve may be achieved by depositing 1.0 ml of solution in the buccal tissues adjacent to the third molar, where the nerve crosses the external oblique line of the mandible (Fig. 6.25).

Unless there is local pathology, it is preferable to infiltrate alongside the tooth being treated.

Infiltration injections

Analgesia of mandibular teeth cannot usually be achieved by infiltration injections because of the thick buccal plates of dense cortical bone. Infiltrations may, however, be used to supplement inferior alveolar nerve blocks or to achieve soft tissue analgesia. However, in the incisor region, the labial plate of bone is thin (the outline of the incisor teeth can sometimes be seen or palpated) and is usually traversed by many neurovascular bundles. Inferior alveolar nerve block analgesia may be deficient at the midline (involving the incisors) due to overlapping nerve fibres from the opposite mental nerve (see Fig. 6.23).

Infiltration injections are usually satisfactory in achieving analgesia of the incisors; if surgery is to be performed, a lingual injection is also required.

The lip is retracted with the thumb and forefinger of the left hand until the mucosa is taut, and the injection site is inspected. The needle penetrates the mucosa in the sulcus just adjacent to the reflection, opposite the tooth

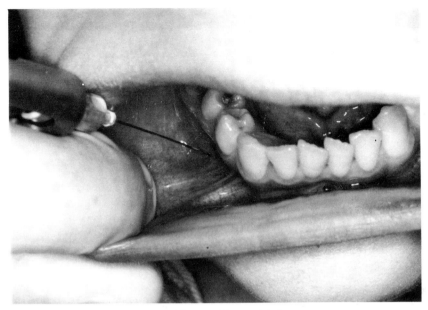

Fig. 6.24 *The mental foramen injection.*

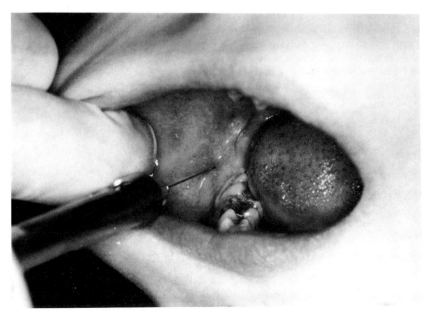

Fig. 6.25 *Analgesia of the buccal nerve.*

to be treated. The syringe must be held at an angle to direct the needle towards the alveolus and not into the labial musculature. The needle should be parallel to the long axis of the tooth, so that the point comes to rest near the estimated position of the apex (Fig. 6.26). It is usual to inject about 1.0 ml of solution, but 0.5 ml is sufficient.

Lingual infiltrations are best delivered into the attached mucosa near the roots of the teeth under consideration—therefore smaller amounts of solution (i.e. 0.5 ml) are injected. Injections into the reflected mucosa spread solution into the floor of the mouth away from the teeth.

Failures of local analgesia

Successful local analgesia depends on the co-operation of the patient, not only to assist the dental surgeon in carrying out accurate injections, but in appreciating the nature of the result. Some nervous patients fail to acknowledge that pain has been adequately abolished and they react to the manipulations of the procedure as if the local analgesic injections had failed to work. Careful patient assessment and management reduce those problems, but some patients need sedation in addition to local analgesia.

However, true failures of analgesia do occur and the following causes may be identified. Inactivity of the analgesic is rare provided the shelf life of storage is not exceeded.

Inaccuracy

This is the most common cause of failure. Unless an injection is carried out with precision, the result cannot be guaranteed. The analgesic solution must be delivered to its target to have an effect. Inaccuracy with infiltration injections is uncommon, but nerve blocks may be more troublesome. The most common reason for inferior alveolar nerve block failures is inaccuracy—and the most common error is injecting too deeply, thus depositing the solution distal to the neurovascular bundle and allowing most of it to diffuse out of the pterygomandibular space away from the inferior alveolar nerve (Fig. 6.22). Clinically this would be apparent by a slow onset of the first symptoms of lip paraesthesia (tingling) and a slow progression to full anaesthesia (numbness). Such poor depth of block is unlikely to give satisfactory pulpal analgesia.

Inadequate field of analgesia

Sometimes several injections may be necessary. For example, although it is usual to achieve pulpal analgesia

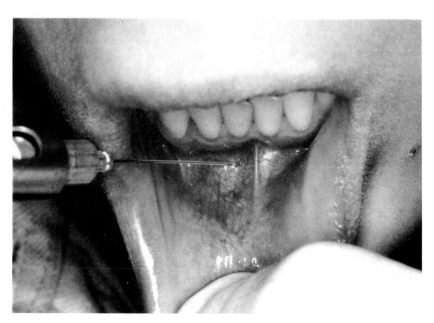

Fig. 6.26 *Infiltration analgesia of the mandibular incisors.*

of an upper first molar by giving a buccal injection only, or of a mandibular tooth from an inferior alveolar nerve block, it is sometimes necessary to give supplementary injections as other adjacent nerves can contribute to the dental plexus.

If the primary injection was considered accurate and produced the expected symptoms rapidly, then selected supplementary injections should be given, e.g. if an inferior alveolar nerve block rapidly induced lip analgesia, but the dentine of a lower tooth remains sensitive, buccal (and sometimes lingual) infiltration injections are required.

If the accuracy of the first 'principal' injection is in doubt, perhaps due to delayed onset or unconvincing symptoms, then it should be repeated.

Inadequate dose of analgesic

The result of an injection is dose dependent. The dose can be altered by adjusting either the concentration or the volume of the injected solution. The concentration of the analgesic solution is predetermined in the cartridge, but the volume is under the control of the operator.

Clinical trials and experience have led to the recommendation that about 1.0 ml of local analgesic solution is required for an infiltration injection (although 0.5 ml may often be sufficient), and 1.5 ml is necessary for an inferior alveolar nerve block. Larger volumes spread over a greater area, and compensate for inaccuracy, but do not necessarily increase the dose delivered at the 'target'.

Repeating an injection is more useful than giving a larger initial volume, because some of the original volume will have dispersed and a second dose localized at the target will increase the concentration of active agents taken up into the nerve structure.

On rare occasions a satisfactory depth of analgesia cannot be achieved with the usual concentrations of analgesic solution. To overcome this problem of 'individual variation', a more potent drug, or a more concentrated preparation of the same drug, may be required.

Local structural problems

Infrequently, difficulty will be encountered with specific injections. It is sometimes impossible to achieve analgesia of upper canine teeth with labial infiltrations, or upper first molars with buccal infiltrations (particularly in adolescents). In such circumstances, nerve block injections may be used or other techniques employed (see later).

In the case of difficulty of analgesia with an upper first molar tooth, it is likely to be due to the bone overlying

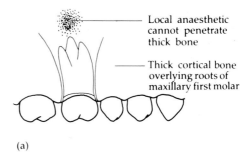

Local anaesthetic cannot penetrate thick bone

Thick cortical bone overlying roots of maxillary first molar

(a)

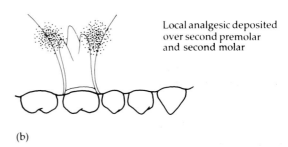

Local analgesic deposited over second premolar and second molar

(b)

Fig. 6.27 *Infiltration analgesia of the maxillary first molar in the presence of a prominent malar buttress of bone.*

the roots being extremely thick due to the malar buttress (Fig. 6.27). In such a situation, an infiltration over the mesial aspect of the second molar, in addition to an infiltration over the second premolar, sometimes gives an adequate result.

On rare occasions, patients are treated for whom one inferior alveolar nerve cannot be successfully blocked. If this is a consistent finding and not due to an inaccurate injection, then alternative methods can be used (see later).

Pathology

Acute inflammation interferes with the success of local analgesia. If analgesic solution is injected directly into inflamed tissues, it may be painful and the resultant analgesia is often inadequate. In theory, injecting into an infected area can spread the infection.

The ineffectiveness of a local analgesic in this situation may be due to combinations of the following

1. Sensitization of the peripheral receptors by the products of inflammation, leading to increased nerve activity.

2. Increased vascularity of the tissues.

3. An alteration of the ionization of the analgesic due to the reduced pH in the tissues (although this is unlikely to be an important factor clinically).

These problems are difficult to overcome immediately. Solutions containing vasoconstrictors *must* be used. The relative effectiveness of the analgesic can be improved by increasing the dose, which can be attempted first by repeating injections. Better results will be achieved by using a more concentrated solution—this is most effective in nerve block analgesia.

An alternative way of managing the problem is to prescribe analgesics and antibiotics for about 5 days. Once the acute inflammation has settled, the usual local analgesics will be adequate. In acute conditions, when the patient is in severe pain, a general anaesthetic may be necessary to complete urgent treatment.

Complications of local analgesia

Untoward responses to treatment may occur during or after the administration of a local analgesic and are not always due directly to the injection. Minor complications of local analgesia are frequently encountered, but serious consequences are very uncommon.

Complications **not** *directly due to the administration of local analgesic*

Psychological

Nervous patients may respond adversely to treatment and their anxiety may be reflected in an increase of heart rate (a rapid pulse), sweating and pallor. This reaction may well be provoked by the anticipation of an injection. A vasovagal response may occur, characterized by a very slow pulse rate and a typical faint—this response is usually less severe when a patient is supine.

Careful patient management and sympathetic handling of the extremely nervous patient may prevent or certainly reduce reactions. Premedication or sedation will be helpful (see Chapters 1 and 4).

Medical

Patients with pre-existing systemic disease may suffer a complication of their disorder whilst receiving dental attention. Diabetic patients occasionally fail to take an adequate meal before treatment, but continue their medication, and this can lead to a hypoglycaemic episode. An attack of angina may be provoked by the stress of dental surgery—not necessarily an injection—and treatment under sedation may be preferable. An epileptic could have a convulsion in the surgery. The specific treatment of these conditions is dealt with elsewhere (Chapters 2 and 4).

Complications related to the administration of local analgesics

Localized

1. *Pain.* Injections can be uncomfortable and, if the patient is tense, more discomfort is likely to be experienced. Needle puncture can be virtually painless if the mucosa is taut, and completely pain free if a topical analgesic is applied.

There may be some mild discomfort during an inferior alveolar block injection, as the needle is directed through the pterygomandibular space. If the needle is inserted inaccurately, and the medial pterygoid muscle is pierced, the procedure will be much more painful (and there will be an increased likelihood of trismus—see below).

If a needle point is sited subperiosteally in error, the delivery of the solution will be more difficult and the patient will experience severe pain as the periosteum is stripped from the underlying bone by the pressure of the fluid. A similarly painful delivery is unavoidable with most palatal injections, where there is little connective tissue.

Direct trauma to a nerve with the needle and injection into a nerve trunk both cause pain (see below).

A rapid injection distends, and sometimes disrupts, tissues and causes pain. The slow delivery of the solution is more comfortable and helps to localize the analgesic, which gives a better result.

Patients sometimes complain of pain after an injection. Local tenderness and occasionally bruising are not uncommon for a day or two. More severe pain, particularly if it increases in intensity, is not usually due to the injection and other (dental) causes should be sought (see below regarding the rare occurrence of infection).

2. *Neurological.* If a needle point touches a nerve, the patient usually responds in a reflex way and afterwards reports a 'sharp pain' or 'electric shock' in the distribution of the nerve. This may occur during an inferior alveolar nerve block injection and the pain is experienced in the lip or the teeth; it is sometimes the lingual nerve which is involved and some patients will state that the needle 'pierced the tongue'. If it is noticed that a patient reacts in this way and it is believed that the needle may have touched a nerve trunk, it must be withdrawn for a few

millimetres to ensure that it is freed, as an injection into a nerve trunk is painful and axons may be damaged resulting in prolonged anaesthesia.

Patients sometimes complain that the injection has 'paralysed their face'. Sensory loss is often misinterpreted as paralysis, but a degree of localized muscle weakness is evident with any infiltration injection as the terminal branches of all nerves are affected. If an inferior alveolar nerve block is given too deeply into the region of the parotid gland, then the main divisions of the facial nerve may be affected, causing a hemifacial paralysis. This is disturbing and the patient will require firm reassurance that the paralysis is temporary. The dental surgeon should assist the patient by covering the eye which cannot be closed fully by using a sterile pad and then ensure that they can return home safely (drivers should be advised to use public transport and to return for their car when facial nerve function has recovered). It is advisable to see the patient later in the day, or at least the following day, to confirm full recovery (see also Chapter 4).

3. *Swelling.* Many patients say that their face feels swollen and this usually is a misinterpretation of their sensory loss. Localized swelling at the time of injection is usually due to the 'pool' of injected fluid, but occasionally local oedema develops. This can be a response to the trauma of the injections, even though this is minimal, or, rarely, due to tissue irritation from the solution. (Symmetrical oedema can occur as an allergic reaction, but this is *rare*—see below.)

Oedema which develops postoperatively may also be the result of trauma from treatment or even self-inflicted injury, such as lip biting. Postoperative swelling may be due to haematoma formation (see below).

4. *Vascular.* Blanching is sometimes noticed during, or immediately after, an injection. Blanching at the point of delivery is due to the pressure of the injection (common in the palate) and to the vasoconstrictor in the solution. Remote areas of blanching in, say, the skin may be due to a reflex vasoconstriction or from local vascular spread of the vasoconstrictor.

An intravascular injection may be delivered accidentally. The results depend on the vessels involved and the amounts injected. There may be responses attributable to vascular constriction or spasm, and local analgesia is likely to be deficient. The systemic effects will be described later.

Haemorrhage can occur as small vessels may be damaged by the needle. Bleeding from the puncture wound arrests spontaneously, but a persistent ooze can be stopped with pressure. Bleeding within the tissues will lead to the formation of a haematoma which may take several weeks to resolve completely. It is wise to prescribe antibiotics to prevent infection developing later. Bleeding in the pterygomandibular space or in the medial pterygoid muscle may cause trismus.

5. *Trismus.* Some limitation of mouth opening after an inferior alveolar nerve block is not uncommon. Oedema or haemorrhage within the pterygomandibular space makes mouth opening uncomfortable for a few days. More significant restriction is caused by direct trauma to muscles of mastication, usually the medial pterygoid. If the patient is disabled by the degree of trismus, it is helpful to prescribe analgesics and possibly diazepam to relieve reflex spasm. If infection is suspected, antibiotics should be prescribed (see below).

Occasionally a serious degree of trismus is encountered. In such cases it is probable that a haematoma has organized, with scar formation within the medial pterygoid muscle. Some advocate forcible opening (under general anaesthetic), but the relief from this procedure is usually limited as scar reforms. A more conservative approach is preferable, but the patient should be referred to a specialist for advice and management.

6. *Infections.* Infection will occasionally develop at the site of an injection. This will be seen as increasing redness, swelling and, later, ulceration—there may even be lymphadenopathy and systemic upset. This complication is treated using appropriate antibiotic therapy.

There have been reports of bony involvement and necrosis, perhaps due to trauma and possibly exacerbated by vasoconstrictors. Such problems are exceedingly rare and therefore the patient should be referred to a consultant for specialist treatment.

7. *Needle fracture.* Since the advent of disposable needles, this complication has been virtually eliminated; when it does occur, it is usually due to a flaw in the needle structure. If sufficient needle is visible, the patient should be instructed to keep quite still whilst the end of the needle is grasped with a suitable pair of forceps, e.g. mosquito artery clip. If the needle is inaccessible and cannot be withdrawn, the patient should be informed and then referred for specialist advice (it is not always necessary to remove a fractured needle).

Systemic (see also Chapter 4)

Systemic responses are due to high levels of analgesic drug or vasoconstrictor in the circulation, and effects usually involve the central nervous system or cardiovascular system. High blood levels can be achieved from either an intravascular injection, producing a 'bolus', or from rapid absorption from the vascular oral tissues.

Mild toxic reactions are fairly common, are usually transient and often unnoticed. Serious toxic effects are rare.

1. *Vasoconstrictor side-effects.* An intravascular bolus of a sympathomimetic vasoconstrictor may cause tachycardia, and general symptoms of dizziness, nausea and panic. Some patients respond in this way to trivial doses and alternative preparations should be selected if this is recognized as a constant reaction.

2. *Local analgesic side-effects.* In most cases severe responses are caused by intravascular injection or overdosage, although sometimes high blood levels can be detected after the recommended amounts of solution have been injected carefully.

The side-effects of local analgesics have already been discussed. The less severe toxic effects are usually short-lived, but, if convulsions ensue, these should be terminated using intravenous diazepam. When serious adverse responses are evident, oxygen must be administered and, if spontaneous respiration fails, then artificial ventilation must be given. The patient must be transferred to hospital immediately (Chapter 4).

3. *Allergic reactions.* As has already been mentioned, allergy to the amide analgesics is *extremely* rare. The local analgesic itself is almost never the provocative agent, and such allergic reactions should become eliminated with improved manufacturing procedures removing 'preservatives' from the solutions. There are few recorded cases of true allergic reactions and all have been delayed responses requiring simple treatment.

If a patient gives a history of 'allergy', it is useful to refer him or her for assessment in order to exclude true allergy, so that local analgesic can be safely employed for painless dental treatment.

Other techniques

Topical analgesia

Preparations are available to produce surface, or mucosal, analgesia. Topical local analgesics are available as pastes or sprays.

It must be remembered that, although the application of a surface analgesic will effectively eliminate the discomfort of the needle penetrating mucosa (which is minimal if a good technique is employed), most pain from injections comes from either depositing the solution too quickly, or from injecting subperiosteally.

The careless application of excess topical analgesic causes its own problem. The spread of analgesic throughout the mouth is distasteful and uncomfortable. The injec-

tion site must be identified and dried, and a small amount of paste applied either on a cotton-wool roll or on a cotton bud (Fig. 6.28).

The spray system delivers a controlled dose of analgesic, and for dental injections a single application is all that is required. As before, the injection site must be clearly seen and dried. Analgesics are rapidly absorbed from the vascular mucosa and in other surgical situations the careless and liberal use of anaesthetic sprays has led to systemic complications.

Jet injection

The delivery of solution under pressure, so that it is driven through the surface into deeper tissues, has been

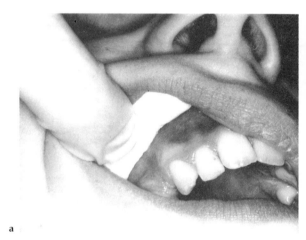

a

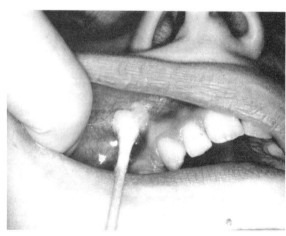

b

Fig. 6.28 *The application of topical analgesic paste.*

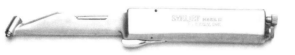

Fig. 6.29 *The Syrijet jet injector.*

exploited in the field of vaccinations. Developments of the system led to the production of an instrument known as the Syrijet (Fig. 6.29) which is spring loaded, has a control to vary the dose injected, and is designed to use a dental local analgesic cartridge. This type of system provides good surface analgesia, but the only other beneficial applications are:

(a) pulpal analgesia of some deciduous teeth can be achieved;

(b) palatal analgesia is possible in adults—avoiding the need for painful injections.

In common with most 'alternative' systems, the instrument is costly and test results were not reliable. At the site of application a painful bruise usually developed, and, if the tip was not held firmly and immobile during the delivery, a laceration could occur. A further problem was that only small amounts of analgesic were used and some dentists were retaining the cartridge to use the remaining solution on other patients. This must *not* be practised as contamination does occur and cross-infection is very likely. Even if only a tiny amount is dispensed, the cartridge must be discarded and the tip of the instrument flushed and sterilized before further use.

Intraosseous injection

On *rare*, and sometimes inexplicable, occasions the standard dental injections fail to produce analgesia of some teeth. In these special, and very uncommon, situations an intraosseous injection may be performed.

Intraosseous injections may be used when the usual methods of applying analgesic consistently fail to induce adequate symptoms, and this technique should *not* be used when initial injections have been given inaccurately (and so are inadequate) or when infection and inflammation interfere with the outcome.

The procedure is simple but a little clumsy (Fig. 6.30). The mucosa is anaesthetized and a small puncture is made with a scalpel. A small sterile bur is used to penetrate the cortical plate, and then, using a short needle, a small

amount of local analgesic is delivered. The resultant dental analgesia is swift and localized to the adjacent teeth. The solution is quickly absorbed so the pulpal analgesia lasts for only a short time (about 10 minutes). Because the solution is taken up extremely rapidly (almost exactly like giving an intravenous injection), it is recommended that only plain solutions (i.e. those without a vasoconstrictor) are used.

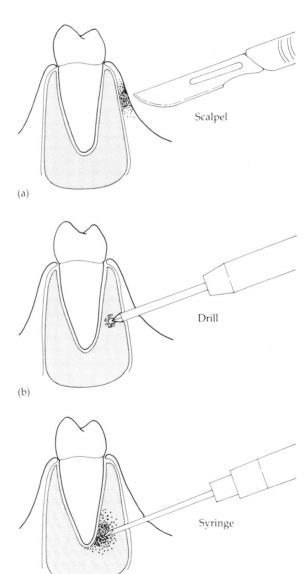

(a)

(b)

(c)

Fig. 6.30 *Diagrammatic representation of the intraosseous injection technique.*

The procedure is uncommonly practised and its application is almost exclusively restricted to the posterior mandibular region. It has probably been completely· superseded by the developments in intraligamental injections.

Intraligamental (intraperiodontal) injections

The direct injection of local analgesic solution into the periodontal tissues is not a new concept, but instruments have recently been developed which have provided technical advances and control to the method. These syringes are provided with protective sleeves into which the dental local analgesic cartridge is inserted. In the event of the glass shattering with the pressure used, the patient is therefore protected.

Several designs of instrument are available, and most depend on a ratchet system to deliver small volumes of solution with each squeeze of the trigger by the operator (Fig. 6.31). The technique is simple but is nevertheless operator-dependent. For convenience and to reduce trauma, a very short and very fine (30 gauge) needle is used.

It is important that the gingival and periodontal tissues are healthy and have no obvious inflammation or infections. The application of a topical antiseptic is recommended by many users, but if, say, povidone-iodine is used, several minutes must be allowed for it to be effective before carrying out the injection.

The fine needle is inserted into the gingival crevice and advanced until firmly seated (Fig. 6.32). The trigger of the instrument is then slowly squeezed to force solution into the periodontal ligament. If resistance is not experienced,

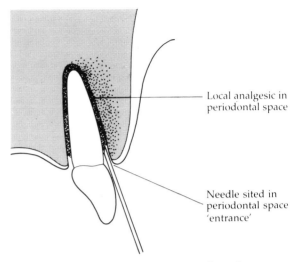

— Local analgesic in periodontal space

— Needle sited in periodontal space 'entrance'

Fig. 6.32 *Diagrammatic representation of the needle site for intraligamental injection.*

it is unlikely that the solution is travelling into the periodontal space, but is probably leaking back out of the gingival crevice.

For a single-rooted tooth, one delivery may be sufficient, but two applications (one mesiobuccally and one distobuccally) will give a more reliable result. For multi-rooted teeth, up to two deliveries per root may be needed.

The resultant analgesia is usually rapid and localized to the tooth injected. However, solution does spread and sometimes adjacent teeth are affected, and occasionally more widespread symptoms may result, e.g. injections in the posterior of the mandible may induce lip paraesthesia.

The main advantages of the techniques are:

(a) the simplicity of the method;
(b) rapid onset of analgesia;
(c) the absence of soft tissue anaesthesia;
(d) the small volume of analgesic used;
(e) the appeal of the system to children—avoiding traditional 'injections'.

[*Note.* It must be stressed again that even if only a small part of a dental cartridge is used, the remaining solution must be discarded and *not* retained for use on other patients.]

There are some disadvantages to this method of local analgesia.

1. It may be painful.

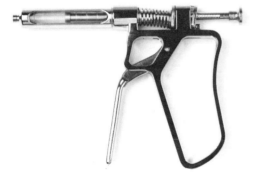

Fig. 6.31 *An intraligamentary injection syringe.*

2. In most cases teeth feel 'high' for about 24 hours, and slightly tender.

3. A small degree of periodontal damage occurs. At the site of injection, tissue damage may involve some resorption of bone and cementum. This is a very small injury which repairs with scar. A single event is of little consequence, but it is thought that repeated use may significantly change the nature of a tooth's supporting tissues.

4. Careless use of the method can dislodge teeth—particularly single-rooted teeth and teeth with incompletely formed roots.

Injudicious use in the primary dentition can lead to damage to the developing permanent successor.

5. It is a form of intraosseous injection—although more convenient than the usual intraosseous procedures.

6. Although analgesia tends to be localized, the solution is not retained in the periodontal space, but is forced into the surrounding alveolar bone. Therefore, although the access is different, this must still be considered an intraosseous injection.

7. The success rate is variable, being highest for single-rooted teeth and in the mandible, and is relatively poor with plain solutions, and even solutions containing adrenaline are not totally reliable.

8. The solution is absorbed rapidly into the bloodstream, and the use of multiple injections on several teeth could well produce high blood levels of analgesic comparable with intravenous delivery.

9. If used where inflammation or infection is present, more significant infection can develop, with the possibility of localized bone involvement. This is of particular importance as some dentists are resorting to this technique when traditional injections fail to anaesthetize a tooth involved in an inflammatory response. *This is not recommended.*

In general practice, intraligamental injections are given frequently for simple restorative treatment, particularly in the mandibular molar region. If it is used carefully and within the recommended limitations, it may prove to be a very successful technique for some patients. It should not be considered as replacing traditional techniques, and should not be thought to be without problems as it can cause quite severe postanaesthetic discomfort.

GENERAL ANAESTHESIA AND SEDATION

The safety and effectiveness of modern local anaesthesia (analgesia) technique makes this the most widely used form of pain control in dentistry. When pain control is by loss of consciousness, a state of general anaesthesia exists. General anaesthesia with its greater risks of complications is reserved for special situations.

Definition and attendant responsibilities

For the purposes of clarification, the General Dental Council has issued the following notice for the guidance of UK registered dentists.

1. Where a general anaesthetic is administered, this should be by a person other than the operator.

2. This second person should be a dental or medical practitioner, appropriately trained and experienced in the use of anaesthetic drugs for dental purposes. As part of a programme of training in anaesthesia, the general anaesthesia may be administered by a dental or medical practitioner under the direct supervision of the said second person.

3. Where intravenous or inhalational sedation* techniques are to be employed, a suitably experienced practitioner may assume the responsibility of sedating the patient, as well as operating, provided that as a minimum requirement a second appropriate person is present throughout. Such an appropriate person might be a suitably trained dental surgery assistant or ancillary dental worker, whose experience and training enable that person to be an efficient member of the dental team and one who is capable of monitoring the clinical condition of the patient. Should the occasion arise, he or she must also be capable of assisting the dentist in case of emergency.

4. Neither general anaesthesia nor sedation should be employed unless proper equipment for their administration and adequate facilities for the resuscitation of the patient are readily available, with both the operator and his staff trained in their use.

5. *A dentist who carried out treatment under general anaesthesia or sedation without fulfilling these conditions would amost certainly be considered to have acted in a manner which constitutes infamous or disgraceful conduct in a professional respect.*

* Simple sedation is defined in the Report of the Working Party on Training in Dental Anaesthesia (Wylie Report, 1981) as follows: 'A technique in which the use of a drug or drugs produces a state of depression of the central nervous system enabling treatment to be carried out, but during which verbal contact with the patient is maintained throughout the period of sedation. The drugs and techniques used should carry a margin of safety wide enough to render unintended loss of consciousness unlikely.'

Indications for general anaesthesia

1. Anxious or mentally handicapped unco-operative patients, where simple sedation is inadequate for any form of treatment. The very young often require general anaesthesia when their understanding and tolerance do not permit dental procedures when conscious.

2. Oral surgery, where the complexity or length of operation makes the procedure intolerable for a conscious patient. Such operations are usually performed in hospital operating theatres.

3. Where local analgesia cannot be given because of sepsis in the area or bleeding tendency.

4. When multiple extractions or periodontal surgery in different quadrants of the jaws are to be performed at a single appointment. A single anaesthetic may be preferable to multiple procedures under local analgesia over a period of time.

Contraindications for general anaesthesia and intravenous sedation

General anaesthesia or sedation in a dental surgery is contraindicated in the following circumstances.

1. If the patient has had food or drink within 4 hours. Whilst vomiting during induction of or recovery from anaesthesia or sedation is not common with modern techniques, the risk of inhalation of vomit still makes this a most stringent rule to be observed, except in dire emergency.

2. If there is inability to abide by the General Dental Council regulations given above, in that an experienced anaesthetist may not be available, the necessary resuscitative and emergency equipment may not be available, or recovery facilities are inadequate.

3. If *any* significant medical contraindication exists (Chapter 2). Out-patient general anaesthesia or sedation in a dental surgery should only be undertaken in those deemed to be totally medically fit. In particular, degenerative heart conditions such as congestive cardiac failure, coronary thrombosis or hypertension are absolute contraindications. Similarly, respiratory diseases present special problems which should only be dealt with by professional anaesthetists in hospital. Respiratory obstruction, such as occurs in Ludwig's angina (a serious complication which may accompany spreading cellulitis originating from a dental abscess), is a dangerous state requiring specialist hospital attention (Chapters 4 and 9).

Endocrine, haematological, liver and kidney diseases, and patients receiving any medications including alcohol, present special management problems, for whom out-patient general anaesthesia or sedation should not be considered. Sickle cell disease and other types of anaemia must also be remembered (Chapter 2).

4. If a patient has no responsible adult escort to convey him or her home, no treatment should be considered. Following out-patient general anaesthesia or sedation, a patient must not be allowed to drive a vehicle, work with machinery, make important decisions or undertake any other responsibility until totally recovered (i.e. for 24 hours).

Pre-anaesthetic checks for out-patient general anaesthesia and sedation (see also Chapter 7; Fig. 6.33)

1. Ensure the identity of the patient and the site and nature of operation.

2. A detailed full medical history must be obtained and any contraindications noted. Make sure consent has been obtained.

3. The patient should have an empty bladder and stomach, with no food or drink intake within the previous 4 hours. Dentures should be removed.

4. A responsible adult should be present to escort the patient home safely.

5. An appropriately trained anaesthetist and nurse must be available to administer the anaesthetic. Intravenous sedation may be administered by a suitably experienced operator in the presence of an appropriately trained assistant.

6. All anaesthetic plus resuscitation equipment should be in first-class order and properly serviced. Emergency drugs should be available and their expiry date checked as valid for use. In particular, emergency oxygen should be available in adequate quantities as well as apparatus for providing positive pressure ventilation of the patient if necessary.

7. For general anaesthesia, effective throat packs should be available. A suitable system is the sterilizable 'V' pack system (Fig. 6.34).

8. Efficient suction must be available to maintain a clear airway. It is also sensible for standby foot-operated suction equipment to be available in case of electrical or mechanical failure.

Consent (Table 7.1)

Fully informed consent must be obtained from the patient in writing before the anaesthetic or sedation and operation commence. This must include a clear statement of any risks or possible sequelae which might forseeably arise, e.g. lip or tongue anaesthesia following removal of impacted mandibular third molars or possible drug effects e.g. muscle pains (p. 170).

Preparation for GA

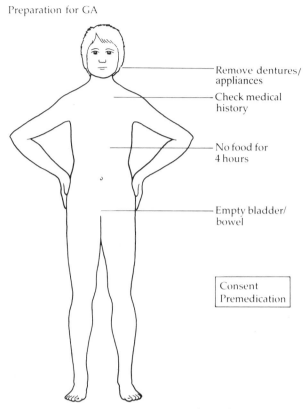

- Remove dentures/ appliances
- Check medical history
- No food for 4 hours
- Empty bladder/ bowel

Consent
Premedication

Fig. 6.33 *Preparation for general anaesthesia.*

The Defence Societies in the UK provide suitable forms which must be signed by the patient (or parent or guardian of a person under the age of 16 years) as well as the surgeon performing the operation. This applies equally to out-patient dental surgery general anaesthetics as it does to hospital-performed operations (see p. 181).

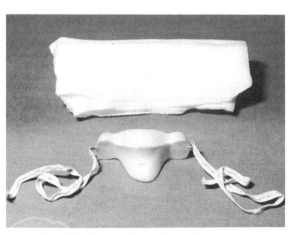

Fig. 6.34 *Gauze and foam V types of throat pack.*

Premedication for out-patient general anaesthesia
(see also Chapter 7)

Prior to operation in hospital, most patients receive premedication which allays fear and often has other beneficial effects such as reducing salivary and bronchial secretions. However, this is rarely necessary for out-patient general anaesthesia, as the anaesthetics are of short duration and the operation simple and quick to perform. Nevertheless, extremely nervous patients occasionally do benefit from premedication such as oral diazepam (5 mg the night before and again 30 minutes preoperatively or temazepam 30 mg orally). It must be noted that the use of diazepam 30 minutes before operation *should not involve swallowing more than 10 ml of fluid*; otherwise the stomach is not considered sufficiently empty for general anaesthesia to proceed.

Gases and vapours

Certain laws of physics explain the behaviour of gases and vapours and these are relevant to understanding the application of such agents for analgesia or anaesthesia.

A gas is a substance which exists in a gaseous state at room temperature and atmospheric pressure. A vapour is the gaseous phase of a substance which, at room temperature and pressure, exists as a liquid. The **critical temper-**ature of a gas is the temperature at which it may be liquefied by pressure. The **critical pressure** of a gas is the pressure at which it liquefies. The relevant values for oxygen are: critical temperature $-116°C$, and critical pressure 138 bar (2000 pounds per square inch, p.s.i.); whilst for nitrous oxide the corresponding figures are: $36.5°C$ and 52 bar (750 p.s.i.). Thus, nitrous oxide stored at a pressure of 55 bar (800 p.s.i.) in cylinders is in a liquid state at room temperature, whereas oxygen stored at 137 bar (1980 p.s.i.) is still in a gaseous state. Cylinder pressure gauges respond to the gaseous phase, and therefore, when an oxygen cylinder is half empty, the gauge registers as such. In contrast, when the nitrous oxide cylinder is half empty, enough liquid remains to produce a vapour pressure effect on the gauge and it is only when the cylinder is more than 4/5 empty that the gauge begins to fall (Fig. 6.35). Therefore, once the nitrous oxide gauge reading begins to fall it will not be long before the cylinder runs out.

Gases and vapours dissolve in liquids, depending upon the pressure of the gas and the temperature of the liquid. The higher the gas pressure, the more goes into solution, but the higher the liquid temperature, the *less* gas it can absorb. Thus oxygen and carbon dioxide dissolve in blood and body fluids. Gases in solution may diffuse across a permeable membrane according to the concentration gradient and the molecular weight of the gas. Despite the greater solubility of carbon dioxide in blood compared with oxygen, the pressure gradient of carbon dioxide is less than that for oxygen across the blood–pulmonary epithelium–alveolar air junction. Oxygen (mol. wt 32) diffuses more rapidly than carbon dioxide (mol. wt 44). It is possible, therefore, with inadequate ventilation, to provide adequate oxygenation of a patient, yet fail to eliminate carbon dioxide.

If at the conclusion of nitrous oxide/oxygen administration, a patient breathes air (containing only 20% oxygen), nitrous oxide rapidly passes into the alveolar air to be exhaled. This causes a fall in the alveolar air oxygen content leading to hypoxia (diffusion hypoxia). However, if 100% oxygen is administered after nitrous oxide administration ceases, diffusion hypoxia is prevented.

The rate of induction of an anaesthetic agent depends upon the rate of equilibration of alveolar air–gas composition with the gas composition delivered by the anaesthetic apparatus. The rate of equilibration depends upon the agent's blood solubility and therefore its rate of movement across the alveolar membrane into the circulation. The higher the concentration and flow rate of gases from the anaesthetic machine, the more rapidly the blood/alveolar air equilibration occurs. The alveolar con-

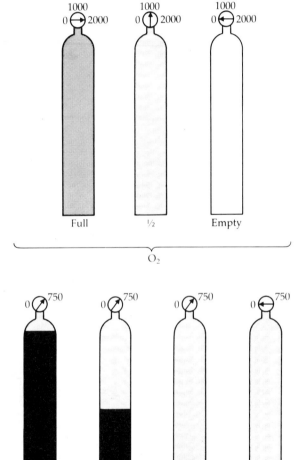

Fig. 6.35 *Relationship between cylinder contents and gauge readings.* (O_2 = oxygen; N_2O = nitrous oxide)

centration equilibrium also depends directly upon the rate of ventilation of lungs.

The **partition coefficient** of a gas is the ratio of the amount of agent dissolved in blood compared with the amount of agent present in the lung alveoli at equilibrium state. The greater the partition coefficient, the greater the agent's solubility in blood, and the longer it takes for equilibration to develop between blood, alveolar air and the concentration of gases delivered. This increases the induction (and recovery) time. Disease of the lung tissue affects the diffusion rate of gases from alveoli to blood. The cardiac output and flow rate of blood through the lungs will also play an obvious role in reaching equilibrium. Once in the blood circulation, the differing *tissue* affinities for different agents affect the rate of equilibration too. Most inhalation agents have similar solubilities in blood and tissue, but all inhalation agents are relatively fat soluble. Halothane is an exception since it is three times more soluble in brain and muscle than in blood. Induction is slightly slower as it takes longer to saturate these tissues to reach an equilibrium state, and recovery time is slightly prolonged by the slow release of halothane from the tissue sites. Once all the body tissues are saturated by administering relatively large amounts of inhalation agents, the amount required to maintain this state is much smaller.

Gases and vapours used in general anaesthesia

Nitrous oxide

Nitrous oxide is a sweet-smelling, colourless, non-irritant gas which is heavier than air (specific gravity 1.5). In the UK it is supplied in blue cylinders at a pressure of 55 bar (800 p.s.i.). The cylinders are fitted with a pin-index locating system to ensure that they are fitted to the correct gas-line of an anaesthetic machine. Nitrous oxide has a partition coefficient of 0.47, indicating its poor solubility in blood. This leads to rapid pulmonary equilibration between blood and alveolar gas, with rapid induction and rapid recovery. It has low anaesthetic potency but good analgesic effects, is administered with at least 30% oxygen and requires additionally more potent agents to achieve surgical anaesthesia.

Nitrous oxide has virtually no adverse effects upon the heart, pulse rate or blood pressure. Respiration is little affected. Muscle relaxation is not profound and there is little effect on salivary or bronchial secretions. Nitrous oxide is neither inflammable nor explosive, but will support combustion in the absence of oxygen due to it breaking down into its component nitrogen and oxygen.

Combustion is possible when exposed to grease or oil under pressure and therefore no grease or oil is used anywhere in the gas delivery system.

Multiple repeated exposure to nitrous oxide/oxygen sedation is not without problems. In such circumstances neurological symptoms may develop. This is because nitrous oxide oxidizes cobalt, an important co-factor in enzyme systems of the body, and can lead to vitamin B_{12} deficiency. The effects are similar to those seen in sub-acute combined degeneration of the cord. Chronic exposure to nitrous oxide, such as occurs if exhaled gases are allowed to accumulate in an operating area, has also been associated with adverse effects (see Chapter 10). A scavenging system is indicated.

Nitrous oxide may produce hallucinogenic effects, which are sometimes erotic. It is for this reason that general anaesthesia should always be administered in the presence of a third party who, when females are anaesthetized, should also be female.

Oxygen

Oxygen is a colourless, tasteless, odourless, non-inflammable gas needed to maintain life. When exposed to debris, grease or oil under pressure, it forms an explosive mixture, making it important that these agents are not contaminants of the oxygen supply and delivery system. When supplied, the cylinder outlet is sealed to prevent debris entering during transit. The gas is supplied in black cylinders which have a white top, and a pin-index location system. The gas is at a pressure of 137 bar (1980 p.s.i.).

Adequate oxygenation of a patient is a vital component of general anaesthesia. There are two principal factors governing oxygenation of body tissues:

(a) cardiac output, and
(b) the oxygen content of blood, representing both the haemoglobin content and the degree of oxygen saturation.

It has been shown that an anaesthetized patient requires *more* oxygen than a conscious patient breathing normal atmospheric air (containing 20% oxygen). The effect of anaesthetic agents is to disrupt ventilation, making a minimum 30% oxygen content of inspired anaesthetic or analgesic mixture advisable.

Trichlorethylene (Trilene)

Trichlorethylene is a cheap, colourless liquid which enjoyed popularity some years ago but has been surplanted by the introduction of halothane, enflurane and isoflurane. It contains a blue dye to distinguish it from other volatile agents. It has a high blood/gas partition coefficient, being relatively soluble in blood. This makes alveolar equilibration slow, and induction slow. It has powerful analgesic properties, with little vasomotor depression. It produces poor muscle relaxation and affects the cardiovascular system producing bradycardia and ectopic cardiac arrhythmias. The myocardium is sensitized to increased carbon dioxide and catecholamine levels. Rapid shallow breathing sometimes occurs (tachypnoea), requiring reduction in the trichlorethylene concentration delivered, otherwise ventilation of the patient will become insufficient. Recovery (like induction) is slow and there is significant postanaesthetic nausea and vomiting. Most inspired trichlorethylene is exhaled from the lungs during recovery, with only a small proportion being metabolized by the liver.

Halothane (Fluothane)

Halothane is still the most widely used adjuvant to nitrous oxide/oxygen for providing surgical anaesthesia. It is a colourless, volatile liquid which has a boiling point of approximately 50°C, readily producing a vapour which is dispensed into the delivery system from a vaporizer in the anaesthetic machine (Fig. 6.38). This has the facility to control the concentration of halothane delivered, usually 1.5–4%.

Halothane has a characteristic smell because of the thymol preservative it contains. It is stored in amber bottles as exposure to light causes its decomposition into volatile acids. In mixtures up to 50% in oxygen it is not inflammable or explosive, but if halothane vapour meets an open flame, toxic fumes of bromine are produced. Halothane has a partition coefficient of 2.36 which, though greater than that of nitrous oxide, still represents relatively poor solubility in blood. For this reason there is rapid equilibration between the alveolar and blood concentrations of halothane. This produces rapid induction of anaesthesia. Similarly, after anaesthesia, the poor solubility of halothane in blood means it is readily released into the lungs and exhaled. Rapid recovery ensues, but it takes many days for halothane to be completely eliminated from the body. Halothane metabolic products are found in urine in the postanaesthetic period, and it has been estimated that between 10% and 25% of inspired halothane is metabolized by the body. Also, there is an increase in serum bromides following prolonged halothane anaesthesia which may produce postoperative de-

pression. The pharmacological effects of halothane include:

Cardiovascular system. The main effects of halothane upon the cardiovascular system are:
 peripheral vasodilatation,
 hypotension,
 myocardial depression and increased irritability,
 bradycardia,
 arrhythmias.

These effects are directly related to the inspired concentration of halothane and the depth of anaesthesia. The bradycardia results from an increase in vagal tone and is not prevented by atropine premedication. The fall in blood pressure results from the peripheral vasodilatation, myocardial depression and the vagal bradycardia. The myocardium shows increased irritability, especially to carbon dioxide and catecholamines, and therefore arrhythmias are often found during halothane anaesthesia, particularly where the respiratory depressive effects have led to carbon dioxide accumulation and fear or anxiety have produced increased endogenous catecholamine release. However, during light anaesthesia for dental procedures, surgical stimulation has regularly been reported to result in a blood pressure *rise*, and hypotension has not been a problem. The arrhythmias produced in some dental cases have been directly related to manipulation of teeth (e.g. the actual removal of a tooth) causing trigeminal stimulation. Such cardiac irregularities may be prevented by the supplemental use of local anaesthesia in the area to be operated on. Adrenaline-free local anaesthetic solutions are advocated since halothane predisposes to myocardial sensitivity to catecholamines.

Respiratory system. Halothane produces dilatation of the bronchi, beneficial especially in asthmatics. It is non-irritant to the pulmonary mucosa and does not increase bronchial or salivary secretions. The *rate* of respiration increases, but the *depth* decreases. Effective saturation of the blood with oxygen under these conditions is ensured by increasing the inspired oxygen concentration to 30%. However, carbon dioxide elimination may be impaired and, as already stated, this may result in cardiac arrhythmias due to increased myocardial irritability inherent with halothane anaesthesia.

Central nervous system. Halothane has weak analgesic properties but usefully complements the properties of nitrous oxide in this respect. However, it produces good muscle relaxation, facilitating good access during oral and dental surgery. It readily produces deep surgical anaesthesia. It has a depressor effect on the vasomotor and respiratory centres.

Other effects. The incidence of postanaesthetic nausea and vomiting is low with halothane. Shivering is frequently seen however, the cause of which is not entirely clear, though the peripheral vasodilatation may cause loss of body heat and a fall in temperature. During shivering the oxygen requirements of the body increase and increased oxygen should be administered.

The effect of halothane on *liver function* has been a major controversy over recent years. A small percentage of patients are particularly sensitive to halothane and develop 'halothane hepatitis'. Following a second exposure, especially within a 4-week period, the hypersensitivity reaction results in pyrexia, eosinophilia, jaundice and acute hepatic necrosis which may be extensive enough to cause death. *Repeated administrations of halothane, especially within a 4-week period, therefore, are to be avoided* (p. 30).

Enflurane (Ethrane)

Enflurane is non-inflammable, has a boiling point of approximately 56°C, and readily vaporizes at room temperature. It is an expensive agent, which is administered, like halothane, using a special vaporizer incorporated into the anaesthetic gas circuit. The vaporizer has the facility to control the concentration of enflurane delivered, which is usually 2–5%. It has a musty odour and, unlike halothane, does not decompose when exposed to light, and it contains no additives or preservatives. During induction of anaesthesia using enflurane, the concentration is only slowly built up, making the actual induction time for enflurane somewhat slower than for halothane.

Enflurane does, however, have the disadvantage of inducing marked electrocardiograph changes and, rarely, produces overt epileptiform fits, for which reason it is contraindicated for epileptics.

The cardiovascular effects of enflurane are sometimes significant, in that there may be a *sudden* drop in blood pressure. The myocardium is not adversely affected and arrhythmias are uncommon. The respiratory system does show marked depression with enflurane anaesthesia, which may lead to carbon dioxide build-up causing a fall in peripheral resistance, and a release of endogenous adrenaline which fails to combat the fall in blood pressure but produces bronchodilatation. Enflurane produces good muscle relaxation. During recovery, 97.5% of the inspired enflurane is exhaled, with only 2.5% being metabolized, mainly in the liver. Enflurane as the adjuvant for nitrous oxide anaesthesia in dental out-patients is gaining popularity. Recently, however, enflurane has been reported to be occasionally associated with halothane-type jaundice.

Isoflurane (Forane)

Isoflurane is an isomer of enflurane. It is a colourless liquid, with a mildly pungent smell, and vaporizes readily at room temperature. It is dispensed from a vaporizer similar to those used for halothane and enflurane. It does not decompose on exposure to light and contains no preservatives. It is more expensive than halothane. It is the least soluble of all the volatile anaesthetic agents in current use, with a blood/gas partition coefficient of 1.4, and theoretically isoflurane could produce rapid induction of anaesthesia. However, because of its pungent odour it is added only slowly to anaesthetic mixtures and therefore the induction time is comparable to that seen with enflurane or halothane. Recovery is rapid. Isoflurane produces minimal depression of the myocardium or cardiac output. There is a slight increase in heart rate, with consequent decrease in stroke volume. Peripheral resistance is lowered, but with usual anaesthetic concentrations (1.5–3.5%) there is little effect on blood pressure. Myocardial irritability and arrhythmias are not common. The depressive effect upon the respiratory system is less than with enflurane but greater than with halothane. Over 98% of inspired isoflurane is exhaled unmetabolized.

Inhalation general anaesthetic machines

Anaesthetic machines are designed according to two basic systems:

(a) intermittent flow machines (McKesson; Walton),
(b) continuous flow machines (Boyle).

Intermittent flow machines

In 1910 McKesson introduced the first intermittent flow nitrous oxide and oxygen anaesthetic machine. Shortly afterwards the Walton machine became available in the UK. Both types are now rarely used.

The intermittent flow machines enjoyed popularity for many years for out-patient dental general anaesthesia but were only suitable for short operative procedures. The basic principle was that 100% nitrous oxide was administered until narcosis was achieved, mainly by anoxia. Then, up to 20% oxygen was added to the gas mixture to maintain anaesthesia. Valves controlled the release of gas to the patient and were arranged such that delivery occurred only during inspiratory effort. Apart from the unacceptable anoxia, many disadvantages centred around these machines which were not overcome by subsequent modifications to enable trichlorethylene or halothane vaporizers to be incorporated into the delivery circuit.

The disadvantages of intermittent flow may be summarized as follows.

1. The gases were delivered by narrow-bore tubing which introduced unnecessarily high resistance to breathing, and it was important not to have a reservoir bag in the circuit.

2. The vaporizers which were later used were not temperature compensated, which meant that accurate control of a vaporizing anaesthetic agent was impossible, as the latent heat of vaporization effect caused the temperature of the liquid to fall.

3. The accuracy of the nitrous oxide/oxygen mixture control was poor and required regular frequent servicing to maintain any reliable degree of accuracy. As servicing is expensive, regular maintenance was rare in most dental surgeries.

4. The machines did not lend themselves for ready adaptation to allow exhaust gases to be scavenged in order to prevent pollution of the operating area (see Chapter 10).

Intermittent flow machines are now out of favour.

Continuous flow machines

Continuous flow (Boyle's) machines have now replaced intermittent flow machines for both out-patient anaesthesia and operating theatre anaesthesia. The machine carries a supply of nitrous oxide and oxygen, either from cylinders in the surgery or via a pipeline from bulk storage cylinders. Each gas passes through a valve with an adjustable control (Fig. 6.36): a flow rate of 6–8 litres per minute is suitable for adults and 4–6 litres per minute for children. The percentage of oxygen delivered should never be allowed to fall below 30%. The volatile agent used as an adjuvant (e.g. halothane, enflurane or isoflurane) is delivered from a vaporizer which is tempera-

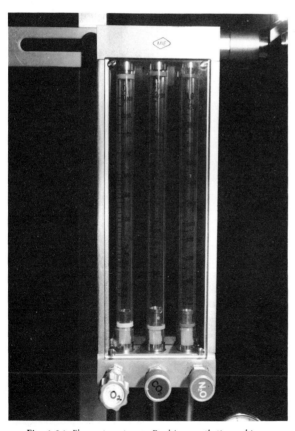

Fig. 6.36 *Flow rate meters on Boyle's anaesthetic machine.*

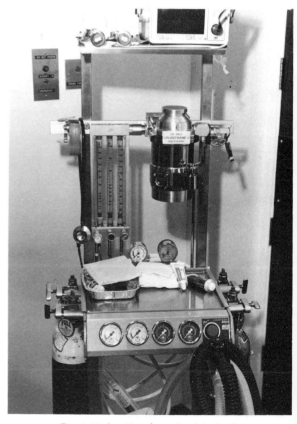

Fig. 6.37 *Insertion of vaporizer into circuit.*

The basic pattern of the Boyle's machine has been modified for delivering nitrous oxide/oxygen mixtures only, for the purpose of producing analgesia and sedation (relative analgesia (RA)—p. 178). With these machines it is impossible to administer less than 50% oxygen to the patient.

A further modification is a machine which has only one flow meter. This is provided to control the flow rate of an Entonox mixture to the patient. Entonox is a manufactured mixture of 50:50 nitrous oxide:oxygen used for relative analgesia. It is supplied in cylinders with a blue body plus a quartered white and blue top, at a pressure of 137 bar (1980 p.s.i.). The physical properties of these two gases at this pressure mean that, provided the room temperature is above 7°C, the nitrous oxide/oxygen ratio delivered remains at a constant and safe 50:50 (see p. 178).

Anaesthetic equipment

Apart from an adequate supply of nitrous oxide, oxygen and volatile agents, and a Boyle's machine, general anaesthesia should never be administered unless the following additional equipment is available.

1. All resuscitative drugs (within their expiry dates), syringes and needles necessary to manage any emergency (see Chapter 4). A Boyle's machine provides the necessary facility to deliver oxygen under pressure, should this be necessary.

2. Endotracheal and orotracheal tubes of sizes 3–9 mm.

3. Laryngoscope (Fig. 6.40).

4. McGill forceps (Fig. 6.41).

5. Catheter mount (Fig. 6.42).

6. Oropharyngeal airways of sizes 00–3 (Fig. 6.43) and nasopharyngeal airways of sizes 3–9 mm (see Fig. 6.44).

Intravenous general anaesthetic agents

The agent most commonly employed is the ultra short-acting barbiturate methohexitone (Brietal Sodium). The previously used agent thiopentone (Pentothal; Intraval Sodium) is now not favoured because of its greater tendency to produce laryngeal spasm and because it causes a severe irritant reaction if inadvertently injected extravascularly. Inadvertent intra-arterial injection of any barbiturate, particularly thiopentone, may produce dangerous vasospasm leading to gangrene.

The use of methohexitone in out-patient dental general anaesthesia is generally restricted to producing a

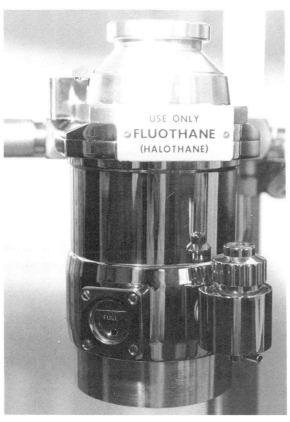

Fig. 6.38 *Halothane vaporizer.*

ture compensated and has a reliable concentration control which regulates the percentage content finally delivered to the patient (Figs 6.37 and 6.38).

The gas/vapour mixture is usually delivered to the patient by a Bain's circuit (Fig. 6.39) which consists of a reservoir bag close to the machine gas mixture outlet, a length of double-lumen corrugated tubing and a delivery mask (full-face or nasal). There is an expiratory valve positioned for convenience close to the anaesthetic machine, through which the expired gases are conveyed by a second flexible pipe to the atmosphere outside the operating area or to a scavenging system. This scavenging prevents pollution of the air in the surgical area with anaesthetic gases, which may produce toxic or teratogenic effects in exposed personnel, including spontaneous abortion in females. The machines have a built-in safety device to warn of oxygen supply failure, when a loud audible warning operates and the supply of other anaesthetic gases is automatically cut off. The patient then breathes atmospheric air.

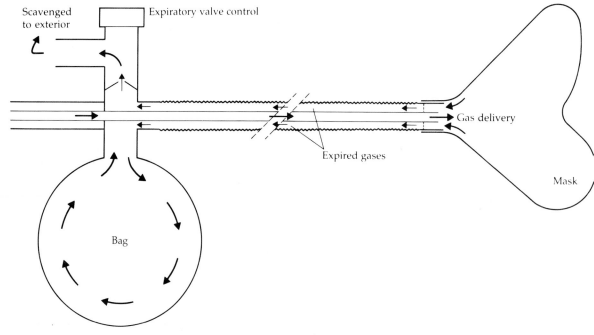

Scavenged to exterior

Expiratory valve control

Gas delivery

Expired gases

Mask

Bag

Fig. 6.39 *Bain's circuit.*

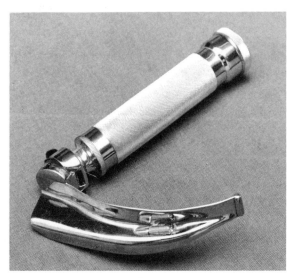

Fig. 6.40 *Laryngoscope.*

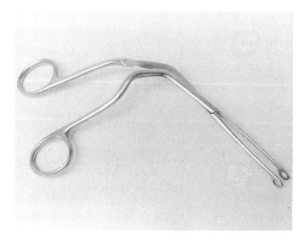

Fig. 6.41 *McGill forceps.*

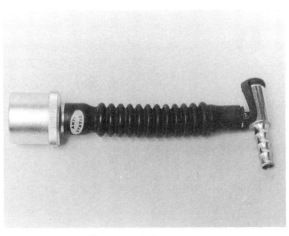

Fig. 6.42 *Catheter mount.*

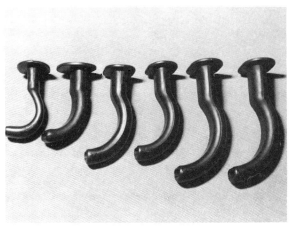

Fig. 6.43 *Oropharyngeal airways.*

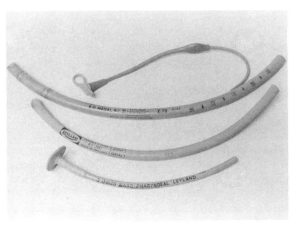

Fig. 6.44 *Nasopharyngeal tubes.*

rapid induction of anaesthesia, which is then maintained by inhalation agents based upon nitrous oxide and oxygen with a volatile agent.

Prolonged 'light' anaesthesia produced by repeatedly administering increments of methohexitone can be achieved, but the technique is not without danger. Barbiturates such as methohexitone are potent, potentially dangerous drugs with marked respiratory depressive effects which, over a prolonged period, can seriously impair ventilation of the patient. Furthermore, there is no analgesic effect from barbiturates, which may even increase pain sensitivity. The patient's movements as a reaction to pain make dental procedures difficult to perform. Attempting to abolish these reactions by increasing the level of analgesia with additional injections of methohexitone, inevitably produces general anaesthesia with loss of the patient's protective reflexes, and with dental work in the mouth this leads to serious hazard to the airway. Further, hypoventilation, which is readily produced by this agent, is a state which even the most experienced anaesthetist finds a difficult recognition and management problem. *Several deaths have occurred using the incremental methohexitone technique in dental practice, and whilst the absolute numbers may be small, it serves to emphasize that intravenous barbiturates are the most dangerous drugs available in dental anaesthesia.* Combining incremental methohexitone administration with powerful centrally acting intravenous analgesics—such as nalbuphine (Nubain)—has been advocated by some to overcome the lack of pain control afforded by methohexitone alone, but the combination of powerful drug 'cocktails' produces unpredictable depressive effects upon the cardiovascular and respiratory systems, which may provide a formula for disaster and must have little place, if any, in the current safe management of any dental out-patient. Far safer and effective sedation techniques are available which are equally acceptable to the majority of anxious patients.

Methohexitone should *not* be used for patients who suffer from epilepsy as it may precipitate fits, and as with all barbiturates, including methohexitone, must *not* be administered to those suffering from porphyria (Chapter 2).

Methohexitone is prepared as the soluble sodium salt and is supplied as a white hygroscopic powder in a multi-dose glass container. It is dissolved in sterile water to produce a 1% solution. Depression of the cardiovascular system is produced and there is reduced cardiac output with peripheral vasodilatation due to central depression of the vasomotor centre. There is a resultant fall in blood pressure. Similarly, there is a marked depressive effect on the respiratory system. Rapid injection may temporarily cause cessation of breathing (apnoea), and laryngospasm is not uncommon. Muscle relaxation is not produced by anaesthetic doses of methohexitone. Postanaesthetic nausea and vomiting are infrequent but hiccoughing is not uncommon. Recovery from anaesthesia is rapid compared to other barbiturates. The biotransformation and metabolism of the administered methohexitone are at the rate of 25% per hour.

Muscle relaxants

Muscle relaxants may be used in general anaesthesia to paralyse the muscles of respiration and larynx to facilitate intubation and to relax skeletal muscles, thus facilitating surgery. They are used predominantly for in-patient general anaesthesia. They are administered intravenously and are of two types: depolarizing and non-depolarizing.

Depolarizing muscle relaxants

The action of these drugs is to cause an initial depolarization at the neuromuscular junction resulting in muscle contraction, but repolarization is prevented and muscle relaxation is then produced. The initial depolarization and muscle contraction often lead to postanaesthetic muscle pain, termed Scoline pain, which subsides after a few days. Suxamethonium (Scoline: Anectine) is the only commonly used drug in this group. The paralysis lasts between 2 and 5 minutes and recovery is by metabolism of suxamethonium by serum pseudocholinesterase enzymes. In patients who lack pseudocholinesterases, the recovery from suxamethonium takes hours rather than minutes, necessitating artificial ventilation of the paralysed patient until the suxamethonium effects have worn off since there are no antagonists available. The absence of plasma cholinesterase may be genetically determined (Scoline sensitivity) or result from liver disease or burns (Chapter 4).

Non-depolarizing (competitive) muscle relaxants

These drugs block the action of acetylcholine released at neuromuscular junctions by occupying the receptors on the post-synaptic membrane. There is no initial depolarization or muscle contraction. The two most commonly used drugs in this group are alcuronium and pancuronium, which are based upon the classical action of curare. Gallamine, vecuronium, and atracurium are also in this group. The duration of action of this type of muscle relaxant is longer than the depolarizing type: alcuronium causes relaxation for approximately 20 minutes, pancuronium for 30 minutes. Newer agents such as atracurium

have advantages of metabolism independent of liver and kidneys.

Non-depolarizing muscle relaxants may be antagonized and their effects reversed by the use of anticholinesterases, such as neostigmine, which overcome or reverse the blockade by increasing the concentration of acetylcholine in the post-synaptic membrane. However, since anticholinesterases also produce bradycardia and an increase in salivary and bronchial secretion—effects mediated by increasing acetylcholine concentrations—atropine (which blocks muscarinic actions of acetylcholine) is given first before neostigmine is used.

Procedure for out-patient inhalation general anaesthesia (see Chapter 7 for in-patient procedures)

Most out-patient general anaesthetics are given for short operations upon children. These young patients may well be frightened and consideration must be given to the pleasant design of waiting areas. Children should be amused and occupied by playing with toys etc.

The pre-anaesthetic checks should have been carried out as given on page 156. Immediately prior to operation, all the required operative equipment should be available and sterilized ready for use. Necessary radiographs should be placed visible on a screen, and the patient's name and nature of the operation should be verified before anaesthesia commences. A check should be made that consent has indeed been obtained. If applicable, orthodontic appliances, dentures, etc. should be removed.

The very young do not tolerate intravenous injections well, and induction is most often achieved by inhalation methods. The young child is escorted into the surgery with a parent who may sit beside the child seated in the dental chair, or the child may sit on the parent's lap in the dental chair. Only the anaesthetist should talk to the child. Most anaesthetists have a personal, gentle form of talk to calm, soothe and reassure the patient, so that the strangeness of the equipment and situation is not frightening. Strange objects can be likened to familiar items in the child's repertoire. For example, the anaesthetic gas delivery pipe may be likened to a spaceman's breathing tube, and the gas may be described as 'magic wind'. Reluctance to inhale may be overcome by asking the child to blow the wind away gently, a process which inevitably leads to inhalation, yet comforts a frightened child. As the specific gravity of nitrous oxide is greater than that of air, the delivery tube from the anaesthetic machine need not be fitted with a mask. A high flow of pure nitrous oxide may be delivered into the anaesthetist's cupped hand held below the child's nose or mouth.

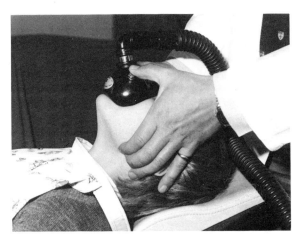

Fig. 6.45 *Using an anaesthetic face mask for a child to ensure patency of the airway.*

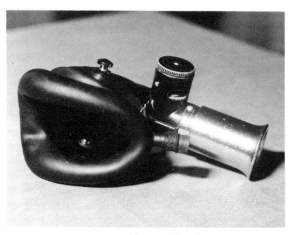

Fig. 6.47 *Goldman nasal mask.*

When the child becomes drowsy a face mask may be used to deliver the anaesthetic, and at this point the oxygen content is introduced at 30% minimum. As the reservoir bag distends and deflates with breathing (a visible sign of a patent airway), vapour agents such as halothane, enflurane or isoflurane may be slowly added into the mixture. The mask is held on to the child's face whilst the angle of the mandible is held forward and the patient's neck extended, thereby maintaining the patency of the airway (Fig. 6.45).

At this stage the parent should be escorted to the waiting room. The child is then laid onto the dental chair in a supine position, to prevent postural hypotension. A seat belt may be secured across the child's lap. Disabled children may most conveniently be stabilized for anaesthesia in the dental chair with the aid of a bean-bag (Fig. 6.46). The depth of anaesthesia is adequate for surgery when the breathing pattern becomes automatic, the eyelash reflex is lost and the pupils of the eyes are fixed and central.

When anaesthesia is adequate the face mask is changed for a nasal mask (Goldman mask—Fig. 6.47) and, with muscles relaxed by the vapour adjuvant, the mouth may be opened. When the anaesthetist indicates, a mouth prop is inserted. The rubber types (e.g. McKesson gag—Fig. 6.48) are less traumatic than the metal 'scissor' type.

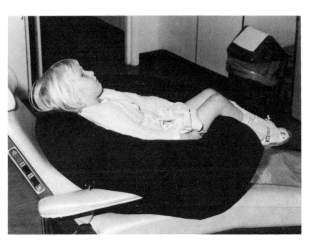

Fig. 6.46 *Use of a bean bag to stabilize small or disabled patients.*

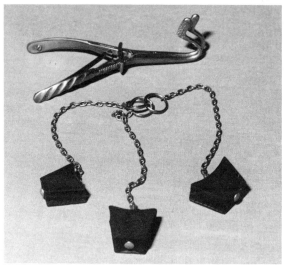

Fig. 6.48 *McKesson rubber props (below), and a metal mouth prop (above).*

A throat pack is carefully placed to protect the airway and to hold the tongue forwards without obstructing the airway. Gauze or sponge throat packs may be used for this purpose. The 'V' pack system is most efficient. Tooth removal (or other procedure) is then carried out by the operator.

Throughout the operation the anaesthetic reservoir bag is periodically observed as a check of efficient breathing by the patient as well as a check that the mask is making an efficient seal onto the face. Constant observation of the patient's chest movements and listening to the breathing pattern are necessary to detect respiratory obstruction.

As soon as the operation is completed, the anaesthetic is stopped and 100% oxygen is delivered for 2 minutes. The patient is turned onto one side in the tonsillar posi-

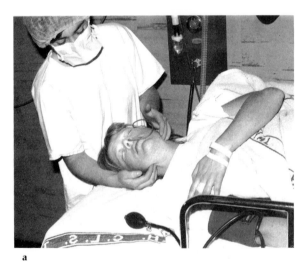

a

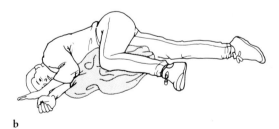

b

Fig. 6.49 *The tonsillar position for maintenance of the airway during recovery.* The postoperative period is the most dangerous time for the patient *since he can asphyxiate if the airway is not kept patent.*

tion (Fig. 6.49) so that fluid and debris fall forward out of the mouth and do not obstruct the airway. *The postoperative period is potentially hazardous unless the patient is carefully monitored to ensure the airway is patent.* The pack and prop are removed and the mandible is held forward to maintain the airway. An absorbent gauze pack held with a cord hanging out of the mouth, so that the pack can readily be removed if necessary, is placed over any bleeding tooth sockets in such a way that the airway is not obstructed. The patient is transferred to the recovery room where, still in the tonsillar position, recovery is supervised by a trained supervisor. Children may be carried from the operating room to the recovery area in a head-down attitude; adults may be transferred by lifting onto a stretcher. A pillow should be placed beneath the shoulder to promote a head-down attitude of the patient, lying on one side. This ensures that blood or saliva drains from the mouth and does not hazard the airway. When the patient awakes, all packs must be removed. Patients are discharged home with their escorts only when able to walk unaided.

Postoperative instructions regarding care of the surgical area, control of haemorrhage and the procedure to be adopted in the event of an emergency should be given to the escort. A prepared information sheet is the most convenient way to confirm this information (Figs. 6.50 and 6.51). Practitioners should offer a contract telephone number.

Throughout the anaesthetic and recovery periods, great care must be taken to ensure the patient comes to no harm. The medical state of the patient is primarily the responsibility of the anaesthetist, but the remainder of the patient's welfare is the joint responsibility of the surgeon and anaesthetist. Crushing of the patient's lips, tongue or cheeks with gags or forcep handles, and damage to teeth and crowns must be consciously avoided. It is all too easy for a patient's limb to fall to one side of the dental chair unobserved and be bruised or crushed by the operator's movements or by movements of the dental chair. The design of the dental chair and surrounding equipment chosen for general anaesthesia should take these possibilities into account (see also Chapter 8).

During induction of inhalation anaesthesia, and during recovery, it must be remembered that the auditory sense is the last to disappear and the first to return. Noisy preoperative or clearing-up procedures are magnified such that seemingly quiet noises become deafening for the patient. Stormy induction or recovery results. Further, conversation between operator and staff will be vividly remembered. One must be cautious of one's remarks during these periods when the patient *appears* unconscious.

BRISTOL DENTAL HOSPITAL
INSTRUCTIONS TO PATIENTS AFTER
TOOTH EXTRACTION

After a tooth has been extracted the socket will usually bleed for a
short time. This bleeding stops because of the formation of a healthy
clot of blood in the tooth socket. These clots are easily disturbed
and if this happens more bleeding will occur. To avoid disturbance
of the clot please follow these instructions.

1. After leaving the hospital do not rinse out your mouth for 24 hours,
   unless you have been told otherwise by the dentist.

2. Do not disturb the clot in the socket with your tongue or your
   fingers.

3. For the rest of the day take only food which requires no chewing.

4. Do not chew on the affected side for at least 3 days.

5. Avoid unneccessary talking, excitement or exercise.

6. Do not take any alcoholic drinks or very hot drinks for the rest
   of the day.

7. Do not sit in front of a fire or in over-heated rooms.

If the tooth socket continues to bleed after you have left the Dental
Hospital, do not be alarmed as much of the liquid which appears to be
blood is saliva. Make a small pad from a clean handkerchief or cotton
wool, place over the socket and close the teeth firmly on to it.
Keep up the pressure for 15–30 minutes. If the bleeding still does
not stop, seek dental or medical advice (Dental Hospital or Royal
Infirmary).

Fig. 6.50 *Instructions to patients after tooth extraction (to be given to patient or patient's escort).*

BRISTOL DENTAL HOSPITAL

CARE OF YOUR MOUTH AFTER 24 HOURS (Following tooth extraction)

Your mouth will heal more quickly if you keep it clean and use <u>hot
salt mouth baths</u>. Dissolve a teaspoonful of table salt in a tumbler
of hot water (about the same temperature as a hot cup of tea). Take
a mouthful and tilt your head so that the hot salt-water bathes the
affected area. After about $\frac{1}{4}$ minute, spit out and repeat the bathing
until you have used the whole tumblerful. If possible, the hot salt
mouth baths should be used three times daily for three days, after meals.

Brush your teeth with toothpaste in the normal way. The affected area
can be cleaned by wiping with cotton wool moistened with the hot salt-water
if it is too tender to be brushed.

Discomfort and mild pain are common after tooth extraction and may be
relieved by the 'pain killer' which you would normally use. Paracetamol
tablets BP, one or two every four hours, are recommended for adults.
Children may take Paracetamol syrup, the dose depending on their age
(follow instructions on the container.).

You should seek the advice of the Dental Hospital or Royal Infirmary if
you have pain which is severe or persists for more than 24 hours.

Fig. 6.51 *Care of mouth after extractions.*

Complications of inhalational or intravenous general anaesthesia (see also Chapter 4)

Airway obstruction

This situation rapidly leads to hypoxia which, if sufficient, causes cardiac arrest and brain damage or death. Obstruction is detected by failure of the reservoir bag on the anaesthetic machine to inflate and deflate regularly. The patient will be seen to use the accessory muscles of respiration. Such muscular activity produces a typical 'see-saw' type of chest movement when, as the patient attempts to inspire, the chest is drawn in rather than expanding. Cyanosis may eventually be detected. The cause might be one of the following.

1. Improper placement of the throat pack or allowing the mandible to become retruded and the tongue to fall against the posterior pharyngeal wall. The remedy is to correct the throat packing and to hold the mandible forward whilst extending the neck to reopen the airway.

2. Laryngeal spasm—sometimes encountered following methohexitone induction or due to irritation from blood or secretions which have leaked around the throat pack. The combination of barbiturate laryngeal sensitivity *and* irritation, which includes normal operative manipulation, makes laryngeal spasm likely. Management is to stop the operation, administer oxygen and suck out the mouth and/or airway. Should the spasm fail to relax, endotracheal intubation following muscle relaxation with suxamethonium is indicated.

3. Inhalation of foreign objects. If the obstruction cannot be readily removed, this eventuality requires immediate expert hospital management. Oxygenation of the patient is essential—by tracheostomy if necessary, such as when a foreign body is impacted at the level of the vocal chords.

Respiratory depression

This may be due to excessive anaesthetic and is corrected by administering 100% oxygen via a full-face mask. The expiratory valve on the mask is closed and, by compressing the reservoir bag, forced ventilation of the patient is performed until normal breathing restarts.

Hyperventilation

Hyperventilation due to anxiety during induction causes excessive carbon dioxide to be discharged from the blood. The carbon dioxide drive to the respiratory centre is, therefore, temporarily lost, and breathing stops. This situation soon corrects itself spontaneously.

Light anaesthesia

Light anaesthesia may cause a partly narcotized patient to breath-hold as a result of fear. As anaesthesia deepens, automatic breathing ensues.

Cardiac arrest (see Chapter 4)

Adverse reactions to anaesthetics (Table 6.1 and Chapter 4)

Table 6.1
Possible adverse reactions to anaesthetic, sedative and related drugs

Drug	Possible adverse reaction
Benzodiazepine	Unmask depression (weepiness and sadness)
	Exacerbate glaucoma
Opiates	Nausea
Droperidol	Anxiety
	Extrapyramidal effects
Atropine	Dry mouth
	Exacerbates glaucoma
Hyoscine	Dry mouth
	Exacerbates glaucoma
	Confusion in the elderly

Anaesthetic and related agents

Drug	Possible adverse reaction
Suxamethonium	Muscle pains—especially if patient exercises postoperatively
	Rarely—malignant hyperthermia
	Rarely—prolonged apnoea
Tubocurare	Hypotension/bronchospasm
Halothane	Shivering
	Hepatitis
	Arrhythmias
	Rarely—malignant hyperthermia
Enflurane	Shivering
	Convulsions
	Rarely—malignant hyperthermia
Nitrous oxide	Transient deafness from diffusion of gas into the middle ear, rarely
Opiates	Respiratory depression
Naloxone	Hypertension
Methohexitone	Convulsions
	Laryngeal spasm
	Respiratory depression
Diazepam	Thrombophlebitis
	Respiratory depression if given rapidly
Midazolam	Respiratory depression if given rapidly

Intravenous injections

Intravenous injections may be necessary for:

(a) induction of general anaesthesia prior to maintenance with gas/vapour/oxygen mixtures;
(b) sedation of a very anxious patient, e.g. to allow dental treatment;
(c) administration of therapeutic drugs such as intravenous antibiotics or in the management of emergencies, e.g. administration of steroids for the management of a steroid crisis or anaphylaxis.

The most common sites used for intravenous injections are the veins on the *lateral* aspect of the cubital fossa at the bend of the elbow, or the veins on the back of the hand. The large veins of the cubital fossa are generally more suitable for administering intravenous sedation agents which may be irritant and cause thrombophlebitis of the small veins of the back of the hand. The anatomy of the veins of the cubital fossa is variable, but a common pattern is illustrated in Figure 6.52.

The site for injection must be carefully chosen. The selected vein may be clearly visible beneath the skin but in any event should be palpated to check for the absence of pulsations, thereby avoiding intra-arterial injection. A butterfly needle (Fig. 6.53) may be used if it is desired to maintain access to the circulation over more than a very short period of time; for example, a butterfly needle inserted into a vein on the back of the hand is a common method of administering methohexitone for rapid induction of general anaesthesia. The needle is left in situ during operation as a ready means of access for the administration of emergency drugs if this becomes necessary.

Syringes for intravenous use often have an eccentrically placed nozzle which enables the syringe needle to lie parallel to the skin surface above the vein to be entered. The veins may be deliberately dilated by the application of a tourniquet or sphygmomanometer cuff at a pressure intermediate between the systolic and diastolic blood pressures, to make venepuncture easier. The skin is then cleansed with an antiseptic such as an isopropyl alcohol wipe (Fig. 6.54), and with the needle bevel facing upwards and the skin slightly tensed distally over the vein, skin penetration is made approximately 2 cm distal to the intended point of entry of the needle into the vein (Fig. 6.55). Aspiration of blood confirms correct positioning of the needle and *after* removal of the tourniquet the injection proceeds *slowly* with the syringe held parallel to

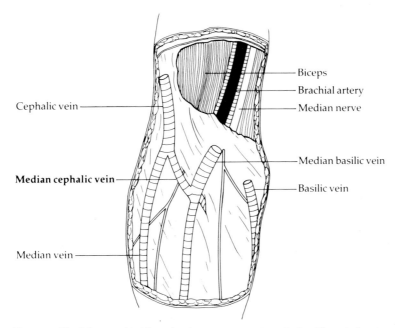

Cephalic vein

Median cephalic vein

Median vein

Biceps
Brachial artery
Median nerve

Median basilic vein

Basilic vein

Fig. 6.52 *The right antecubital fossa showing a common pattern of veins. The cephalic vein is very suitable for intravenous injections.*

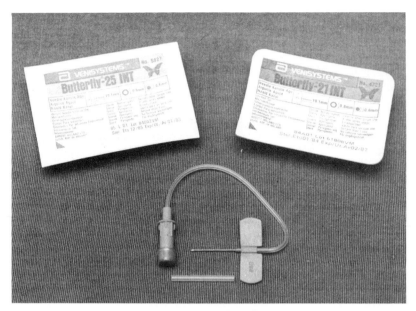

Fig. 6.53 *Butterfly needle.*

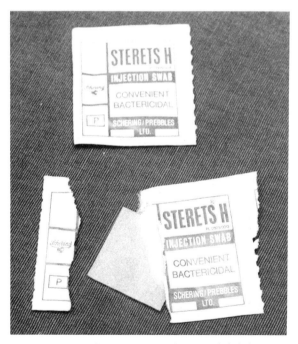

Fig. 6.54 *Skin preparation swab (isopropyl alcohol).*

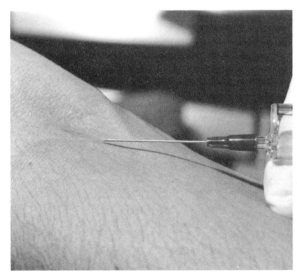

Fig. 6.55 *Skin penetration: syringe and needle are at about 28° to the skin surface.*

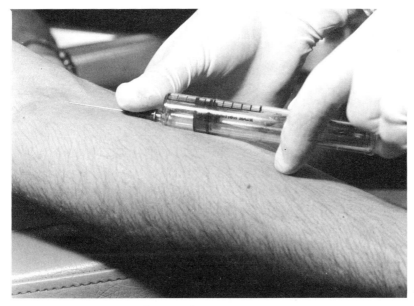

Fig. 6.56 *Intravenous injection.*

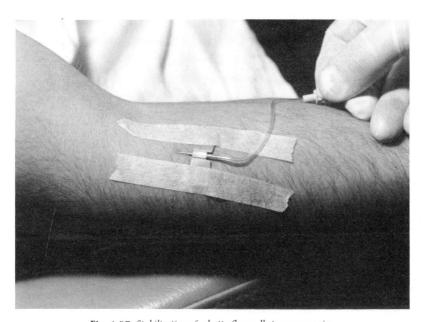

Fig. 6.57 *Stabilization of a butterfly needle in an arm vein.*

the arm and stabilized with the left hand (right-handed operators—Fig. 6.56). Constant observation is required to detect any inadvertent extravascular injection being made. Butterfly needles should be stabilized by the use of micropore tape across the butterfly wings parallel to, and either side of, the needle (Fig. 6.57). After needle removal, the injection site should be compressed for a few moments to arrest haemorrhage and then covered with an adhesive dressing.

Drugs for intravenous sedation

Assessment of fitness to receive intravenous sedation is by the same criteria used for general anaesthesia (see page 156).

Diazepam

Diazepam is a benzodiazepine anxiolytic agent which has been used for dental sedation since 1961. It is a colourless crystalline powder, insoluble in water, and available in amber-coloured glass ampoules as a 5 mg/ml solution dissolved in a propylene glycol (Valium (Roche) Fig. 6.58) or in clear glass ampoules as a solution dissolved in soya-bean oil emulsified in water (Diazemuls (Kabi-Vitrum) Fig. 6.59).

A propylene glycol preparation of diazepam should not be mixed with other drugs or diluted, otherwise the diazepam precipitates out of solution. Furthermore, propylene glycol is irritant to the delicate intimal lining of veins, and intravenous use is occasionally associated with pain on injection and sometimes phlebitis or thrombo-

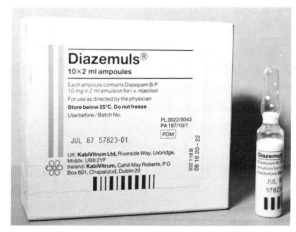

Fig. 6.59 *Diazemuls—for intravenous injection.*

phlebitis of the injected vein. Avoiding injections into small veins, especially those of the back of the hand, reduces, but does not eliminate, the incidence of these postoperative complications. Diazemuls, however, does not cause thrombophlebitis.

The kinetic and biotransformation properties of propylene glycol or soya-bean emulsion preparations of diazepam are similar. Following intravenous administration, there is not a linear relationship between the dose given and the plasma level achieved. Further the plasma level does not correlate directly with the therapeutic effect: there is great individual variability in response to intravenous benzodiazepines. The dosage required for sedation is determined only by slow administration of increments of diazepam to allow dose titration of an individual response to produce the desired level of sedation. After a few minutes, most patients become placid and drowsy, with slurring of speech. The satisfactory dosage end-point for sedation with diazepam is judged by three signs:

(a) ptosis (drooping of the eyelid—Verril's sign—Fig. 6.60),

(b) slurred speech,

(c) delayed response to answering questions.

Once sedated, local anaesthesia (analgesia) is used to control pain in the normal way. The amnesic effect of diazepam usually makes this an experience which is not remembered and therefore overcomes needle phobia. After 10–15 minutes the patient is usually drowsy but can be aroused and found to be comfortable and co-operative. Apparently unresponding patients should not

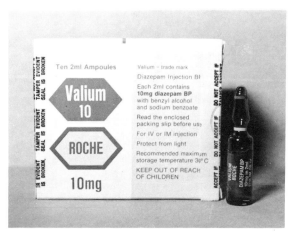

Fig. 6.58 *Diazepam for injection.*

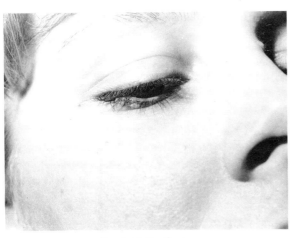

Fig. 6.60 *Verril's sign.*

have the maximal sedation dose for adults of 20 mg exceeded under any circumstances as a useful sedative effect is unlikely and complications such as respiratory depression become more likely. *Benzodiazepines, such as diazepam, if given in sufficient dosage, will produce general anaesthesia.* The average adult dosage for sedation is 10–15 mg, but for particularly susceptible patients, notably

the elderly, even 5 mg may be sufficient to produce *general* anaesthesia. It is for this reason that injections should be made very slowly indeed, and the dose/response carefully titrated. It is also for this reason that not less than 4 hours preoperatively the patient should have only a very light meal. If general anaesthesia does result inadvertently, inhalation of vomit will not present such a serious management problem as it would had the patient eaten recently.

Once injected, diazepam disappears from the circulation, first by a rapid phase of tissue redistribution, followed by a very prolonged elimination phase. Diazepam is metabolized however, mainly by the liver, into several sedating compounds (Fig. 6.61), the most important of which is desmethyldiazepam. Whilst the elimination half-life of the injected diazepam is biphasic and between 24 and 48 hours, the desmethyldiazepam has the much longer corresponding figure of 51–120 hours. The very prolonged recovery time from intravenous diazepam sedation is due to the long elimination time of desmethyl-diazepam. Since these metabolites enter breast milk, mothers who breast feed should not receive diazepam.

Postoperatively, the patient should rest for at least 1 hour until sufficiently recovered to leave the surgery with an escort. The patient must be escorted home by a re-

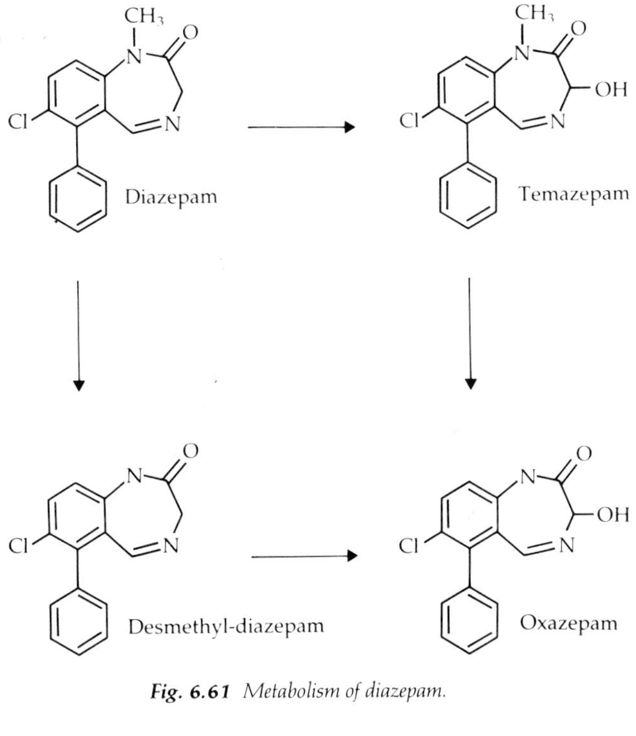

Fig. 6.61 *Metabolism of diazepam.*

sponsible adult and not permitted to drive, make important decisions, or perform any other responsible duties, such as working with machinery, for at least 24 hours or even longer if feeling drowsy. Exceptionally, this period could be for up to 5 days postoperatively.

Diazepam has no analgesic properties, but produces a feeling of well-being and dissociation from the surroundings. Amnesia is marked. An operating time of up to 1 hour is usually achieved. Diazepam has respiratory depressant effects which are potentiated by centrally acting opiate-based drugs such as pentazocine, morphine, pethidine and nalbuphine. Very rarely, diazepam alone causes apnoea, especially if injected rapidly, but a real danger exists with drug combinations, especially in patients with respiratory disease. Alcohol potentiates the depressant effects of diazepam and it should be avoided in the 12 hours preoperatively and for at least 24 hours postoperatively. Drug interactions otherwise are rare with diazepam, *except* for cimetidine, an agent used to control peptic ulceration. This drug delays the elimination of diazepam and may prolong recovery. It is a commonly prescribed drug which should be asked about specifically.

The sedative effects of diazepam can be reversed, at least partially by flumazenil (p. 116).

Midazolam

Midazolam (Hypnovel (Roche) Fig, 6.62) is a benzodiazepine suitable for dental out-patient sedation. Like diazepam, it has poor analgesic properties and is used in conjunction with conventional local anaesthesia (analgesia). The unique chemical structure of midazolam confers a number of physicochemical properties which dis-

tinguish it from other benzodiazepines. It has great advantages over diazepam in that it is soluble in water, thereby allowing a parenteral formulation which avoids troublesome solvents such as propylene glycol; it has a more rapid onset of action; and it has a more rapid rate of recovery without the disadvantage of sedative metabolites.

It is presented as a sterile liquid in colourless glass ampoules which contain 10 mg of midazolam in 5 ml of aqueous solution. Midazolam causes little or no local irritation by intravenous administration. Like all benzodiazepines, it has anxiolytic, hypnotic, anticonvulsant, muscle relaxant and anterograde amnesic effects. The amnesic effects of midazolam often, but not always, parallel the degree of drowsiness produced. Some respiratory depression is caused via a central nervous system effect which, as with diazepam, may manifest as apnoea. However, apnoea seems to be related to rapid rates of injection which, therefore, should be avoided. With normal dosages, cardiovascular effects are minimal, with a 5% and 10% drop in systolic and diastolic blood pressures respectively, and an 18% increase in heart rate.

Like diazepam, the depressive effects of midazolam are dangerously intensified by alcohol and by centrally acting opiate-derived analgesics. Such combinations are best avoided. Patients should avoid alcohol in the 12-hour preoperative period and for 24 hours afterwards. Lactating mothers should not breast feed for at least 4 hours after receiving midazolam since the drug enters the milk.

Biotransformation of midazolam (Fig. 6.63) is carried out by the hepatic microsomal oxidative enzyme systems to metabolites which have only minor pharmacological effects, in contrast to the powerful effects of the metabolites of diazepam.

Onset of the clinical effects of intravenously administered midazolam is rapid due to its high lipid solubility and rapid entry into brain tissue. Recovery is equally rapid due to the high rate of metabolic clearance and rapid elimination, but although the duration of activity is short, working times in excess of 30 minutes are produced.

The average intravenous dose required for sedation is 0.07 mg/kg body weight, with a usual total administration of between 2.5 mg and 7.5 mg for the average adult patient. The clinical effects of midazolam, again like all benzodiazepines, are variable from individual to individual and even in the same patient treated at different times. At the desirable end-point, the patient will be drowsy with slurred speech, response to command will be maintained and laryngeal reflexes will be present. Very slow administration of small amounts (0.25–0.5 ml mida-

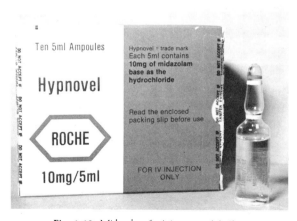

Fig. 6.62 *Midazolam for intravenous injection.*

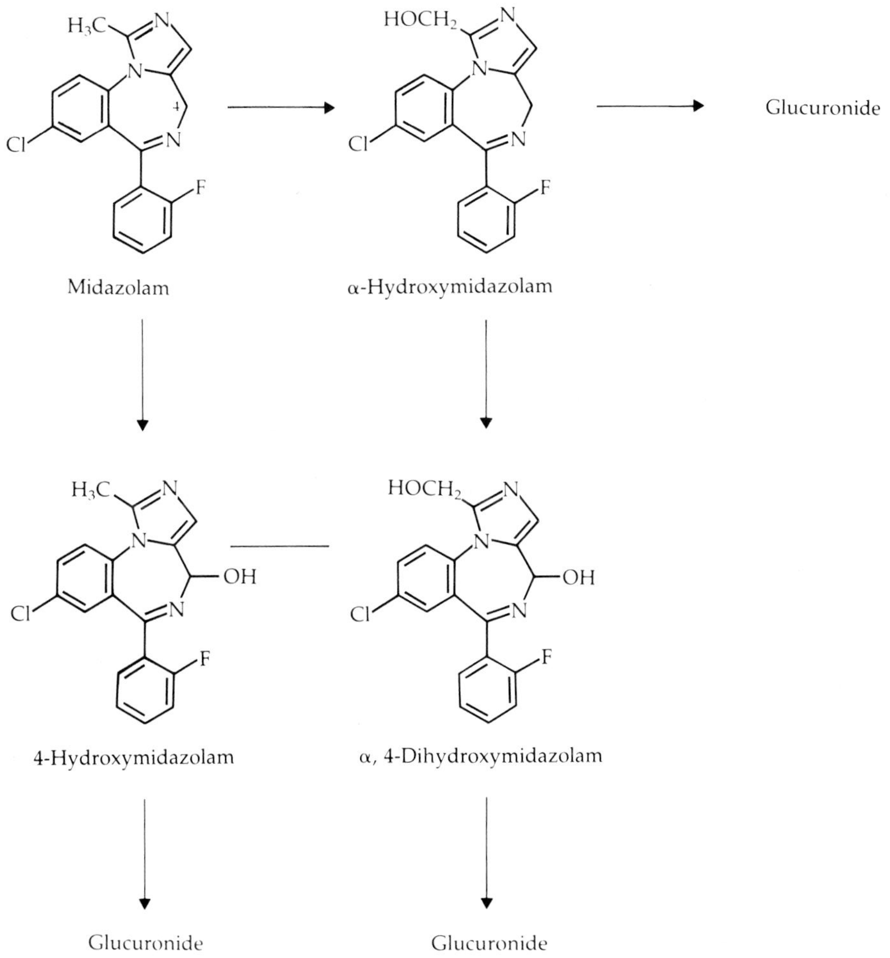

Fig. 6.63 *Metabolism of midazolam.*

zolam solution) over 3–5 minutes is necessary to titrate the response of the patient. Ptosis is *not* an end-point indication for effective sedation with midazolam; indeed, when this occurs it indicates onset of general anaesthesia.

However, midazolam does have a wider margin of safety than diazepam in that inadvertent general anaesthesia is less likely provided ptosis is not sought. The elderly are particularly susceptible to the effects of benzodiazepines: a total dose of 2.5 mg midazolam is often more than adequate for sedation. Although patients sedated with midazolam appear much less sleepy than with diazepam, operators used to using diazepam should not attempt to produce the same degree of sleepiness with midazolam since otherwise overdosing will occur. Flumazenil can at least partially reverse the sedative effects of midazolam (p. 116).

When the patient has recovered sufficiently to leave the surgery, by resting for at least 1 hour, the fact that he or she is likely to have impaired reflexes should be explained to the escort, who should also be instructed to ensure that the patient avoids driving or controlling machinery or making important decisions or drinking alcohol for at least 24 hours postoperatively. Due to the more powerful amnesic effects of midazolam compared with diazepam, it is important that the special postoperative instructions are given both to the patient and to the adult escort.

Orally administered benzodiazepines

The oral route for administering drugs such as diazepam or temazepam for sedation during dental treatment has not met with great success. The variable absorption from the gastrointestinal tract coupled with the variable response to plasma levels of drug have often meant either failure due to inadequate sedation or dangerous overdosing. Children may anomalously become hyperactive rather than sedated by diazepam.

Recent trials with sublingual temazepam have shown that effective plasma levels of this drug, equivalent to intravenous injection, may be obtained within 40 minutes of exposure, but this interesting technique has yet to be justified as reliably useful in dental practice.

Relative analgesia

Relative analgesia utilizes the analgesic and mild amnesic effects of a mixture of nitrous oxide, oxygen and air. The technique was first described by Harry Langa, an American dentist, in 1968. It has proved highly effective for the management of some anxious dental patients and is particularly successful with children. Many procedures may be completed without additional analgesia, but some may also require local analgesia injections.

Relative analgesia is remarkably safe and simple, with very rapid recovery, well suited to ambulant dental patients. The contraindications for relative analgesia are few, but include severe emphysema, chronic bronchitis and open pulmonary tuberculosis. The common cold (coryza) is also a contraindication as the nasal congestion makes delivery of the gases difficult.

A special delivery apparatus is required (Fig. 6.64) and care must be taken to scavenge expired nitrous oxide from the operating room to the exterior when relative analgesia is in use since chronic exposure of dental personnel to small amounts of nitrous oxide has been linked with disease (Chapter 10).

Four zones of general analgesia have been described with the use of nitrous oxide, each dependent upon the percentage of nitrous oxide administered. Zones 1 and 2 represent 'relative analgesia': beyond that is general anaesthesia.

Zones of analgesia

1. *Moderate analgesia (6–25% nitrous oxide)*. The patient feels euphoric, with a sometimes pleasant tingling feeling in the mouth, fingers and toes. There is some sensory loss involving touch, hearing and peripheral proprioception, and visual acuity may be impaired.

2. *Dissociation analgesia (26–45% nitrous oxide)*. In this zone there are definite signs of the effects of nitrous oxide in which the patient feels detached from the surround-

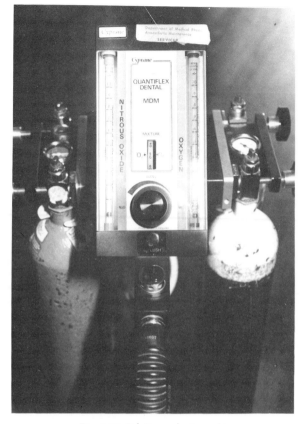

Fig. 6.64 *Relative analgesia machine.*

ings, light-headed and has poor concentration with some amnesia. Conversation with the patient is possible, and there is positive response to instructions. Analgesia in this zone is good, and it is the ideal state for relative analgesia.

The correct depth of analgesia must be constantly judged by assessing whether the patient is able to maintain sensible verbal contact with the operator, respond to instructions and hold his mouth open without the use of props.

Zones 3 and 4 are to be avoided and do not represent relative analgesia—rather general anaesthesia.

3. *Analgesic anaesthesia (46–65% nitrous oxide)*. At this stage the patient is entering a state of general anaesthesia and this is *not* relative analgesia. The patient shows loss of conversational sense and fails to respond to instructions such as to hold the mouth open.

4. *Light anaesthesia (66–80% nitrous oxide)*. With this concentration of nitrous oxide, general anaesthesia ensues.

Technique of relative analgesia

Though machines of different types and manufacture are available for RA, they all possess common requirements for an effective and safe technique, particularly for 'fail-safe' devices such that, should the oxygen supply fail, the nitrous oxide supply is automatically cut off and a valve in the nasal mask permits the patient to breathe room air. The oxygen flow rate in the delivery system cannot be reduced to a level less than 3 litres per minute, and nitrous oxide will only flow after the oxygen supply is at least at this minimal rate. Flow rates of nitrous oxide and oxygen are readily visible at any time on flow meters incorporated into the machine. The level of nitrous oxide being delivered is controlled by an accurate graduated mixing valve or flow control. The gases are delivered by a nasal mask (Fig. 6.65).

Patients, especially children, should be completely familiarized with the relative analgesia equipment before treatment is started. In particular, fear of the nasal mask should be overcome and patients should be taught to position this themselves. The expected feelings of tingling or light-headedness should be carefully explained so that alarm is not introduced to an already frightened patient. With time and care, even the most unwilling patient may be brought to have confidence in the technique, which will then often be requested at future appointments. It may be wise to devote at least a session to this initial familiarization, the patient sitting comfort-ably in the dental chair. The first treatment session should be short and simple.

Before commencing a treatment session, the regularly serviced apparatus should first be checked to ensure it has an adequate oxygen and nitrous oxide supply. When the machine is turned on, oxygen will automatically flow at the predetermined level of 3 litres per minute, and the reservoir bag should be allowed to fill with oxygen. The patient, with assistance if necessary, positions the nasal mask and is advised to breathe normally *through the nose*. The oxygen flow rate is increased until the reservoir bag fills, but does not overdistend as the patient exhales. Increments of 10% nitrous oxide are then introduced into the mixture at 1-minute intervals until the patient reaches the second zone of analgesia. The percentage of nitrous oxide required will vary but, by slowly titrating the patient's response, the correct level will be determined. The patient should *not* receive more than 40% nitrous oxide under any circumstances. High gas flow rates will be required if the patient mouth breathes. The dental operation begins when the correct level of sedation is achieved. The patient continues to breathe the final nitrous oxide/oxygen mixture, but must be constantly observed during treatment to detect oversedation. Failure of the patient to respond to instructions or to hold the mouth open is a sign of oversedation and the nitrous oxide level should be reduced immediately. At the end of sedation, the patient should breathe 100% oxygen for 2 minutes (see page 168).

After a further 15 minutes breathing air, the patient should be able to leave the surgery. An escort is not essential for a normal adult patient.

FURTHER READING

Allen W. A. (1981). Enflurane for dental extractions. *Br. dent. J.*, **151**: 51–53.

Barer M. R., McAllen M. K. (1982). Hypersensitivity to local anaesthetics: a direct challenge test with lignocaine for definitive diagnosis. *Br. med. J.*, **284**: 1229–1230.

Barker I., Bulchart D. G. M., Gibson J. *et al.* (1986). IV sedation for conservative dentistry. *Br. J. Anaesth.*, **58**: 371–377.

Cathermole R. W., Verghese C., Blair I. J. *et al.* (1986). Isoflurane and halothane for outpatient dental anaesthesia in children. *Br. J. Anaesth.*, **58**: 385–389.

Cawson R. A., Curson I., Whittington D. R. (1983). The hazards of dental local anaesthetics. *Br. dent. J.*, **154**: 253–257.

Dundee J. W. *et al.* (1980). Midazolam: a water-soluble benzodiazepine. *Anaesthesia*, **35**: 454–458.

Editorial (1980). Halothane and hepatitis. *Lancet*, **i**: 24–25.

Gustanis J. F., Peterson L. J. (1981). An alternative method of mandibular nerve block. *J. Am. Dent. Ass.*, **103**: 22–26.

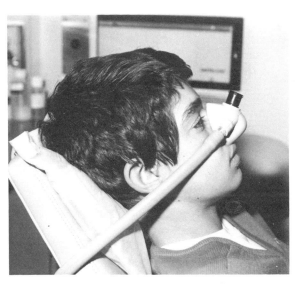

Fig. 6.65 *Administration of relative analgesia.*

Lindsay S. J. E., Yates J. A. (1985). The effectiveness of oral diazepam in anxious child dental patients. *Br dent. J.,* **159**: 149–153.

McGimpsie J. G. *et al.* (1983). Midazolam in dentistry. *Br. dent. J.,* **155**: 47–50.

Seymour R. A. (1985). Prescribing analgesics. *Br. dent. J.,* **159**: 177–181.

Scully C. (1985). *Handbook for Hospital Dental Surgeons.* London: British Dental Journal.

Scully C., Cawson R. A. (1987). *Medical problems in dentistry,* 2nd edn. Bristol: Wright.

Woolgrave J. (1983). Pain, perception and patient management. *Br. dent. J.,* **154**: 243–246.

Wylie Report (1981). *Brit. dent. J.,* **151**: 385–388.

Perioperative management of the dental patient having surgery

Virtually any patient awaiting operation, however apparently trivial the procedure may be, has some anxiety. This anxiety tends to be greater in the very young, in those who have had previous unpleasant hospital experiences, and when general anaesthesia is to be used.

Much of the anxiety can be reduced by careful, confident counselling by staff with full explanation of what is going to happen (Chapter 1). Written information can help supplement this, as can discussion with another patient who has successfully undergone a similar operation recently.

Consent for surgery

It is obligatory that informed consent is obtained from every patient before beginning *any* surgical procedure. Consent is best obtained in writing, particularly when the administration of sedative or general anaesthetic drugs is involved. The exact nature of the consent required varies from country to country depending on local medico-legal factors (Table 7.1), but the basis of informed consent does not alter. *Patients must have a good understanding of their condition, the treatment options available, the most appropriate treatment plan in their individual cases, and the inherent and recognized complications of treatment as well as the sequelae of not proceeding with treatment.* For instance, the patient presenting with an impacted wisdom tooth should be told the likelihood of the tooth giving rise to problems such as infection or damage to adjacent teeth; given an opinion on whether it should be removed or retained; and be made aware of the recognized complications of surgery, such as injury to the inferior alveolar or lingual nerve. It is only after being given this information that the patient can make a balanced judgement and decision whether or not to proceed with surgery.

Table 7.1 ✓
Consent to treatment (UK)

Age of consent	16 years If patient is 16–18 and living at home it is prudent to inform parents also.
Implied consent	Consent to treatment is implied if the patient does not refuse after the practitioner states the treatment he/she intends to give.
Verbal consent	The general type of consent used for most outpatient routine dental treatment given to the fully conscious patient.
Written consent	Operations or general anaesthetics (including intravenous sedation) should only be carried out if informed written consent has been given by the patient or parent/guardian.

A sample of a commonly used consent form is shown in Figure 7.1. Some centres also provide information sheets to help counsel patients in the various procedures involved and sequelae that may follow.

Patients who are to be nursed postoperatively in an intensive care ward, or who are to have a tracheostomy or intermaxillary fixation (their jaws fixed temporarily together), *must* be warned preoperatively.

PREOPERATIVE PREPARATION FOR IN-PATIENTS

Preoperative assessment and investigation

The extent of preoperative assessment and investigation will depend on the nature of the procedure proposed. For example, a patient requiring the simple extraction of a

(i) CONSENT

I .... hereby consent to the
                                given name   surname
following operation(s) ....
                                                              specify operation(s)
being performed upon ....
                                                              * relationship to patient
The nature and effect of the above operation(s) have been explained to me by

Dr. .... I also consent to such further emergency
operative procedures as may be found necessary to be performed during the course of
the operation(s) stated above.

In conjunction with the above-stated operation(s), I consent to the administration of such
anaesthetics as may be considered by the anaesthetist to be necessary or advisable, with the
exception of

....
                              state 'none' or type of anaesthesia
Dated this.. day of . 19 ....

Signed .... *Relationship to the Patient ....

Signature of Witness ....

Fig. 7.1 *Consent form.*

single tooth will need quite different management from a patient undergoing extensive jaw surgery.

The basis of preoperative assessment is the taking of an adequate medical history and careful examination and investigations where required (Chapters 2 and 3). There are few absolute contraindications to surgical treatment, but the treatment plan must be tailored to take into consideration the patient's general medical condition. For patients suffering from significant medical conditions, especially cardiac, respiratory, endocrine, renal and haematological conditions (Chapter 4), consultation with their treating physician should be sought.

In healthy young patients with no relevant medical history, minor oral surgical procedures may be undertaken under local analgesia without the need for laboratory investigations (Chapter 6). However, patients who are to be submitted to a more major procedure or to inpatient treatment under general anaesthesia or sedation, or those who are elderly or who have a relevant medical history, may need some basic investigations. These investigations include the following (see also Chapter 3; Table 7.2).

1. General medical examination, including especially cardiovascular and respiratory physical examination: temperature, pulse, blood pressure and weight measurement, auscultation and percussion of the chest and abdominal palpation.

2. Urine analysis with particular attention to the presence of protein or glucose.

3. A full blood examination reporting haemoglobin concentration and the number and quality of red cells, white cells and platelets.

These investigations should detect any relevant occult medical disorders which will alter either the surgical or anaesthetic management.

The following additional investigations may be indicated.

4. A sickle cell test result should be obtained for all black patients (Chapter 2).

5. An ECG when there is evidence of cardiovascular abnormalities, or in the older patient—who may have undiagnosed ischaemic heart disease.

6. A chest x-ray and respiratory function tests when there are respiratory abnormalities present.

7. Urea and electrolyte measurements for patients with renal disorders or those taking antihypertensive medications.

8. Liver function tests when liver disease or excess alcohol intake is known or suspected.

9. Assessment of haemostasis if the history is suggestive of a bleeding disorder or when there is liver disease (Chapters 2 and 3).

10. Screening for HBsAg and HIV, after counselling, in appropriate cases (Chapter 2).

11. When there is a possibility that blood loss will be significant, the patient's blood should be grouped and an appropriate volume of blood cross-matched for possible transfusion.

When surgery is elective and the need for blood transfusion is anticipated, an autologous blood transfusion may be prepared. This involves the drawing of a unit of blood from the patient 10 and 3 days preoperatively. At the time of operation the patient is transfused with his or her own blood. This technique avoids the problems asso-

Table 7.2
Preoperative investigations for dental in-patients

Investigation	When indicated
Routine investigations	
Physical examination ⎫	
Urinalysis ⎬	All patients
Haemoglobin level ⎭	
Investigations that may be required	
Sickle test	Black patients
Electrocardiogram (ECG)	History of cardiovascular disease
	Patient over 50 years
Chest radiograph (CXR)	Respiratory disease
Urea and electrolyte	Renal disease
levels (U & E)	Patients on antihypertensive drugs
Liver function tests (LFT)	Liver disease
	High alcohol intake
Haemostatic function	Liver disease
tests	Anticoagulants
	Bleeding tendency
Hepatitis or AIDS-virus	High-risk patients (see Chapter 2
screening	and note need for counselling)

ciated with the transmission of infectious diseases, such as HBV and HIV infection (Chapter 2), the occasional difficulties in cross-matching and transfusion, and the depletion of blood bank supplies.

In order that all these preparations can be made, patients for surgery are generally admitted to hospital on or before the day prior to surgery and occasionally on the morning of surgery when the procedure is to be performed later in the day. Patients who cannot sleep on the night before operation may benefit from a hypnotic such as diazepam or nitrazepam. The physician and anaesthetist should be consulted if there are queries as to whether the patient should discontinue any regular medication he/she is taking.

Preparation of the patient for surgery (Fig. 6.33)

Prior to surgery patients should shower and wash, the operative site should be cleansed with a suitable antiseptic solution, i.e. the skin or hair washed with a 5% alcoholic chlorhexidine solution when a skin incision is to be used, or a 0.2% aqueous chlorhexidine mouthwash after tooth-brushing when the incisions are intraoral. These preparations reduce the flora which may give rise to wound infection. Preoperative shaving of the hair may also be required with certain incisions.

The patient should be completely fasted for a minimum of 4 hours before the induction of general anaesthesia or sedation. Preoperative fasting reduces the risk of vomiting and regurgitation of stomach contents which could be aspirated during anaesthesia, giving rise to serious respiratory sequelae, asphyxia, or even death (Chapter 6).

The bladder should be emptied prior to the administration of the premedication, and dentures or appliances removed. The anaesthetist should be warned of the presence of expensive or fragile restorative work in the patient's mouth.

Finally, it is crucially important to check and record clearly the patient's identity and the nature, side and site of operation, and teeth to be removed. Ask the patient his full name and address and what operation *he* understands he is to have. Check that consent *has* been obtained.

Premedication (see also p. 5)

After the patient has been washed and changed into a clean theatre gown, the premedication is given at the appropriate preoperative time.

Commonly used combinations of drugs for premedication include pethidine with atropine; or Omnopon with Scopolamine (papaveretum with hyoscine), given intramuscularly an hour before the induction of anaesthesia. In selected cases an oral sedative such as diazepam or temazepam may be given instead (Chapter 1; Table 7.3).

The principal aims are to provide the following at the time of operation.

1. *Sedation and amnesia.* The patient who is to have a surgical procedure is naturally apprehensive and anxious. The discharge of adrenaline and increased metabolic rate which are responses to anxiety render the patient more difficult to anaesthetize, and more liable to cardiac arrhythmias with inhalational anaesthetic agents such as

Table 7.3
Premedication for dental in-patients

Age	Alternative regimens
Children	Trimeprazine *or* promethazine *or* diazepam *or* atropine
Adults	Omnopon and Scopolamine *or* Morphine and atropine *or* Temazepam and metoclopramide

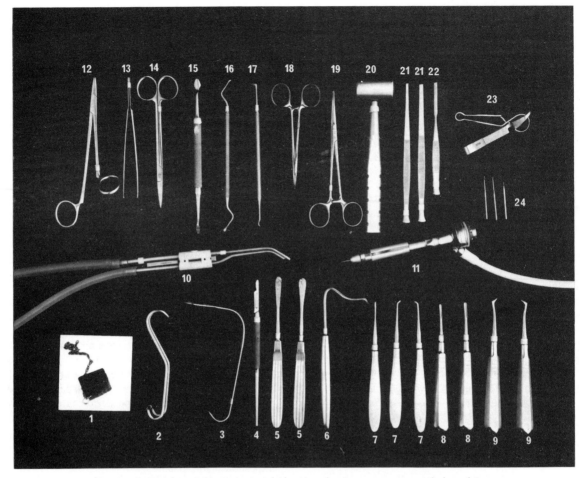

Fig. 7.2 *Basic oral surgical instrument set, laid out in order of use commencing at the lower left.*

1. *McKesson mouth prop.*
2. *Wire cheek retractor.*
3. *Weider tongue depressor.*
4. *Long scalpel handle (pencil shape) with no. 15 BP blade.*
5. *Obwegeser periosteal elevator, small and large.*
6. *Bowdler Henry's rake retractor.*
7. *Warwick James' elevators, straight, right and left curved.*
8. *Coupland's elevators sizes 1 and 2.*
9. *Cryer's elevators right and left.*

Middle row
10. *Essar suction irrigator.*
11. *Dental-air surgical drill.*

Upper row
12. *Ward's needle holder.*
13. *Gillies' tooth forceps 14.5 cm.*
14. *Joseph suture cutting scissors 16 cm.*
15. *Miller bone file.*
16. *Double-ended curette.*
17. *Mitchell's trimmer.*
18. *Halstead mosquito haemostatic forceps.*
19. *Curved forceps 16 cm.*
20. *Surgical mallet.*
21. *Bone-cutting chisels, 3 mm and 5 mm.*
22. *Osteotome 5 mm.*
23. *Towel clips.*
24. *Burs: Ash Toller, Round and Fissure, Jet TC701.*

halothane. Drugs such as papaveretum (Omnopon) are helpful premedicants in this respect.

2. *Analgesia.* When there is preoperative pain, or postoperative pain is expected, an analgesic such as pethidine or papaveretum should be given.

3. *Reduction of bronchial and oral secretions.* These secretions tend to cause a wet operative field, and bronchospasm and laryngospasm. Inhibition of the parasympathetic nerve supply with an anticholinergic agent such as atropine will reduce secretions and vagal parasympathetic activity, thus reducing the likelihood of cardiac arrhythmias. This is especially important in children.

4. *For some patients.*

(a) Antimicrobials may be indicated to reduce the incidence of postoperative infection and morbidity, particularly in surgical procedures such as the treatment of contaminated wounds, removal of impacted teeth, osteotomies (jaw surgery), bone grafts and other major maxillofacial procedures (Table 8.1: Chapter 9). Preoperative antibiotics are also indicated for patients susceptible to infective endocarditis (Chapter 2) and those with reduced host resistance to infections, i.e. diabetics, patients with disorders of white blood cells, and those on systemic corticosteroids and cytotoxic drugs (Chapters 2 and 9).

The drug of choice in these cases is usually benzyl penicillin 600 mg intramuscularly, given with the premedication. Patients allergic to penicillin may be given erythromycin orally, 2 hours preoperatively. In certain cases other antibiotics may be specifically indicated depending on microbiological assessment, or when traumatic wounds are present.

(b) The preoperative administration of hydrocortisone is needed for those patients with adrenal insufficiency, i.e. those having taken systemic corticosteroids recently and patients with Addison's disease (Chapter 2).

(c) Diabetics and patients with other relevant medical conditions may require special care, e.g. diabetes control (Chapter 2).

Instrumentation

Instrument layout

A great variety of instruments is available for oral and maxillofacial surgical procedures. A simplified set as used by the author will be described. This set comprises a basic oral set, which allows most intraoral dentoalveolar operations to be completed (Fig. 7.2). To this basic set, further instruments can be added as required, e.g. extraction forceps (Fig. 7.3), soft tissue set (Fig. 7.4), and fracture wiring set (Fig. 7.5). Special instruments are also required for mid-facial fractures, orthognathic, preprosthetic, periodontal temporomandibular joint, and extraoral tumour surgery.

Following sterilization, the instruments are laid out— for intraoral surgery it is convenient to use a Mayo stand placed over the patient's chest (Fig. 7.6). For major operations where more instruments are required, it is appropriate to have these laid out on a side trolley, with an instrument sister to pass them to the operator.

Sutures and suturing (see also Chapter 8)

The principal purpose of suturing is gently to approximate wound edges to allow healing by primary intention. Various suture materials are available and each has a specific use. Resorbable sutures are generally used to close deep tissues where the suture cannot be removed. The disintegration of these resorbable sutures may elicit an inflammatory response which is generally not significant. Non-resorbable sutures are used for superficial wound closure, i.e. skin and sometimes mucosa.

For routine intraoral mucosal suturing, a resorbable suture such as 3.0 plain gut or 4.0 chromic gut can be used. Plain gut generally resorbs within 5–7 days and chromic gut within 7–14 days in the mouth. The advantage of these resorbable sutures for intraoral wound closure is that they do not require removal, a procedure which may often be unpleasant and painful for the patient. As an alternative to resorbable suture, silk or nylon which are non-resorbable can be used for intraoral mucosal closure. Braided silk, either 3.0 or 4.0, is more comfortable for the patient than nylon as it is softer. Monofilament nylon tends to excite less of an inflammatory response than braided silk, but the suture ends tend to irritate. For skin closure, monofilament nylon is preferred, either 5.0 or 6.0.

Modern suture needles are swaged to the thread, which eliminates the need for threading of suture material through the eye of the needle. Commonly used needle types for intraoral surgery are a 3/8 circle 18.7 mm cutting needle or a 1/2 circle 20 mm taper-point needle. A cutting edge needle is easier to pull through ligamentous tissue such as mucoperiosteum; the round-bodied needle more easily passes through mucosa and leaves a smaller hole.

For intraoral suturing two types of needle holder are commonly used: the non-ratchet type (Ward's) needle holder, with which finger pressure is required to hold the needle in place—this pattern also incorporates a perforation in one beak so that the needle can be passed end on; and the ratchet type (Mayo–Hegar 16 cm) in which the

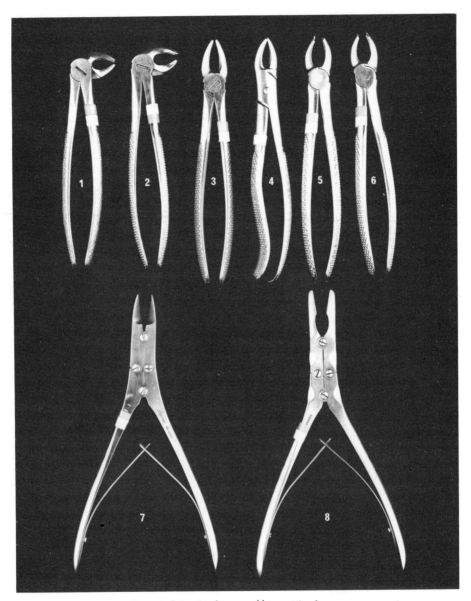

Fig. 7.3 *Extraction forceps and bone-cutting forceps.*

1. *Lower universal forceps Ash Pattern 13.*
2. *Lower hawksbill molar forceps Ash Pattern 22.*
3. *Upper straight forceps Ash Pattern 1.*
4. *Upper universal forceps Ash Pattern 76.*

5. *Upper hawksbill right side Ash Pattern 17.*
6. *Upper hawksbill left side Ash Pattern 18.*
7. *Bone-cutting forceps (side cutting).*
8. *Bone-cutting forceps (end cutting).*

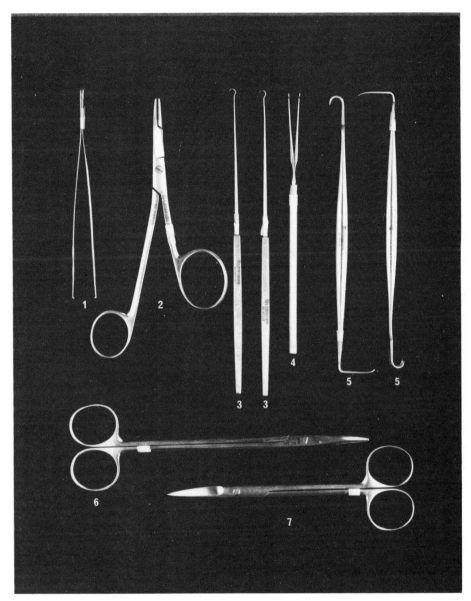

Fig. 7.4 *Soft tissue set.*

1. *Adson tooth forceps.*
2. *Gillies' needle holder.*
3. *Gillies' skin hooks.*
4. *Barsky double skin hooks.*

5. *Kilner cat's paw retractors.*
6. *McIndoe curved blunt-tipped dissecting scissors.*
7. *Joseph curved dissecting scissors.*

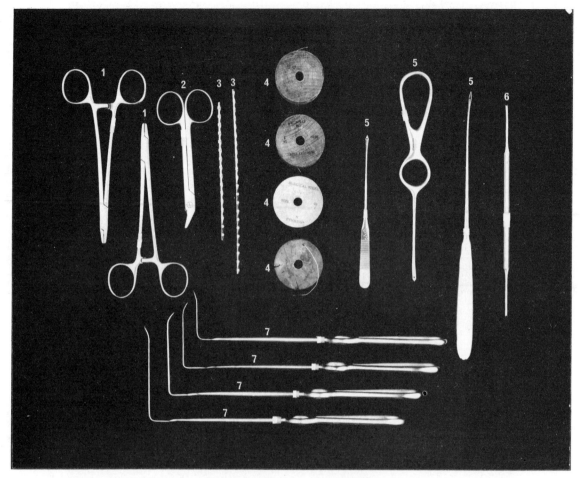

Fig. 7.5 *Mandibular fracture set (wiring).*

1. *Tungsten carbide insert wire-holding forceps.*
2. *Tungsten carbide insert wire cutters.*
3. *Erich arch bars.*
4. *Selection of stainless steel wires 24, 25, 26 and 28 gauge.*
5. *Obwegeser awls, mandibular, peralveolar and circum-zygomatic.*
6. *Ligature director.*
7. *Assorted Langenbeck retractors.*

needle is held without finger pressure. Selection of either one of these types of needle holder depends upon the surgeon's preference. A tooth dissecting forcep (e.g. Gillies 14.5 cm), preferably with tungsten carbide inserts, is used to pick up the wound edge prior to passage of the suture and also to retrieve the needle once it has been passed through the tissues.

The technique of instrument tying of sutures is shown in Figure 8.7 (p. 200). Care should be taken to pass the suture through an equal depth of tissue on either side of the wound to approximate the tissues without tension. If tension is required to bring the edges together, the edges should be released by undermining.

Scrubbing, gowning and gloving

The purpose of scrubbing, gowning and gloving is twofold. The first object of scrubbing is to reduce the

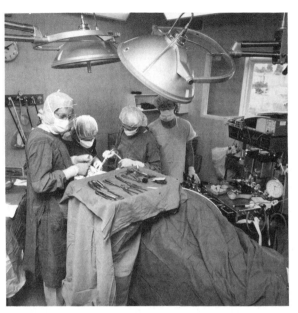

Fig. 7.6 *Patient draped in the operating theatre with instruments laid out on the Mayo stand over the patient's chest.*

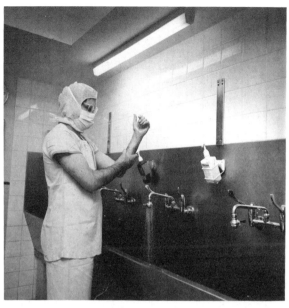

Fig. 7.7 *Surgeon clothed in theatre dress with balaclava and mask, washing to the elbows.*

incidence of wound infection caused by bacterial contamination from the surgeon and theatre staff. The second object is to protect the surgeon from contracting diseases, mainly viral but also bacterial, from the patient. Many viruses, including those which cause hepatitis B and AIDS (see Chapter 2), could be transmitted to surgical staff by contamination with blood, saliva or other blood-contaminated secretions.

Before entering the operating theatre, street clothes are replaced with clean linen trousers and a short-sleeved blouse; conductive rubber-soled shoes or boots should be worn. Hair must be adequately covered with either a cotton or disposable paper cap. Those with a beard should wear a balaclava. A disposable face mask is worn to prevent contamination of the wounds by oral and nasal flora.

The surgical scrub is performed prior to putting on sterile gowns and gloves. The scrub should use either a 5% chlorhexidine solution or povidone-iodine (Betadine). First the hands and forearms are scrubbed for 1 minute with a brush to the elbows, with particular attention to the fingernails. Following the scrub, hands and forearms are washed to the elbows for a further 2 minutes (Figs. 7.7 and 7.8).

The hands and arms are then dried with a sterile towel divided into quadrants, using a clean quadrant for each

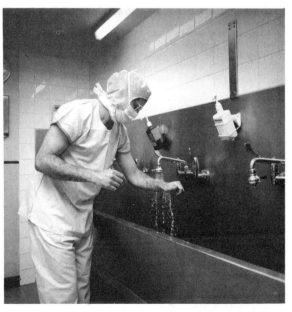

Fig. 7.8 *Rinsing arms, taking care not to contaminate hands.*

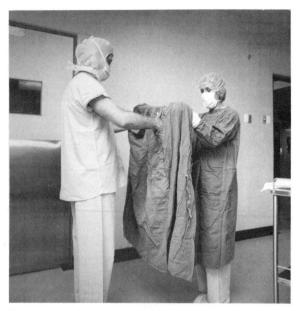

Fig. 7.9 *Surgeon being helped into a sterile gown, taking care not to contaminate the outside surface.*

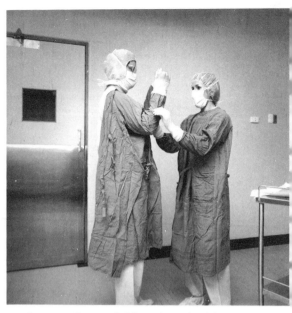

Fig. 7.10 *Sleeves pulled down clear of hands by assistant.*

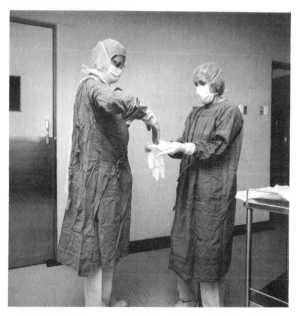

Fig. 7.11 *The surgeon's right hand is inserted into a sterile glove held by the assistant.*

hand and forearm; *scrubbed hands are surgically clean but not sterile.*

A sterile gown is then put on, taking care not to touch any external surfaces (Figs. 7.9 and 7.10). The back and that part of the gown below the waist are considered unsterile. Sterile disposable gloves are then put on with a sterile technique, ensuring no contact between the hand and the external parts of the glove (Fig. 7.11). The gown flap is then turned to protect the surgeon's back.

OPERATIVE MANAGEMENT

Once patients have been premedicated they may become disorientated, and should be confined to bed, preferably with the cot sides up.

The patient is transferred to the operating trolley or table when the theatre is ready, and anaesthesia then induced. Nasal endotracheal intubation is preferred for most oral surgical procedures as then the tube does not get in the way of the surgeon. Oral intubation may occasionally be appropriate, as may open anaesthetic techniques in selected cases, e.g. children undergoing the removal of deciduous teeth.

The oropharynx must be protected at all times to avoid inhalation of debris or instruments from the mouth. When the patients are intubated an oropharyngeal pack is put in position. This is usually a length of moistened gauze or occasionally a preformed sponge. The placement of a pack is in addition to the use of a cuffed tube which is used when indicated. With open anaesthetic techniques an oral pack must be expertly used by the surgeon (see Chapter 6).

Since injuries and abrasions to the patient's eyes are a hazard, protection of the eyes is most essential. The eyelids should be closed and taped, keeping eyelashes clear of the cornea. An antibiotic ointment may be instilled and then packs or shields placed over the eyes. Protection should be adequate to prevent penetration by a sharp instrument (Figs. 7.12–7.15).

Pressure points such as the patient's elbows and heels must be padded to avoid damage while the patient is still on the operating table. Modern operating tables are fitted with foam mattresses to reduce damage to any other pressure points. For long surgical procedures, a heating mattress with circulating warm water should be used to minimize hypothermia (see also p. 196).

Once the patient has been secured safely on the operating table, further preparation of the operative site is undertaken with antiseptic lotions, to reduce bacterial contamination. Chlorhexidine or iodine solutions are generally used: alcoholic solutions may be added for skin preparation. The patient is then draped in a sterile manner (Fig. 7.16).

At the completion of surgery the mouth and oropharynx are sucked out and inspected before removal of the throat pack. The pharynx is then similarly attended to prior to extubation, with particular attention to the posterior nasopharynx where blood clots may be found. All extracted teeth, instruments, packs used etc. should be accounted for before the patient can safely be extubated.

Following extubation, when the patient's cough and other reflexes have recovered sufficiently for him to be able to maintain his airway, he is transferred to the recovery room lying on his side in the head-down or tonsillar position (see Fig. 6.49, p. 168). This is the most dangerous period for the patient, whose airway must be carefully kept clear. Gauze dressings are commonly placed over oral wounds to maintain haemostasis, and also to mop up any further oozing of blood from the wounds, but these dressings must have tapes attached and hanging out of the mouth so that they cannot be lost into the airways. They must also be placed so as not to cause upper airway obstruction. Extraoral dressings are also used over skin incisions, or to support wounds in the chin or under the upper lip.

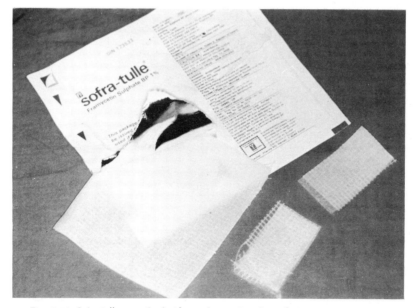

Fig. 7.12 *Sofra-tulle gauze for first layer of protection of eyes during in-patient operation.*

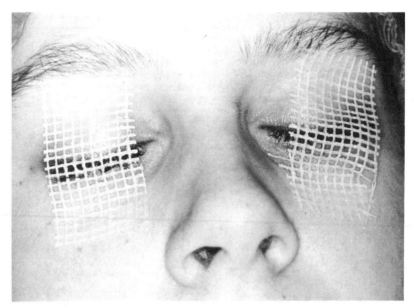

Fig. 7.13 *Gauze in place.*

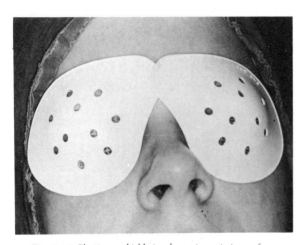

Fig. 7.14 *Plastic eye shields in place—to protect eyes from sharp objects.*

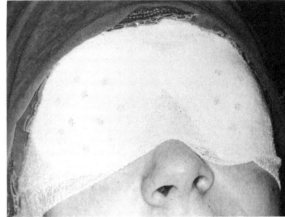

Fig. 7.15 *Eye protection in place.*

POSTOPERATIVE CARE

Recovery phase

During the early recovery phase the patient will begin to regain consciousness and the protective reflexes. The cough reflex and spontaneous breathing must be present before patients are moved from the theatre. It is during these early phases that patients are most vulnerable to respiratory obstruction. In order to assist in the maintenance of an airway, the mandible should be postured forwards as this tends to bring the tongue forward out of the oropharynx and the patient should be on his side in a head-down position, as previously mentioned (Fig. 6.49). Oxygen is generally administered either by mask or intranasal cannula at a rate of 6–8 litres/minute. An oro-

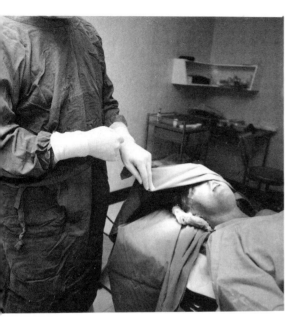

pharyngeal airway may be of use in patients who have not fully regained reflexes (Figs 7.17 and 7.18).

Recovery room care is designed to assist and protect patients until they have fully regained consciousness and protective reflexes. A qualified nurse should regularly observe their breathing pattern and colour (checking for cyanosis), response to command, pulse rate, character and volume, and blood pressure. Observation is continued until the patient is fully conscious and observations stable, at which point he may be returned to the ward.

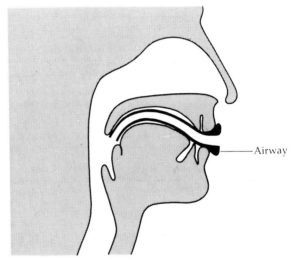

Fig. 7.17 *Oral airway in place.*

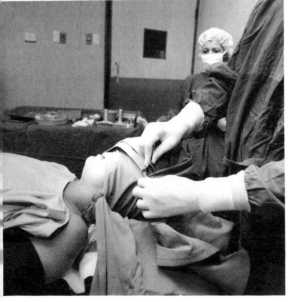

Fig. 7.16 (a) *and* (b) *The head drape is being prepared to allow access to the mouth.*

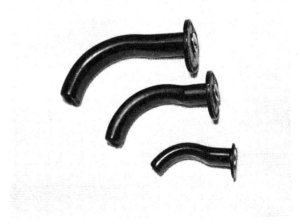

Fig. 7.18 *Airways.*

Any patient whose airway is threatened, for example by oedema or infection in the neck, or whose jaws are wired together, should be closely observed for at least 24 hours—in an intensive care ward if indicated (see below and Volume 2).

Intra- and postoperative medication

Analgesics

Some pain is generally experienced after surgery, and pain control is essential (Chapter 6). During the early postoperative phase, when the patient cannot take oral medications, parenteral drugs such as pethidine, morphine or papaveretum may be required. Once the patient is able to drink and take oral fluids, an oral analgesic such as paracetamol or codeine phosphate is substituted. Aspirin should be avoided because it may cause a bleeding tendency by interfering with platelet aggregation.

As an adjunct to pain control following surgery, a long-acting local analgesic solution such as bupivicaine 1% with adrenaline 1:200 000 may be injected into the operative site immediately *before* surgery. This injection should render the operative area anaesthetic for up to 8 hours, and may well reduce the need for injectable narcotic analgesics postoperatively. This form of pain control is particularly effective for patients who are having their mandibles immobilized.

Antiemetics

Since there is a tendency to nausea and vomiting in the postanaesthetic phase, patients often require an antiemetic drug parenterally. Those most commonly used are metoclopramide, perphenazine or prochlorperazine. However, care should be taken when these drugs are administered, especially to children and adolescents, as even low doses may give rise to side-effects on the extrapyramidal system and to abnormal movements (dyskinesias).

Antimicrobials

Antimicrobials may be continued postoperatively as previously discussed, depending upon operative findings and the patient's progress (Chapter 9).

Corticosteroids

Corticosteroids such as dexamethasone may be used systemically both intraoperatively and postoperatively to re-duce surgical oedema in selected cases, e.g. for patients undergoing maxillary and mandibular osteotomies, or for other procedures likely to cause oedema (Chapter 8).

Hydration and fluid replacement

Depending on the nature of surgery, there may be significant loss of blood and a subsequent fall in blood volume. In such cases it is necessary to replace this lost volume in order to maintain blood pressure and perfusion. Fluids are administered via an intravenous cannula, usually sited in the forearm. The nature of the replacement will depend on the volume lost and may vary from saline and dextrose solutions to artificial plasma volume expanders or transfused blood.

An intravenous infusion will also be required to maintain hydration when patients are unable to take oral fluids in the postoperative phase, and for the administration of antibiotics when treating severe infections. An accurate fluid balance chart should be kept, listing all intravenous and oral input, as well as urinary output or other fluid loss, for example by vomiting.

Nutrition

Most oral surgery patients are able to resume normal eating and nutrition in the early postoperative period. A soft diet is often required for the first 5 days, particularly for patients who are unable to resume adequate oral intake, e.g. those with maxillofacial injuries, jaw osteotomies or those having major tumour surgery.

Some patients will require the placement of a nasogastric tube and nasogastric feeding until they are able to resume an oral intake. In a few cases when nasogastric feeding is inappropriate, total parenteral nutrition may be needed.

Intermaxillary fixation

A special note is needed about intermaxillary fixation (IMF); this type of fixation is commonly used when treating patients with maxillofacial injuries, or following osteotomies of the jaws. In these cases, because the jaws are fixed together, the patient is unable to open his mouth, and special care is required in the early postoperative or recovery phase to ensure that respiratory obstruction or aspiration of vomit does not occur.

1. The placement of a tongue stitch until the patient is fully conscious may assist in bringing the tongue forward out of the pharynx. The tongue stitch is usually of 1.0

black silk, and should be placed in the posterior half of the tongue and brought out between the teeth.

2. Wire cutters, scissors or spanners must be available at the bedside at all times, depending on whether the IMF is applied with wires, elastics or frames. Fixation should be released in case of respiratory obstruction, and staff associated with the patient must know how to achieve this. Various mechanical locks and release mechanisms have been designed for IMF and these may be helpful.

3. It is essential that proper lighting, suction and retractors should be immediately available at the bedside.

4. The placement of a nasogastric tube and intermittent aspiration of stomach contents may reduce the risk of postoperative vomiting. The tube is usually in place on free drainage for 12 hours and suctioned 2 hourly.

5. In certain cases when IMF is applied, it may be prudent to leave the patient intubated for up to 72 hours postoperatively, or to perform an elective tracheostomy if a longer period of intubation is anticipated. Patients with extensive oedema around the floor of mouth, neck and pharynx may well require this type of assistance with airway management, as may those with a combination of injuries of the maxillofacial region, chest and/or head.

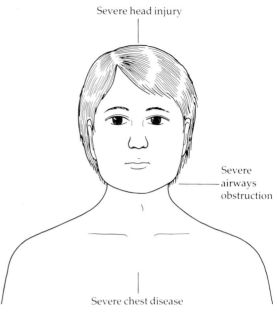

Fig. 7.19 *Indications for tracheostomy.*

Tracheostomy

A tracheostomy is an opening made into the trachea through the neck in order to create an airway when an upper airway obstruction is present or anticipated. The tracheal opening is usually made between the second and third tracheal rings, and a tracheostomy tube is then placed directly into the trachea. The tube can be connected to a breathing apparatus which provides positive pressure ventilation, or, depending on the patient's condition, he may be able to breathe without assistance.

Tracheostomy is rarely indicated in patients undergoing minor oral surgical procedures. The exceptions are those who may develop severe infections in the floor of the mouth and submandibular spaces (Ludwig's angina) which lead to upper airway obstruction. Patients who develop severe oedema or haematoma formation in these surgical spaces may also require tracheostomy to relieve obstruction.

In major oral and maxillofacial surgical procedures tracheostomy is more commonly required. The indications include the following (Fig. 7.19).

1. Patients who have a severe facial injury which may lead to obstruction, either mid-facial or mandibular, or who have a combination of injuries to both jaws.

2. Patients who have a combination of facial injury together with either a head or chest injury. When a chest injury is present the patient may have difficulty with inspiration, as well as with coughing to clear secretions.

The chest problem in combination with a degree of upper airway obstruction, either due to a facial injury or intermaxillary fixation, often requires the provision of a tracheostomy to facilitate breathing. The presence of a head injury, with associated respiratory depression or lack of patient co-operation in coughing and clearing secretions may equally give rise to the need for a tracheostomy in order to clear secretions and prevent obstruction.

3. Patients undergoing major surgery to the tongue, floor of mouth, or neck often require a tracheostomy to maintain an airway. Examples of this type of surgery include cancer resections of the tongue, floor of mouth or mandible.

Once the question of the need for a tracheostomy has been raised, particularly in the injured patient, arrangements should be made to proceed with the provision of the tracheostomy promptly. An elective tracheostomy is preferably performed under general anaesthesia after intubation, but may be performed with local anaesthesia.

The decision to proceed with an elective tracheostomy

is sometimes difficult; however, it is better to err on the side of safety and perform an elective tracheostomy rather than find that the patient obstructs and to preserve his or her life needs an emergency tracheostomy under difficult conditions.

Postoperative ward care

Following return to the ward, patients should be confined to bed for at least 4 hours. Oral fluids are encouraged 4–6 hours postoperatively, as is voiding of the bladder. Day surgery patients may be discharged under the care of a responsible adult once they have drunk and kept down oral fluids and voided urine. *They must remain under the care of a responsible adult for 24 hours, and not drive a motor vehicle, operate machinery or make important decisions for the same period.*

Patients undergoing minor oral surgery are usually discharged on the first postoperative day and, in other cases, the duration of stay will depend on the individual's progress.

Early mobilization is encouraged, particularly in the elderly, to avoid the problems of deep venous thrombosis and pressure sores. Postsurgically patients are advised to refrain from heavy exercise or hard physical work for 5–7 days, and then slowly to resume their normal activities.

Oral hygiene must be maintained using a soft toothbrush and 0.2% aqueous chlorhexidine mouthwashes. Fixation and splints should be checked daily.

FURTHER READING

Burn J. M. B. (1978). Perioperative care. *Brit. J. Hosp. Med.,* **19**: 425–429.

Evaskus D. S. (1980). General principles and techniques of surgery. In *Oral and maxillofacial surgery,* Vol. 1 (D. M. Larkin, Ed.) pp. 255–291. St Louis, Miss.: Mosby.

Kirk R. M. (1978). *Basic surgical technique,* 2nd edn. Edinburgh: Churchill Livingstone.

Norman J. (1980). Use of anaesthesia: preoperative assessment of patients. *Brit. med. J.,* **1**: 1507–1508.

Scully C. (1985). *Handbook for Hospital Dental Surgeons.* London: British Dental Journal.

Chapter
8
Prevention and reduction of operative trauma and complications of surgery

PSYCHOLOGICAL AND PHYSIOLOGICAL ASPECTS

The management of trauma begins when a patient crosses the threshold of a dental practice. Fear of dentistry in general, and surgical procedures in particular, is already initiating responses to their intrinsic adrenaline as patients take their seats in the waiting room (Chapter 1). However, the welcome of a warm and comfortable room, and cheerful, understanding staff does much to dispel anxiety. It is reassuring for a patient to be attended to quickly and efficiently, and the appointment should be scheduled with this in mind, in order to avoid the distressing experience being prolonged by delay in the waiting room. A policy of accommodating emergency minor oral surgery at the end of the working day should be resisted. Operator fatigue can lead to intolerant behaviour, and whereas an incomplete restorative operation is usually amenable to a temporizing procedure if time runs out, leaving a partially removed tooth after a failed extraction is far more troublesome and painful for the patient.

Minor oral or periodontal surgery in general dental practice should never be undertaken without previous experience, or without adequate instrumentation. Anxiety in a practitioner which is related to concern with potential failure will quickly communicate itself to staff, a parent when present and, most important, to the patient.

As the patient enters the surgery, all should be ready, with instruments as inconspicuous as possible. The practitioner should place the patient in a dominant position, preferably with the dental chair raised and the practitioner seated at a lower level in order to calm him. The fearful patient may chatter uncontrollably, and this is usually a favourable sign, as it is the strong, silent types who are bottling up their emotions who are more likely to suffer a vasovagal attack and faint (Chapter 4).

GENERAL ASPECTS

Pain control is important (Chapter 6). In general dental practice, local analgesia is the method of choice, although it may be supplemented by tranquillizing or anaesthetic drugs, and the administration of a painless local analgesic is often rightly regarded by the patient as a characteristic of a caring operator. Equally important is a courteous and thoughtful approach to the patient and gentle handling of oral soft tissues. Patients are readily concerned if the operator is rough during cheek retraction or procedures such as placing a saliva ejector, using an aspirator, or inserting and withdrawing cotton-wool rolls for moisture control. It is all too easy to lacerate or bruise the mucosa during these manipulations (see p. 168). Rotating and sharp instruments must always be used with great care.

Atraumatic operating is facilitated by good access, good suction, and a good light. The degree of access through the oral commissure may be limited, increasing the difficulty, and in many patients the coronoid process lies immediately lateral to the maxillary third molar when the mouth is wide open. Paradoxically, this area may be more easily displayed when the mouth is partly closed.

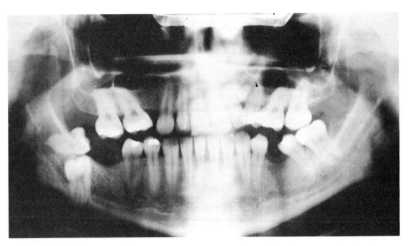

Fig. 8.1 *Removal of the lower right molars is clearly a hazard to the inferior alveolar nerve.*

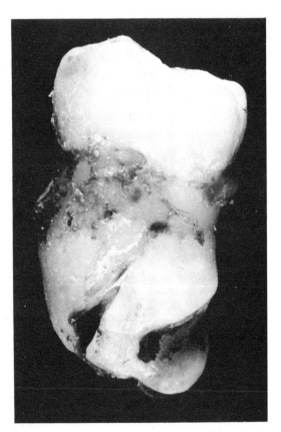

Fig. 8.2 *The inferior alveolar nerve perforated the root of this third molar.*

CONTROL OF SURGICAL TRAUMA

In the removal of teeth, it is impossible to avoid violence to the periodontium and supporting bone, but bruising and crushing of soft tissues should be minimized and great care should be taken of important anatomical structures at risk. These include the inferior alveolar, lingual and mental nerves, as their recovery from bruising, let alone severance, can be very protracted (Figs. 8.1 and 8.2). The location of blood vessels is relevant; for example it is possible to sever the facial artery in the depth of the lower buccal sulcus by a badly designed incision in the molar region. Anatomical spaces can be sites into which teeth or dental fragments are all too easily displaced. The most important of these are the antrum (for maxillary molars and premolars) (Volume 2), and the lingual space (for mandibular third molars and deeply buried premolars). In addition, the maxillary third molar can be lost into the buccal pad of fat, or even into the infratemporal fossa.

INCISIONS

Where incisions are needed in mucoperiosteum for the raising of flaps, they should be of adequate length (long incisions heal just as quickly as short ones) to allow easy access and delivery of the tooth, and minimize the risk of displacement of the tooth into an inappropriate space. In addition, a large flap is less likely to be traumatized by re-

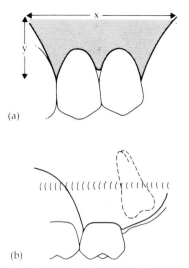

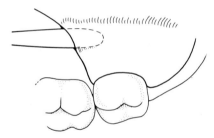

Fig. 8.3 *Flap design: (a) the base x must be greater than the height y; (b) should spare the interdental papilla.*

Fig. 8.4 *Raising a flap with a periosteal elevator.*

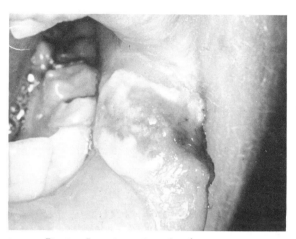

Fig. 8.5 *Burn at commissure from hot instrument.*

traction. The incision should be based on bone whenever possible, and the scalpel should be carried down to bone so that raising of the flap is facilitated. A periosteal elevator is placed in the incision and pressed hard against the bone beneath an area of loose soft tissue; it is advanced subperiosteally until the attached mucoperiosteum can be lifted away from the neck of an adjacent tooth, without tearing or bruising (Figs. 8.3 and 8.4).

Incisions for soft tissue biopsies should also be of sufficient length to obtain an adequate specimen representative of the lesion in question.

RETRACTION

Retractors should be properly designed (see Chapter 7), and the assistant should be taught to use them gently.

The angle of a retractor is often more important than the force of retraction. Sensitive anatomical structures such as the lingual and mental nerves must be protected from bruising, traction and severance. The commissure of the mouth is particularly vulnerable to sharp edges on retractors, and care should be exercised in selecting instruments that are appropriately curved to diminish trauma, further helped by lubrication with an emollient such as a preparation based on lanolin or even just vaseline. Damaged retractors should be discarded lest they lacerate tissue. The angle of the mouth is also the site of damage from overheated handpieces, or instruments hot from the autoclave, and burns have occasionally resulted (Fig. 8.5).

BONE REMOVAL

Extraction of teeth is discussed in Volumes 3 and 4. This section considers bone removal in relation to surgical procedures.

Bone removal should be carried out with a sharp chisel or with a bur specifically designed for oral surgery (see Chapter 7). The wound should be constantly irrigated with sterile normal saline or sterile water when a bur is being used. The surgical bur should be run at a speed of about 20 000 r/min for maximum efficiency, and should be used gently to 'wipe away' bone and to avoid the instrument catching and running uncontrollably into soft tissue. The air rotor should *not* be used once a flap is raised, because of the dangers of surgical emphysema and infection from the non-sterile water supply. Surgical emphysema can also be caused by the air/water syringe,

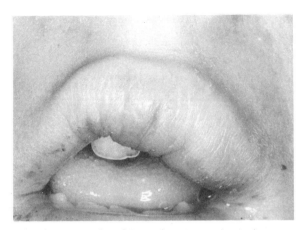

Fig. 8.6 *Surgical emphysema after using an air rotor in an apicectomy.*

which also should be avoided once a flap is raised (Chapter 10 and Fig. 8.6). Once adequate bone has been removed, removal of the tooth or root can ensue with forceps or elevators.

CLOSING THE WOUND AND SUTURING
(see Chapter 7)

Non-viable bone fragments should then be detached, bone edges smoothed and the wound irrigated with sterile normal saline. Where bone is displaced, but still attached to periosteum, it should be compressed into a satisfactory position, which helps to prevent bleeding from the site of fracture. Adequate apposition of flaps is obtained with gut or silk sutures (Figs. 8.7 and 8.8), and haemostatic gauze (oxidized cellulose—Surgicel) may be used to arrest bleeding from bone. Attention should be paid to the ends of the incision where a vessel may be partially incised and commence bleeding some hours later. Haemostasis must be ensured.

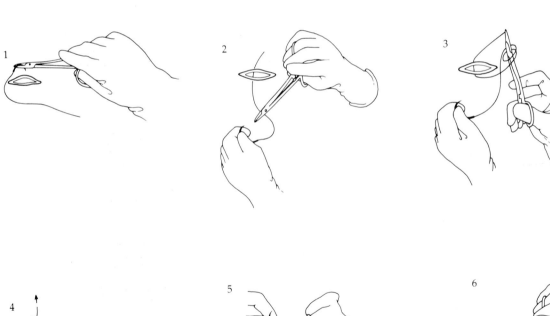

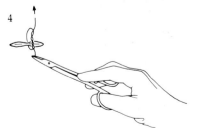

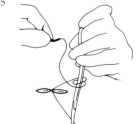

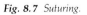

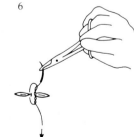

Fig. 8.7 *Suturing.*

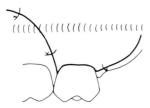

Fig. 8.8 *Sutured flap.*

Table 8.1 (see also p. 228)
Indications for antimicrobial cover for surgery

Patient predisposed to infective endocarditis

Major surgery, e.g. osteotomies, cancer surgery

Immunocompromised patient, e.g. with AIDS or diabetes

Where there has been radiotherapy affecting the jaw

Previous history of 'dry socket' (Volume 2)

When all is done, the patient is congratulated on his or her fortitude, and provided with appropriate medication. Patients should always be given written instructions including advice on how to proceed in case of postoperative bleeding or infection. *An out-of-hours telephone number to contact the practitioner is essential.*

OEDEMA AND ITS CONTROL

Post-surgical oedema arises usually from physical trauma or infection. Both are reduced by attention to the points discussed above, and by an aseptic technique. An antimicrobial cover is indicated in some circumstances (Table 8.1).

Modern dental practice has eliminated most of the old-fashioned caustic agents that could induce oedema, but the use of formaldehyde in root-filling materials persists. Although generally used without complication, a number of litigants have been successful when a rotary spiral root-filling instrument has pumped the caustic material into the inferior alveolar canal, with resultant intractable labial anaesthesia (see Fig. 10.5, p. 237).

Oedema is a particular problem following third molar removal (Fig. 8.9). It can be minimized by careful technique, but it is impossible to remove an impacted tooth without a degree of violence to the tissues. Paradoxically, the removal of a deeply buried third molar in the 30–40-year-old male may often produce minimal swelling, in contrast to the marked response to an easy removal in a

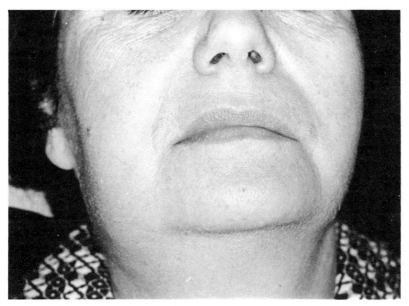

Fig. 8.9 *Postoperative oedema after removal of a lower third molar.*

late-teenage female. It is likely that trauma to bone in this circumstance is less important than trauma to soft tissue, and it is possible that young females have some intrinsic susceptibility to greater swelling.

The prevention of oedema is difficult. In the past, ice packs were placed over the angle of the jaw, but it is unlikely that the temperature of the tissues below the skin was lowered much, and the method has largely been abandoned. Some authorities recommend the use of parenteral corticosteroids such as dexamethasone in divided doses on the day of operation, which certainly reduces early swelling. However, oedema seems to appear a day or two later. Others have recommended the use of non-steroidal anti-inflammatory drugs (NSAID) to minimize oedema. The simplest of these is aspirin, but since this produces a bleeding tendency, newer drugs such as indomethacin and ibuprofen are better. Unfortunately, all NSAIDs can produce some bleeding tendency (Chapter 2).

The best policy to reduce oedema is, undoubtedly, to improve the surgical technique to minimize trauma, and to pay attention to the arrest of bleeding at the end of the procedure.

It is important to differentiate between the almost invariable oedema due to tissue damage, and haematoma due to postoperative bleeding confined within the tissues (Fig. 8.10), or infection.

Haematoma is usually more tender than simple postoperative oedema. Ideally, a haematoma should be evacuated but, in the circumstance of third molar removal, the haematoma is diffuse within the tissues (Fig. 8.11) and not amenable to drainage. Therefore, treatment should be re-

stricted to antibiotic therapy to prevent infection. Efforts to prevent haematoma formation include sometimes a delay for a few minutes before suturing, leaving sutures a little loose to discourage the collection of blood, and careful haemostasis.

Infections are usually characterized by a tender swelling, fetor, and sometimes suppuration and constitutional disturbances. Pus should be drained and antimicrobials given (Chapter 9).

POSTOPERATIVE BLEEDING AND ITS CONTROL

Most postoperative bleeding is of local aetiology only. Anxiety, however, appears to increase the level of fibrinolysins in blood and saliva, and potentiates bleeding. Rarely there is a systemic bleeding tendency (see also Chapter 2).

The practitioner should give clear instructions to the

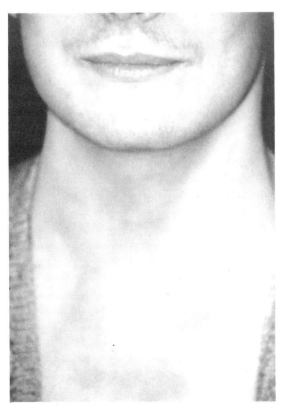

Fig. 8.11 *Haemorrhage may track down subcutaneously under gravity to reach the chest wall.*

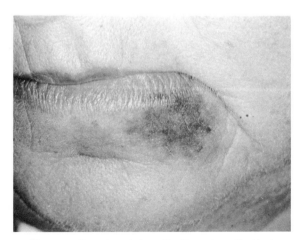

Fig. 8.10 *Haematoma in lower lip after postoperative bleeding.*

patient on the correct course of action to take if bleeding is persistent, which should include access to a hospital with a dental service if the dentist is not available. It should be borne in mind that dental bleeding is not always a minor matter, and it is often a cause of some discord between medical and dental practitioners when patients, for lack of proper instructions, consult their doctor or a hospital doctor for help.

Prevention is a counsel of perfection. Most bleeding diatheses can be excluded by taking a careful history, and nowadays very nearly all patients who suffer from a bleeding tendency are aware of the fact, and need hospital care. Various long-term drug therapies, including anticoagulants, and anti-inflammatory drugs will interfere with the natural arrest of bleeding, and if in doubt, the patient's general practitioner should be consulted. The patient who denies that he is taking aspirin may be using a proprietary aspirin-containing drug with an uninformative name.

Pathological local causes of postoperative bleeding include pre-existing inflammation, which should be eliminated by antibiotic therapy (if the infection is acute) and measures such as oral hygiene. Anatomical causes of postoperative bleeding relate to the ability of vessels to retract, and the morphology of the tissues in certain situations to render suturing difficult or impossible.

The general principle of arrest of haemorrhage is to apply pressure to the bleeding point so that coagulation can occur in the capillary bed. Where small vessels are bleeding, they should be allowed to retract. When minor oral surgery is carried out under local anaesthesia, the use of a vasoconstrictive agent clouds the issue, because the presence of a torn vessel can be masked at the time of surgery, and it is only some hours later that the vasoconstrictor wears off, vessels relax, and bleeding starts. Assuming that the patient does not have a bleeding tend-

ency such as a coagulation disorder, when pressure from suturing might divert bleeding into deeper tissues, the simple remedy is to insert sutures until the bleeding stops. The application of sutures should attempt to compress the soft tissue against bone, and where this is not possible, it may be necessary to construct a splint. For example, where a vessel is bleeding in the palate following exposure of an impacted canine, or where an epulis has been removed, leaving a bleeding point which is inaccessible to a suture, a splint will be useful. A dressing of zinc oxide paste (or Coe-pak) is placed under the splint so that it exerts additional pressure on the bleeding point. If bleeding continues, it is advisable to explore the wound to eliminate the possibility of a partially torn vessel, and where bleeding from bone is not arrested by haemostatic gauze, sterile beeswax should be applied.

All figures for this chapter are by courtesy of Professor C. Scully.

FURTHER READING

Doran B. R. H., Quayle A. A. (1985). The care of patients following oral surgery. In *Surgery of the mouth and jaws* (J. R. Moore, Ed.) pp. 829–850. Oxford: Blackwell Scientific.

Gillbe G. V., Moore J. R. (1985). Complications of extractions. In *Surgery of the mouth and jaws* (J. R. Moore, Ed.) pp. 395–408. Oxford: Blackwell Scientific.

Guralnick W. C., Laskin D. M. (1980). NIH consensus development conference for removal of third molars. *J. oral Surg.*, **38**: 235–236.

Nitzan D. W. (1983). On the genesis of the dry socket. *J. oral maxillofac. Surg.*, **41**: 706–710.

Rood J. P., Danforth M. (1981). Metronidazole in the treatment of dry socket. *Int. J. oral Surg.*, **10**: 345–347.

Scully C. (1985). *Handbook for Hospital Dental Surgeons*. London: British Dental Journal.

Chapter
9   *Infection*

This chapter deals mainly with general aspects of infection and with surgical infections; prevention of cross-infection is discussed in some detail in Chapter 2 in relation to viral hepatitis and AIDS.

SOURCES AND TRANSMISSION OF INFECTION

Sources of infection

Micro-organisms are present as a normal flora in many sites on the body including, for example, the nose, large intestine, vagina and mouth. The oral flora is usually non-pathogenic and termed **commensal** (Tables 9.1 and 9.2). Occasionally, organisms from the commensal flora can cause harmful **endogenous** infection. *Streptococcus viridans* species, for example, are implicated not only in dental caries and in odontogenic infections but also in infective endocarditis (Chapter 2); *Actinomyces israelii* causes actinomycosis (p. 227). If host defences are impaired, as in immunocompromised patients, then organisms that are usually commensal may become **opportunistic pathogens**: *Candida albicans* is a notorious opportunistic oral pathogen in, for example, AIDS (Chapter 2).

Many infections are **exogenous**, transmitted almost invariably from humans but occasionally from animals, or other reservoirs. The infection may be contracted from a patient who is obviously ill from the particular infection, e.g. viral hepatitis (Chapter 2), or may be contracted from a convalescing person or from one who is asymptomatic but still a **carrier** of the micro-organism (e.g. hepatitis B virus: Chapter 2). Viral infections are almost invariably exogenous and at least 50% of patients infected have **subclinical (asymptomatic)** infection. Most viruses are eventually destroyed and removed from the body, but some remain as **latent** infections (e.g. herpes simplex virus: Volume 2) which may be reactivated, and some

viruses cause chronic infection (e.g. carriage of hepatitis B virus: Chapter 2).

Infections transmitted to humans from domestic pets and from farm and other animals are known as **zoonoses** (Table 9.3). Animal excreta are the source of some infective agents in soil: tetanus, for example, is caused by spores of *Clostridium tetani*, often derived from horse manure. Food, including milk, is a major source of infections derived from infected animals, the excreta of animals or humans, human skin or mucous membranes, soil or other reservoirs. Important infections transmitted in food include viral hepatitis and, where milk is unpasteurized, brucellosis and tuberculosis (Table 9.4). Water is a potential source of infection where it is contaminated with excreta or untreated. It is most unwise to drink untreated water in some countries (or ice!) since it can be a source of a number of infections including viral hepatitis (Table 9.4).

Transmission of infection

Transmission of infection can be from person to person (Fig. 9.1); environment to person; or animal to person.

Person to person

Person to person transmission is usually horizontal transmission between individuals by direct spread through the physical contact of touch or sexual intercourse, by blood transmission, or by airborne spread through the respiratory tract or conjunctiva.

Staphylococci, streptococci and Gram-negative bacteria, as well as viruses such as herpes simplex, are commonly transmitted by touch. Transmission can be significantly controlled in dental practice by hand-washing and by wearing rubber or latex gloves.

Sexual transmission is the route for various bacteria, fungi and viruses that are often not robust enough to survive outside the body and can usually be transmitted

Table 9.1
Main Gram-positive oral bacterial flora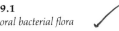

	Group	Organism	Alternative nomenclature
Gram positive	Cocci	*Streptococcus mutans* *milleri* *sanguis* *mitis (mitior)* *salivarius*	*Streptococcus viridans*
		faecalis	enterococcus
		Staphylococcus aureus *epidermidis* *salivarius*	*Micrococcus mucilagenous*
		Peptostreptococcus species	
	Actinomycetes	*Actinomyces israelii* *naeslundii* *odontolyticus* *viscosus* *meyeri*	
		Rothia dentocariosa	*Nocardia dentocariosa*
		Bacterionema matruchotti *Arachnia propionica* *Propionibacteria acnes* *Corynebacterium* species	
	Asporogenous rod-shaped	*Lactobacillus casei* *acidophilus* *plantarum* *fermentum* *salivarius* *brevis*	

only by intimate mucosal contact. Syphilis, gonorrhoea, non-specific urethritis, herpes simplex virus, papillomaviruses, hepatitis viruses and human immunodeficiency viruses (HIV) are all spread by this route. Transmission can be significantly reduced by avoiding promiscuity, and by using condoms.

An increasingly important route of person to person transmission is *transmission via injections or the transfusion of unscreened blood and blood products*. Intravenous drug abuse is a major factor in this type of transmission. Infections that can be transmitted in this way include pyogenic cocci and Gram-negative enteric bacteria as well as *Candida albicans* and a range of viruses (particularly hepatitis B virus (HBV); non-A, non-B hepatitis; delta agent; HIV; Epstein–Barr virus (EBV) and cytomegalovirus (CMV) (see Chapters 2 and 10, and Volume 2). Infection can be reduced by using sterile disposable needles and

syringes, by screening blood donations to exclude these agents, by heat-treating blood products, and by reducing the frequency of transfusions.

Respiratory transmission is important in the direct spread of tuberculosis, diphtheria, scarlet fever and many viral infections such as rubella and mumps. Infections may enter through the respiratory tract or sometimes the conjunctivae. Interestingly, the common cold is now known to be spread from person to person by touch rather than by coughs and sneezes.

The aerosols from dental equipment contain microorganisms when used in the mouth. The use of rubber dam and the wearing of an efficient face mask and protective eye wear can markedly reduce the risk from this potential source of infection during operative procedures.

Human bites can cause infection, especially localised mixed infection with *streptococci, staphylococci, Corynebac-*

Table 9.2
Main Gram-negative oral bacterial flora

	Group	Organism	Alternative nomenclature
Gram negative	Cocci	*Neisseria flavescens* *mucosa* *sicca* *subflava*	*Neisseria pharyngis*
		Branhamella catarrhalis	*Neisseria catarrhalis*
		Veillonella alcalescens *parvula*	
	Bacilli	*Haemophilius influenzae* *parainfluenzae* *actinomycetemcomitans*	*Actinobacillus actinomycetemcomitans*
		Bacteroides gingivalis *melaninogenicus* *denticola* *ruminicola* *oralis* *corrodens* *ochraceus* *loescheii*	*Bacteroides melaninogenicus* *Eikenella corrodens* *Capnocytophaga ochraceus*
		Fusobacterium nucleatum *planti*	
		Leptotrichia buccalis *Selenomonas sputigena*	*Spirillum sputigena*
	Spiral and curved	*Campylobacter sputorum*	*Vibrio sputorum*
	Spirochaetes	*Treponema vincentii* *buccale* *denticola* *macrodentium* *mucosum* *orale* *scoliodontum*	*Borrelia vincentii* *Borrelia buccale*

terium and *Bacteroides* species; and may transmit systemic infection such as syphilis and hepatitis B.

Indirect spread of infection, person to person, can occur through the respiratory tract from organisms in dust, e.g. *Mycobacterium tuberculosis* and *Streptococcus pyogenes*. It is possible, though there is little evidence, that the aerosols produced during the use of dental equipment could transmit organisms in the water supply (e.g. bacteria such as *Legionella* species). The various infections spread by the ingestion of contaminated food and water are other examples of the indirect spread of infection.

Transmission of infection from mother to fetus or neonate is known as vertical transmission and is seen in con-

genital syphilis and congenital rubella, CMV, hepatitis B, HIV infection, *Toxoplasma gondii* and other infections (Volume 2).

Environment to person

Environment to person transmission includes spread by dust, droplets, food or water. Wounds resulting from trauma, especially those contaminated with soil, may be contaminated by *Clostridium tetani* (the cause of tetanus) or *Clostridium perfringens* (a cause of gas gangrene). Surgical wounds may be contaminated by these or by any of a number of other organisms, especially staphylococci in

Table 9.3
Examples of zoonoses related to animals

Animal host	Organism	Disease in humans
Cat	*Toxoplasma gondii*	Toxoplasmosis
	Chlamydia	Catscratch fever
	Microsporum catis	Ringworm
	Toxocara catis	Toxocarosis
Dog	*Brucella canis*	Brucellosis
	Toxocara cani	Toxocarosis
	Rabies virus	Rabies
Pig	*Trichinella spiralis*	Trichinellosis
	Brucella suis	*Brucellosis*
Cattle	*Coxiella burnetii*	Q fever
	Mycobacterium bovis	Tuberculosis
	Brucella abortus	Brucellosis

the hospital environment (nosocomial infections). This type of transmission can be reduced by careful wound toilet, asepsis during operation and the changing of dressings and, in the case of tetanus, by immunization with tetanus toxoid.

Animal to person

Animal to person transmission causes a range of infections, a classic example being rabies (see Table 9.3).

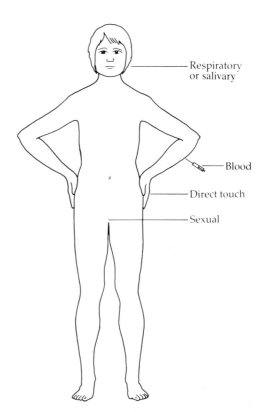

Fig. 9.1 *Sources of infection from humans.*

Table 9.4
Some infections spread by food and drink

Organism	Food and drink vehicle	Source of organism
Staphylococcus aureus	Animal products, e.g. processed meat, cream	Skin and nares of food handlers
Salmonella spp.	Improperly cooked chicken, milk	Hands of handler, battery chickens, rodents, flies, infected excreta
Vibrio parahaemolyticus	Shellfish	Sewage outfall
Brucella spp.	Milk/cheese	Cattle, goats, sheep
Cholera vibrio	Water	Infected excreta
Polio virus	Water	Infected excreta
Hepatitis viruses	Water/shellfish	Infected excreta
Entamoeba	Water	Infected excreta
Giardia	Water	Infected excreta

HOST RESPONSE AND IMMUNIZATION

Infection can only take hold where there is a susceptible host. Some agents, such as mumps virus, are highly infectious and infect most persons if they are appropriately exposed. Others, such as herpes simplex virus, are somewhat less infectious but are harmful especially when the host defences are impaired, e.g. when the patient is immunocompromised.

Defensive factors include:

(a) intact mucous membranes and skin,

(b) intact mechanical and non-specific chemical defences, e.g. saliva, tears, respiratory mucus, gastric juices,

(c) intact immune mechanisms (Volume 2), which have specificity and memory.

Any breach of mucous membranes or skin renders the host more liable to infection. Wound infection, such as a dry socket that can follow tooth extraction, is a good example of this.

Decrease in salivation (xerostomia—such as occurs with some drugs and salivary gland disease) renders the host liable to oral infections (Volume 2), especially caries, candidosis and sialadenitis.

Immune mechanisms may be impaired especially in AIDS and because of immunosuppressive drugs such as corticosteroids. Such immunocompromised persons are prone to opportunistic infections with *Candida albicans* and herpes viruses (Chapter 2; Volume 2) and some malignant neoplasms. It is possible that at least some malignant neoplasms have a viral aetiology: EBV, for example, is associated with some types of Burkitt's lymphoma (Volume 2) and nasopharyngeal carcinoma.

In contrast, it is possible to bolster immunity against some organisms by immunization actively using vaccines, or passively by giving immunoglobulins or immune serum (containing specific antibodies) from immune persons.

Active immunization is the act of stimulating antibody production by administering live, attenuated, or dead micro-organisms or their products (Table 9.5). Inactivated toxins (toxoids) of tetanus and diphtheria are administered by injection for the active immunization of children against those infections. Immunization against poliomyelitis can be achieved either with an injection of inactivated vaccine (Salk vaccine), or with a live attenuated virus (Sabin vaccine) given orally, though the latter is the most effective. Immunization against tuberculosis uses the Bacille Calmette–Guérin (BCG), an attenuated mycobacterium. Hepatitis B surface antigen is inactivated and used for immunization against HBV (Chapter 2).

Immunization has tremendous advantages in conferring protection against some very serious infective diseases and has reduced the mortality and morbidity from diphtheria, tetanus, polio and hepatitis B in particular. All persons should be immunized against diphtheria, tetanus and polio. Dental staff should be immunized also against hepatitis B virus and tuberculosis; and all females against rubella (German measles) since rubella infection can

Table 9.5
Common vaccines

Vaccine indicated for	Vaccine against	Type
*Infants and pre-school children**	Diphtheria	Toxoid
	Tetanus	Toxoid
	Pertussis (whooping cough)	Inactivated bacterium
	Measles	Live attenuated virus
	Poliomyelitis	Live attenuated virus (Sabin)
Older children	Tuberculosis	Bacille Calmette–Guérin (BCG: live attenuated bacterium)
	Influenza	Inactivated virus
Females	Rubella (German measles)	Live attenuated virus
Adults		
	Influenza	Inactivated virus
	Hepatitis B	Inactivated HBsAg (also recombinant vaccine available)

* DPT = combined diphtheria, pertussis, and tetanus vaccine.
  MMR = new combined measles, mumps and rubella vaccine.

damage the developing fetus. There is, as yet, no vaccine against HIV.

Adverse reactions to immunization are uncommon and usually minor. Localized inflammation and tenderness, and mild fever, may occur. Live viral vaccines may occasionally produce a mild form of the illness they are designed to prevent. In pregnancy, there is a danger that viruses used in live vaccines will cross the placenta to infect the fetus, and pregnancy is therefore a contraindication to vaccination with live viruses. Patients who are immunocompromised may also be at risk from vaccination with live viruses which may produce severe and sometimes fatal infections.

More worrying is the possibility that vaccine strains of virus can occasionally revert to virulent forms—this has occasionally happened with poliovirus immunization.

DISINFECTION AND STERILIZATION

Disinfection and sterilization play an important role in preventing transmission of infection, especially in the dental surgery. Disinfection is a term which implies removal of most pathogenic micro-organisms (usually by chemicals), as opposed to sterilization which is the destruction of *all* micro-organisms (usually by heat). Equipment introduced into a patient's body (especially if causing a breach in skin or mucous membranes) must be sterilized. Objects such as working surfaces etc. can simply be disinfected.

Aseptic techniques are essential in dentistry not only to reduce wound infection but particularly to prevent the transmission of, and cross-infection with, bacterial pathogens such as *Treponema pallidum*, *Mycobacterium tuberculosis* and *Clostridium tetani*, and viral pathogens such as herpes viruses, hepatitis viruses and human immunodeficiency viruses (HIV) (see p. 43).

The following are particular areas where sterilization and disinfection are needed.

1. Sterilization of instruments, solutions to be injected, and surgical dressings (and avoiding subsequent contamination of these).
2. Disinfection of the hands of operating staff, and the use of gloves whenever mucous membranes or body fluids are touched.
3. Disinfection of the mucous membranes or skin at the site of operation or injection.
4. The use of protective clothing, masks and possibly glasses, where operative procedures are being performed and splatter or aerosols created.

5. Air filtration where surgical operations are being performed.

Prevention of cross-infection in a hospital environment will usually be controlled by a Cross-Infection Committee that governs central policy. There will often be a Central Sterile Supplies Department (CSSD) to which all dirty instruments are sent for sterilization, sterile packing and despatch back to the clinic.

In dental practice, disposable items should be used where possible and sterilization carried out with an autoclave (see p. 44). Staff should be educated in cross-infection control. Sterile instruments should be stored in sterile trays until required and *not* in disinfectants, which rapidly become contaminated.

Once used, instruments should be washed to remove blood and other debris before being autoclaved. Sharp instruments such as needles, scalpel blades and endodontic instruments should be discarded into rigid waste containers, produced specifically for biohazard waste disposal. Non-sharp waste should be placed in suitable impervious plastic bags for disposal.

Sterilization of instruments and dressings

Mechanical cleansing

Mechanical cleansing of instruments is a required preliminary to remove gross debris, which insulates against heat sterilization or chemical disinfection. The person cleaning the instruments should wear heavy duty rubber gloves and take care to avoid needlestick injuries (see p. 43). The instruments should be brushed with a stiff brush after soaking for a few minutes in a disinfectant such as 2% glutaraldehyde. Ultrasonic cleaning is a suitable method of removing debris from small items such as burs, but does not sterilize. The washed instruments should then be rinsed with hot water, drained, and placed in a container for sterilization.

Autoclaving

Sterilization by moist heat (autoclave) is quicker than by dry heat (hot-air oven). Boiling water for 30 minutes, which does not sterilize since it does not kill spores or reliably kill viruses such as hepatitis B virus, *is now an obsolete technique*.

Commonly autoclaves operate at 121°C at 15 lb/in² for 15 minutes holding time or 134°C at 32 lb/in² for 3 minutes holding time. The complete cycles take 50 minutes or 15 minutes, respectively, and therefore 134°C 32 lb/in² is preferred.

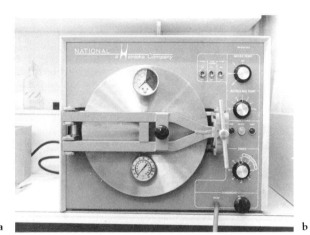
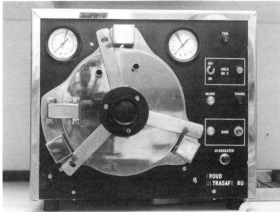

a   b

Fig. 9.2 *(a) and (b) Autoclaves.*

The autoclave produces steam which gives up its latent heat on condensing on objects and thus coagulates and denatures microbial proteins, killing the organisms. The autoclave is loaded with instruments, allowing sufficient space to permit steam circulation and penetration of the load, and the autoclave is then sealed. The cycle is automatically controlled and consists of displacement (or evacuation) of air and its replacement by steam at the required operating temperature and pressures for the required time. The inflow of dry filtered air at the end of the cycle allows for drying of the contents (Fig. 9.2).

To check that the cycle has been effective, an indicator such as Bowie–Dick autoclave tape that changes colour at the required sterilization temperatures should be fastened on the outside of each dental tray. The appearance of brown lines on the tape confirms that sterilization has taken place (Fig. 9.3) Alternatives are Brownes tubes that turn from red to green when sterilization is complete.

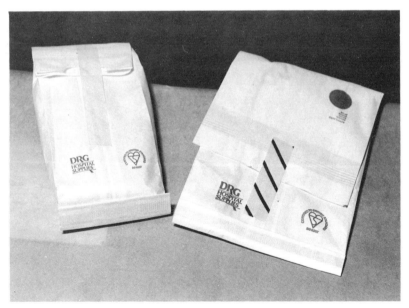

Fig. 9.3 *Autoclave tape. The tape is cream coloured (left), but brown lines appear if the correct autoclave conditions for sterilization have been fulfilled (right).*

Microbiological indicators of sterilization are tubes or strips containing spores of *Bacillus stearothermophilus* which are killed only at temperatures above 120°C.

Heat sterilization

Less satisfactory, since sterilization is slower, are hot-air ovens which take 1 hour at 160°C, or 30 minutes at 180°C, to kill pathogens. An additional 1–2 hours is required to allow heating up, and 30 minutes for cooling. Hot-air ovens are useful where glassware needs to be sterilized, but will char paper points, cotton wool, etc.

Other methods of heat sterilization now have little application in dentistry, but a hot glass bead or salt sterilizer, provided it reaches 218°C, is useful for sterilizing endodontic instruments and can do so within 10–15 seconds.

Other methods of sterilization

Other physical methods of sterilization are mainly restricted to hospital practice and include gamma irradiation and ethylene oxide gas. Disposable needles and plastic equipment are often effectively sterilized by the manufacturer, using cobalt 60 irradiation. Ethylene oxide gas usefully sterilizes heat-sensitive equipment but the gas is toxic and explosive and therefore used only in hospital and industrial sterilizing departments.

Disinfectants

Liquids are effective only as disinfectants rather than as sterilizing agents, though glutaraldehyde is perhaps the exception. There is a wide range of disinfectants available, each with disadvantages and advantages (Table 9.6), but current dental practices can be satisfactorily carried out with relatively few, viz. glutaraldehyde, chlorhexidine and isopropyl alcohol (see below).

In general, disinfectants work most effectively if there is the minimum of organic matter present on the instrument, if the pH of the solution is correct, if the solution is freshly prepared, and as long as no inactivators are present. For example, rubber inactivates chlorhexidine.

Glutaraldehyde is a useful agent and is the preferred disinfectant against pathogenic viruses and other agents likely to be encountered in dentistry (see Fig. 2.32, p. 45). A 2% solution of glutaraldehyde in 70% isopropanol is highly effective, non-corrosive, and after about 3 hours almost achieves sterilization. *Mycobacterium tuberculosis*, however, is very resistant to glutaraldehyde and 10–12 hours are required to kill spores.

Other preparations of glutaraldehyde have certain advantages (Chapter 2).

Chlorhexidine is highly active against Gram-positive but less so against Gram-negative bacteria. Chlorhexidine combined with acetyl pyridinium chloride, or alcohol, can be useful for disinfecting working surfaces but its expense tends to restrict its use to that of an antiseptic for skin or mucous membranes. Chlorhexidine, 4% in detergent, is a useful surgical scrub for hand preparation (Hibiscrub: Fig. 9.4).

Chlorhexidine 0.2% aqueous solution (Corsodyl) is one of the few agents effective against the formation of dental bacterial plaque (although it does not remove existing plaque). It is adsorbed to hydroxyapatite, salivary mucin deposits and plaque, and effectively controls plaque as well as other organisms such as *Candida* species. The disadvantages of unpleasant taste and staining of the teeth are relatively minor compared with the significant antiplaque effect).

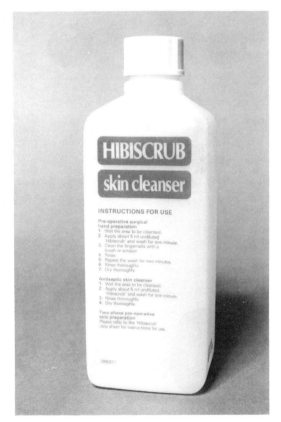

Fig. 9.4 *Chlorhexidine-containing hand cleansers are popular and effective.*

Table 9.6
Disinfectants and antiseptics

	Advantages or disadvantages	Trade name	Use: disinfection of
Disinfectants			
Glutaraldehyde 2%	Actively virucidal and sporicidal	Cidex, Asep, Totacide	Instruments, surfaces
	Acid and buffered phenol forms more active	Sporicidin	
Hypochlorite 10%	As above but corrosive to metals	Chloros, Domestos, Milton	Non-corroding instruments, surfaces
Formaldehyde	Virucidal and sporicidal	Formalin	Heat-sensitive equipment, fumigating rooms
Chlorhexidine (alcoholic)	Active mainly against Gram-positive organisms	Hibitane Hibiscrub	Surgical scrub
Phenols	Poorly virucidal or sporicidal	Clearsol, Hycolin, Stericol, Izal, Jeyes fluid	Bacterial contaminants of laboratory wear
Cresols	" " "	Lysol	" " "
Antiseptics			*Use:*
Chlorhexidine 0.2% (aqueous)	Effective antiplaque agent	Corsodyl	Mouthwash
Ethyl alcohol 70%	Ineffective in mouth		Skin preparation
Isopropyl alcohol 70%	Ineffective in mouth		Skin preparation
Iodine 2% in alcohol	Sensitizes, corrosive to metal		Preoperative skin preparation
Povidone iodine	Less potent than iodine	Betadine	Surgical scrub, mouthwash
Hexachlorophane	Toxic if absorbed in infants	Phisohex	Soaps
Parahydroxybenzoic esters	May sensitize	Parabens	Preservative in LA
Hydrogen peroxide 3%	Cleanses also by frothing		Mouthwash for oral infections
Phenol 1.5%	Mild antiseptic		Mouthwash
Cresols (e.g. parachlorophenol)	Irritant		Endodontics

Other agents

Iodophors are organic complexes that liberate their iodine, but they are said not to produce iodine sensitivity. The complex with polyvinyl pyrolidone (povidone iodine: Betadine) is popular as a mucosal and skin antiseptic. Parachlorophenol, camphorated parachlorophenol and creosote (mixed phenols) are used in endodontics as root canal disinfectants. Sodium hypochlorite 1–2% is useful for disinfecting dentures, as it is candidacidal, and for irrigating root canals. Hypochlorite is an effective alternative to glutaraldehyde as a virucidal agent but is corrosive to metals.

Disinfection of the hands of operating staff, and the use of gloves (see also Chapter 2)

Current recommendations for the protection against

cross-infection are quite definite that *gloves should be worn by all dental health care personnel when contacting blood, saliva, or mucous membranes, i.e. at all times when treating all patients.*

Gloves can be worn with few, if any, problems, though some complain of difficulty using endodontic and other fine instruments. Neurosurgeons, ophthalmic and other surgeons, however, manage to operate when wearing gloves.

Gloves perforate readily with use, especially when wires are handled as, for example, in oral surgery or orthodontics. Handwashing should, therefore, precede and follow the wearing of gloves.

Chlorhexidine-containing compounds such as Hibiscrub are popular for handwashing. Before surgical procedures, the hands should be washed thoroughly and the nails scrubbed for about 1 minute and then rinsed. The lathering and rinsing should be repeated three times before drying the hands on sterile towels (see Chapter 7).

Preparation of skin and mucosa before injections or incisions

Skin is routinely cleansed before injections with a solvent antiseptic such as 70% alcohol, though this is more ritualistic than realistic since only surface contaminants are removed and organisms rapidly appear from sweat pores and elsewhere. Before skin incisions, however, the area should be shaved if necessary and cleansed with repeated applications of alcoholic chlorhexidine or povidone iodine.

Alcoholic solutions of iodine or chlorhexidine are appropriate for the preparation of mucosa before injections, but again this is more ritualistic than realistic. Before surgery, the use of a 0.2% chlorhexidine mouthwash by the patient is probably as effective in reducing oral micro-organisms as are any of the commonly used antiseptics.

SURGICAL INFECTIONS

Surgical infections of the head and neck are usually bacterial, pyogenic (pus-forming) infections, the majority of which have an odontogenic aetiology. Most arise from necrotic pulps, some from infected periodontal pockets or around partially erupted teeth.

Pyogenic infections in the head and neck are often fairly trivial, albeit causing substantial pain, but may be life-threatening because of the hazard of airway obstruction and the proximity of vital structures. Rarely, even

minor infections such as a boil on the upper lip may spread (by emissary veins) to infect the cavernous sinus and cause cavernous sinus thrombosis and death if not treated. Odontogenic infections in the normal host are rarely responsible for haematogenous spread of infection elsewhere: infective endocarditis is one exception (Chapter 2).

In all infections the outcome depends on the balance between host factors, including the immune response, and bacterial factors such as the virulence of the micro-organism. Surgical drainage and antimicrobials are the main means of tipping the balance in favour of the host.

Host defences (Volume 2)

The major defence against pyogenic infections is mechanical and afforded by the intact mucosa and skin. Saliva may also play a role by mechanically cleaning the mucosa.

Resistance to infection is impaired if there are breaches in the mechanical defences or if tissue vascularity or immune responses are reduced (see above). Radiotherapy to neoplasms in the head and neck can cause xerostomia (dry mouth), reduces vascularity and predisposes to mucositis and bone infection (Chapter 2). Immune responses may be reduced in old age, and in any debilitating disease, especially in diabetes mellitus, alcoholism, white blood cell dyscrasias (e.g. leukaemia) and AIDS. Patients may also have been deliberately immunosuppressed with drugs, for example to prevent rejection of kidney transplants (Chapter 2).

Any impairment of host defences may not only predispose to infection but the latter is also more likely to spread and persist.

Microbiology of surgical infections in the head and neck

A mixture of three or four species of bacteria is often involved in orofacial infections of odontogenic origin (i.e. infections are usually **polymicrobial**). Anaerobes predominate and are isolated from virtually all dentoalveolar infections; aerobes are isolated from about one-third of infections (Table 9.7). Most infections originate from the oral flora.

Anaerobes such as the Gram-negative microorganisms bacteroides and fusobacteria appear more commonly in severe infections (Table 9.7). The pathogenicity of anaerobes is probably related to lipopolysaccharides, other capsular material and bacterial enzymes. Aerobes, especially *Streptococcus milleri* (a viri-

Table 9.7
The predominant flora isolated from orofacial surgical infections

Infection	Organisms implicated	
	Most commonly	Others
Dental abscess	*Bacteroides species* *Fusobacterium species* *Streptococcus viridans*	*Peptostreptococcus species* *Peptococcus species* *Actinomyces species* *Veillonella parvula*
Fascial space infections	*Bacteroides species* Peptostreptococci	*Staphylococcus species* *Streptococcus viridans* *Klebsiella species* *Escherichia coli* *Pseudomonas aeruginosa*
Pericoronitis	*Bacteroides melaninogenicus* *Bacteroides gingivalis* *Fusobacterium species* *Streptococcus viridans*	
Osteomyelitis	*Bacteroides species* *Staphylococcus aureus*	*Streptococcus viridans* *Bacteroides species* *Capnocytophaga species* *Peptococcus* *Actinomyces*
Wound infection	*Streptococcus viridans* *Bacteroides species* *Staphylococcus aureus*	*Streptococcus faecalis* *Eikenella corrodens*
Sinusitis	Pneumococci *Haemophilus influenzae*	*Streptococci species* Anaerobes
Suppurative sialadenitis	*Streptococcus viridans* *Staphylococcus aureus*	

dans streptococcus), are also found more commonly in severe than mild infections. Aerobes may, by reducing the available oxygen, enhance proliferation of anaerobes.

Most orofacial infections respond to penicillin, but occasional organisms, especially *Bacteroides* species, may, by producing beta lactamase, cause failures. Metronidazole is then usually effective. Many of the organisms implicated in orofacial infections are, or readily become, resistant to erythromycin (see below).

Pathology

Pyogenic bacteria usually excite an acute inflammatory response characterized clinically by the four cardinal signs of inflammation—swelling, heat, redness and pain—which occur mainly as a result of increased blood flow and vessel permeability consequent on complement activation (Volume 2). The local immune response leads to enlarged tender cervical lymph nodes because of reactive hyperplasia (Volume 2).

Release of chemical mediators from leucocytes (such as interleukin-1 or endogenous pyrogen), and bacterial toxins, or the entry of bacteria into the bloodstream will cause systemic disturbance. Pyrexia (fever), malaise and slight tachycardia are not uncommon in patients with any infection but are usually cause for little concern. However, if the pyrexia and tachycardia are high or are associated with sweating and rigors, the patient is described as 'toxic' and should be admitted to hospital. The absence of fever is not always a safe sign since it may be absent in Gram-negative septicaemia and in some elderly or immunocompromised patients. Profound shock and death may ensue from a Gram-negative septicaemia.

Two different clinical patterns of infection occur—the cellulitic and the abscess-forming. Cellulitic infections, which are classically caused by streptococci, produce little pus but spread rapidly through the tissues, which become tense and brawny. An abscess, on the other hand, is a circumscribed collection of pus (necrotic tissue, leuco-cytes and micro-organisms) surrounded by a localized inflammatory response.

Diagnosis of orofacial bacterial infections

Infections are usually diagnosed from the clinical features of pain, redness, heat and swelling. There may be pyrexia (temperature above 37°C orally), tender enlarged re-gional lymph nodes, a raised erythrocyte sedimentation rate (ESR) or plasma viscosity, and a neutrophilia (leuco-cytosis).

Bacteriological samples are indicated in some instances in order to determine the organisms involved and their antimicrobial sensitivities. Such investigations are neces-sary primarily when there is a bacterial infection requiring antibiotic therapy (page 228), viz. odontogenic infections in an ill or immunocompromised patient, fascial space infections, osteomyelitis, suppurative parotitis, suppura-tive lymphadenitis, and some other conditions such as actinomycosis, tuberculosis, syphilis and some cases of acute ulcerative gingivitis.

The following investigations may be useful (see also Chapter 3).

1. *Inspection* of a sample of pus may occasionally be useful, for example by showing the 'sulphur granules' indicative of colonies of *Actinomyces* in actinomycosis.

2. *Direct microscopy* of a smear may be of value if the smear is stained by Gram's method which shows leuco-cytes, cocci and other organisms such as those involved in acute ulcerative gingivitis (Fig. 3.42). Methyl violet can also be useful in examining Vincent's organisms. Ziehl–Nielsen stain is helpful for identifying mycobacteria.

Immunostains can help in identifying some organisms such as *Treponema pallidum*, and dark ground microscopy can also be useful in the diagnosis of syphilis (Volume 2 and p. 91).

3. *Culture* (Fig. 9.5). The laboratory can only report on the micro-organisms that can be cultured from the sample provided. The specimen should therefore be taken before antibiotics are started, be as large as possible (e.g. frank pus should be sent if available rather than a swab), and then sent immediately to the laboratory, or, if there will

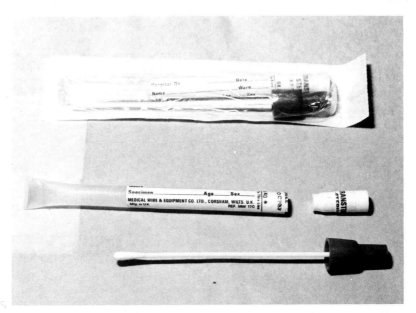

Fig. 9.5 *Microbiology swab. Specimens should be sent immediately to the laboratory: if delay is unavoidable, the swab should be placed in transport medium.*

be any delay, swabs should be sent in transport media which *to some extent* prevent the specimen deteriorating. By definition, most transport media will not protect anaerobes, though 'reduced transport fluids' do have some protective effect.

4. *Serological tests* for bacterial infections are valuable mainly in the diagnosis of syphilis.

Local spread of infection

The common oral bacterial infections such as apical abscesses and pericoronitis fortunately do not usually spread to any great extent. Intrabony pus arising from an apical abscess will usually penetrate the thinnest cortical plate of bone, to emerge usually on the buccal side of the jaws (Figs. 9.6–9.8). Abscesses from upper lateral incisors or palatal roots of first molars may, however, emerge on the palatal side (Figs. 9.9–9.12). Occasionally, abscesses from

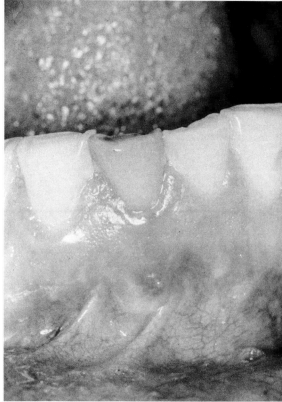

Fig. 9.7 *Apical abscess discharging in the usual site—the buccal vestibule. Apical abscesses are usually a sequel to pulpal death from caries; occasionally from trauma, as shown here by the discoloration of the non-vital lower right central incisor.*

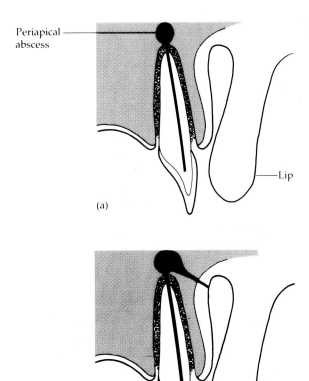

Fig. 9.6 *(a) and (b) Most apical abscesses discharge buccally.*

maxillary posterior teeth discharge into the antrum (Fig. 9.12). Most apical abscesses give rise to only minor soft tissue infections (see below), but facial oedema can be severe (see below and Figs. 9.22–9.26).

Abscesses that discharge below the mylohyoid muscle, or infection from pericoronitis or other infections in the pterygoid area, may spread to the fascial spaces of the neck. The relationship of the muscle insertions and fascia determines the subsequent direction of spread, since pus always follows the path of least resistance. Thus channelled and directed by the fascia and muscles, the pus spreads easily through the soft tissue spaces, which intercommunicate freely (Figs. 9.13–9.15). Fascial space infections not only cause 'toxicity' but may spread intra-cranially via emissary veins, or may cause asphyxia. These serious infections are discussed more fully below (page 226).

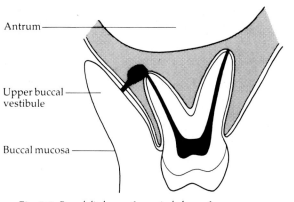

Antrum

Upper buccal
vestibule

Buccal mucosa

Fig. 9.8 *Buccal discharge of an apical abscess from a
maxillary molar.*

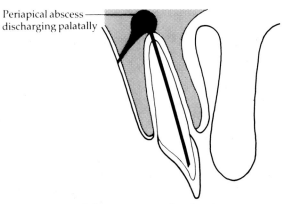

Periapical abscess
discharging palatally

Fig. 9.9 *Apical abscesses from maxillary lateral incisors
may discharge palatally since the roots of these teeth are often
placed palatally.*

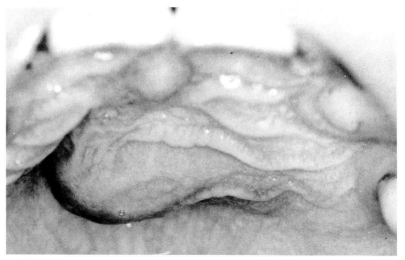

Fig. 9.10 *Palatal abscess from a maxillary lateral incisor.*

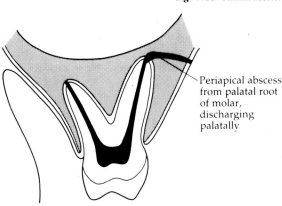

Periapical abscess
from palatal root
of molar,
discharging
palatally

Fig. 9.11 *Apical abscesses from the palatal roots of
maxillary molars may discharge palatally.*

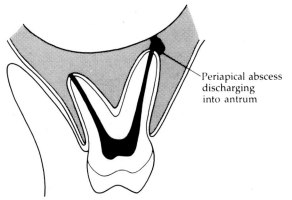

Periapical abscess
discharging
into antrum

Fig. 9.12 *Apical abscesses from maxillary premolars or
molars may discharge into the maxillary antrum.*

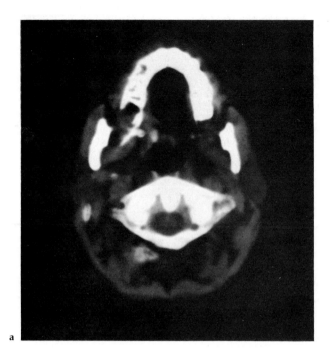

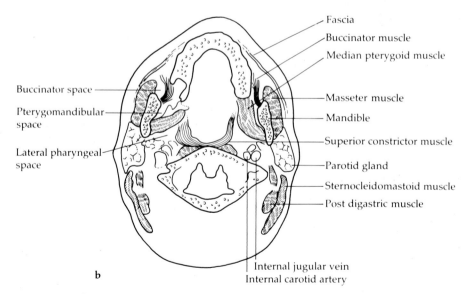

Fig. 9.13 (a) and (b) Spread of infection, especially from the mandibular third molar region, may reach the pterygomandibular space, as shown in this CT scan (at level of maxillary alveolus).

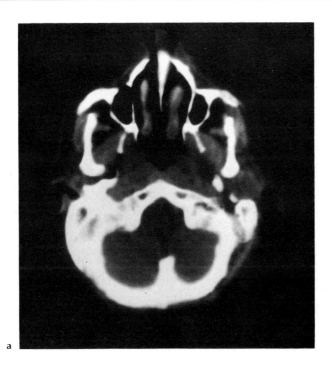

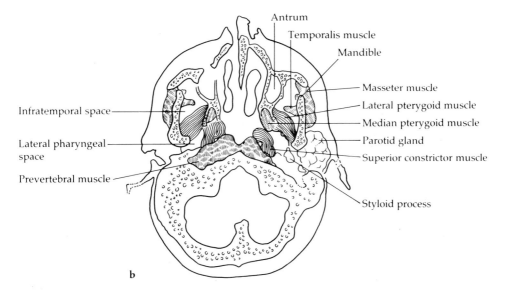

Antrum
Temporalis muscle
Mandible
Masseter muscle
Lateral pterygoid muscle
Median pterygoid muscle
Parotid gland
Superior constrictor muscle
Styloid process
Infratemporal space
Lateral pharyngeal space
Prevertebral muscle

Fig. 9.14 (a) and (b) Infratemporal space infection (CT scan at antral level).

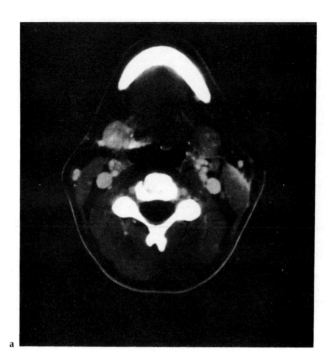

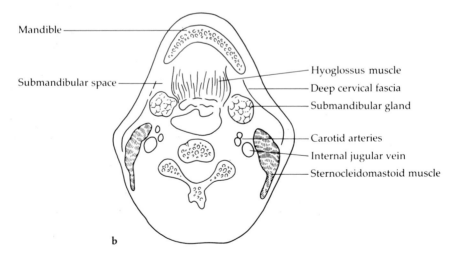

Mandible

Submandibular space

Hyoglossus muscle

Deep cervical fascia

Submandibular gland

Carotid arteries

Internal jugular vein

Sternocleidomastoid muscle

Fig. 9.15 *(a) and (b) Submandibular space infection (CT scan at lower border of mandible).*

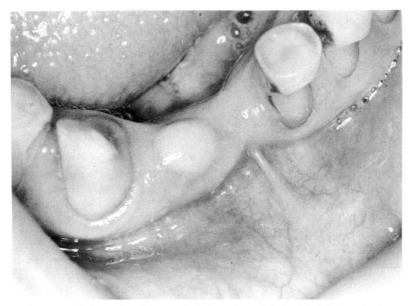

Fig. 9.16 *Discharge of pus from an apical abscess through the tooth socket after extraction.*

Principles of treatment of orofacial bacterial infections (Table 9.8)

Drainage

Infections are best treated by removal of the cause and surgical drainage of pus as soon as an obvious collection forms: a well-known surgical aphorism is 'never let the sun set on undrained pus'. Dental abscesses can be drained through the root canal or by incising a fluctuant abscess or by extracting the tooth (Fig. 9.16). Incisions should be made at the part of an abscess where pus is collecting, avoiding important anatomical structures such as the mandibular branch of the facial nerve in the submandibular region. Drainage should ensure breakdown of all loculi of pus by using Hilton's method (Figs. 9.17–9.18) and, if necessary, to prevent the wound closing before drainage is complete, a corrugated rubber drain is inserted. Palatal abscesses are notorious for closing after incision and therefore an ellipse of tissue should be excised to establish drainage. In cellulitic infections the tense oedematous tissues may cause compression of the airway and, therefore, large incisions with the insertion of multiple drains are needed to decompress the tissue spaces (for example in Ludwig's angina: see below).

At the time of incision, pus is taken for aerobic and anaerobic culture. The importance of anaerobic pathogens has become increasingly obvious with better methods of bacteriological specimen transport and culture.

The source of infection, such as a carious tooth, may also be removed at the time of drainage if this is carried out under general anaesthesia, or under local analgesia after the acute infection has resolved.

Table 9.8 ✔
Treatment of pyogenic orofacial infections

Treatment	Example
Surgical	
Drainage	Incision of abscess
Removal of source	Extraction of infected tooth
Decompression	Wide incision of tissues in Ludwig's angina
Medical	
Antimicrobials	Penicillin, metronidazole
Antipyretics, analgesics	Acetylsalicylic acid, paracetamol
Local heat	Hot salt-water mouthbaths

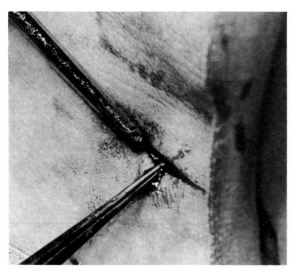

Fig. 9.17 *Skin incision for drainage of an abscess pointing onto the skin.*

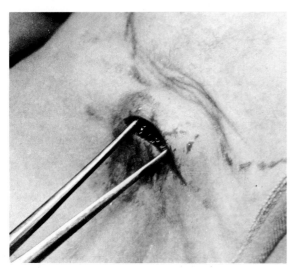

Fig. 9.18 *Hilton's method of opening up tissue to drain locules of pus.*

Antimicrobial therapy (see p. 228 and Tables 9.8 and 9.9)

If the infection is localized and the pus drains well, and the patient is otherwise well, antimicrobials are not always required. Antimicrobials, however, are indicated particularly for infections in ill, toxic or immuno-compromised patients; where fascial spaces are infected; and in osteomyelitis (see below). Antibiotics should not be used to treat established pus since, although the

organism may be eradicated, the pus can remain as a sterile swelling—an antibioma.

Rational selection of an antibiotic depends upon the antibiotic sensitivity of the pathogenic bacteria but, since bacterial culture results are seldom immediately available, empirical therapy is often started on a 'best guess' basis, based on knowledge of the micro-organisms usually implicated and their antimicrobial sensitivities. Fortunately, virtually all odontogenic infections are still caused by organisms sensitive to penicillin and to metronidazole, though there are marked exceptions. These two antimicrobials have a fairly narrow spectrum and are preferred to the broad-spectrum, less specific alternatives. Antibiotic selection also requires that the patient has no adverse reaction or allergy to the drug (see below and Chapter 5).

The commonest route for antibiotic therapy is oral, because of convenience and cost and the fact that intramuscular injections are painful. Higher blood levels are obtained with oral amoxycillin (a broad-spectrum penicillin) than with other forms of oral penicillin but, in severe infections, where the patient is toxic and needs high blood levels of antimicrobials urgently, or where gastrointestinal absorption is impaired, antibiotics are needed by intravenous or intramuscular injection (see below and Chapter 5).

The duration of antibiotic therapy is assessed on the response achieved. Poor response of an infection to antibiotics may be because the micro-organisms are not sensitive to the antibiotic; because dosage is inadequate; because there is failure to achieve a therapeutic blood level; because of development of bacterial resistance; or because pus is still present.

Other measures

Local heat from saline mouth baths or, occasionally, short-wave diathermy may aid resolution. The non-steroidal anti-inflammatory analgesics such as aspirin are useful to reduce pain and fever but paracetamol is preferred (Chapters 2 and 6). Narcotic analgesics cause respiratory depression, which is undesirable in these patients whose upper airways may already be severely embarrassed by spreading infection.

Minor soft tissue infections

Apical dental abscesses

Most apical abscesses from mandibular and maxillary teeth track to the buccal sulcus where they discharge or can be drained intra-orally. Pus may, in the mandibular

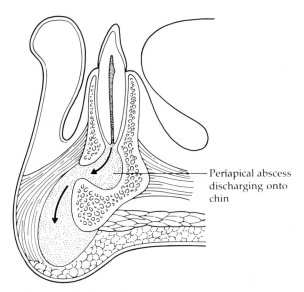

Fig. 9.19 *Rarely, apical abscesses on mandibular teeth discharge inferiorly to the muscle insertions into the mandible and discharge on the skin of the chin or submental region.*

— Periapical abscess discharging onto chin

molar region, be directed anteriorly by the buccinator insertion and can cause confusion as to the source of infection (migratory abscess). Lower incisor abscesses may discharge onto the skin, over or beneath the chin. Less commonly, dental sepsis from other teeth may also give rise to a facial sinus (Figs. 9.19 and 9.20). Palatal abscesses may arise from the palatal root of maxillary molars or upper lateral incisors. Rarely, infection from maxillary teeth may discharge into the maxillary antrum causing sinusitis.

Drainage of dental abscesses can be effected by opening the necrotic pulp, extracting the tooth, or incising a fluctuant abscess.

Periodontal abscesses

These are discussed in Volume 3.

Pericoronitis

Pericoronitis is inflammation of the soft tissues overlying a partially erupted tooth, almost invariably a mandibular third molar. Precipitating factors include poor oral hygiene, trauma from an upper molar, and immune defects. Acute pericoronitis presents with painful swelling of the operculum, halitosis, trismus, fever and regional lymph node enlargement (Fig. 9.21).

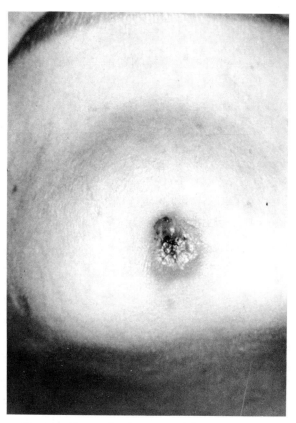

Fig. 9.20 *Sinus on skin, from an apical abscess on a mandibular incisor.*

Early treatment of pericoronitis affecting mandibular third molars includes hot salt-water or 0.2% aqueous chlorhexidine mouthbaths, chlorhexidine gel under the operculum, and grinding or removal of an upper third molar impinging on a swollen gum flap. Antibiotics (penicillin or metronidazole) are used if there is increasing pain, swelling, trismus, fever and lymphadenopathy. When the acute infection has resolved, the tooth involved may need to be extracted (Volumes 2 and 3).

Dry socket

This is discussed in Volumes 2 and 3.

Major fascial space infections

Fascial space infections are summarized below; treatment is on p. 227.

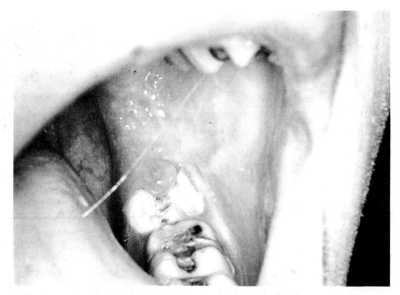

Fig. 9.21 *Pericoronitis related to lower third molar.*

Submandibular space infection (Fig. 9.22)

Anatomy. The mylohyoid muscle lies supero-medially, the hyoglossus postero-medially, the digastric anteriorly and the cervical investing fascia superficially.

Aetiology. Pus tracking lingually from mandibular molars with apices below the mylohyoid insertion: breakdown of submandibular lymph nodes; spread from submental or sublingual space infections; or penetrating wound.

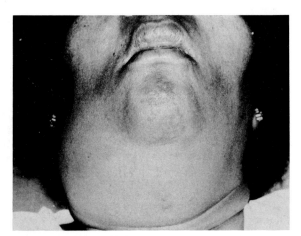

Fig. 9.22 *Submandibular space infection (courtesy of R. P. Ward-Booth).*

Presentation. Submandibular inflammatory swelling, fever, dysphagia, and slight trismus (Fig. 9.22).

Progression without treatment. May cross the midline to the opposite submandibular space or behind the mylohyoid to the sublingual spaces, or progress to Ludwig's angina (see below).

Submental space infection

Anatomy. The mandible lies anteriorly, the mylohyoid muscle superiorly, anterior bellies of digastric muscle laterally, hyoid bone posteriorly and cervical fascia superficially.

Aetiology. Breakdown of submental lymph nodes, or a penetrating wound.

Presentation. Intense, tender swelling under the chin, with dysphagia.

Progression without treatment. Spread to the submandibular space.

Sublingual space infection

Anatomy. The oral mucosa lies superiorly, the hyoglossus and genial muscles medially, and the mylohyoid inferiorly and laterally.

Aetiology. Pus tracking lingually from mandibular teeth with apices above the mylohyoid, or a penetrating wound.

Presentation. Swollen, tender raised floor of mouth with oedematous jelly-like mucosa.

Progression without treatment. May cross midline or spread posteriorly to the submandibular or pterygomandibular spaces.

Pterygomandibular space infection

Anatomy. The vertical mandibular ramus lies laterally, the medial pterygoid muscle medially, and the parotid gland posteriorly.

Aetiology. Pericoronitis; needle track infection (inferior alveolar block injection).

Presentation. Pain, severe trismus, dysphagia and fever.

Progression without treatment. Spread to lateral pharyngeal or infratemporal spaces.

Lateral pharyngeal space infection

Anatomy. The medial pterygoid muscle lies laterally, the superior constrictor medially, the styloid apparatus postero-medially, and the base of skull posteriorly.

Aetiology. Pericoronitis; or spread from pterygomandibular/buccal/submandibular spaces.

Presentation. Pain, fever, trismus, dysphagia, dysphonia and medial displacement of the pharyngeal wall.

Progression without treatment. Spread to the retropharyngeal space and mediastinum. Involvement of the carotid sheath with carotid artery rupture or septic internal jugular vein thrombosis. Spread via the pterygoid plexus to cause cavernous sinus thrombosis.

Peritonsillar space infection

Anatomy. The superior constrictor muscle lies laterally and the pharyngeal mucosa medially.

Aetiology. Tonsillar abscesses; pericoronitis.

Presentation. Pain radiating to the ear, dysphagia, fever, tender swelling involving the soft palate displacing the uvula to the opposite side (this is a quinsy).

Progression without treatment. Spread across the midline with upper airway obstruction.

Buccal space infection (Fig. 9.23)

Anatomy. The buccinator muscle lies medially, the masseter postero-medially, and the platysma laterally.

Aetiology. Apical abscess from maxillary or mandibular molars with apices outside the buccinator insertion.

Presentation. Tender swelling of the cheek, trismus.

Progression without treatment. Posterior spread to

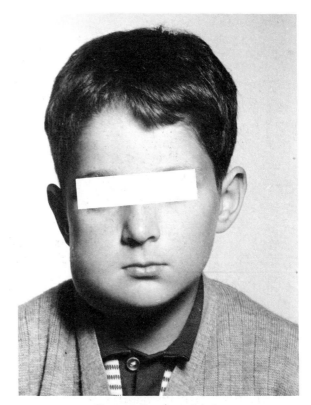

Fig. 9.23 *Buccal space infection.*

the pterygomandibular/lateral pharyngeal/infratemporal spaces.

Infratemporal space infection (Fig. 9.24)

Anatomy. The coronoid process and temporalis muscle tendon lie laterally, and the pterygoid muscles medially.

Aetiology. Infection from upper third molars; needle track infection from posterior-superior-alveolar nerve local analgesic injections; or spread from pterygomandibular/buccal spaces.

Presentation. Pain, extreme trismus, tender swelling above the zygomatic arch (Fig. 9.24).

Progression without treatment. Via the pterygoid plexus to cause cavernous sinus thrombosis. Osteomyelitis of the outer table of skull.

Submasseteric abscess

Anatomy. The vertical mandibular ramus lies medially, the masseter laterally, and the parotid posteriorly.

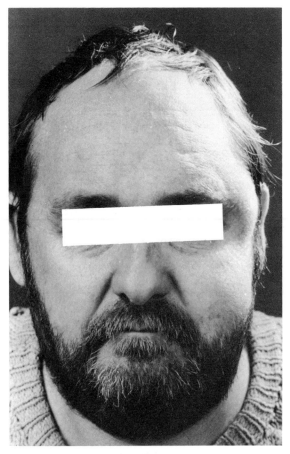

Fig. 9.24 *Inftatemporal space infection on the left.*

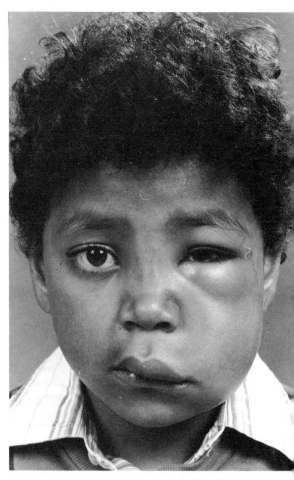

Fig. 9.25 *Canine fossa infection; the oedema also gravitates, so that the swelling involves a large part of the lower left face.*

Aetiology. Pericoronitis, particularly of distally impacted lower wisdom teeth.

Presentation. Intense trismus, minimal tender swelling. Radiographs show masseter muscle lifted away from mandible.

Progression without treatment. Osteomyelitis and sequestration of buccal plate of vertical ramus.

Canine fossa infection (Fig. 9.25)

Anatomy. Anteriorly lies the orbicularis oris muscle, posteriorly the buccinator, superiorly the extrinsic muscles of the upper lip.

Aetiology. Apical infections of maxillary canines and premolars.

Presentation. Swelling, cellulitis of upper cheek, naso-labial fold and lower eyelid (Fig. 9.25).

Progression without treatment. Via the external angular vein to give a cavernous sinus thrombosis.

Ludwig's angina (Fig. 9.26)

Anatomy. Bilateral infection of submandibular and sublingual spaces.

Aetiology. Pericoronitis; spread of submandibular/sublingual infections; penetrating wounds.

Presentation. Bilateral swelling submandibularly, a raised tender floor of mouth and tongue, dysphagia, dysphonia and respiratory embarrassment.

Progression without treatment. Upper airway obstruction and death.

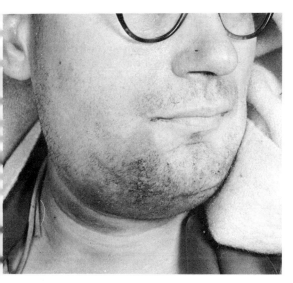

Fig. 9.26 *Ludwig's angina: a dangerous bilateral infection of the sublingual and submandibular spaces.*

Treatment of major soft tissue infections

Deaths from asphyxia, mediastinitis, cavernous sinus thrombosis, carotid artery rupture, and septic thrombosis of the internal jugular vein are possible, but the incidence has fallen with the use of high dose antibiotics. Patients should be admitted to hospital. Drainage should be intra-oral, extra-oral, or 'through and through' i.e. from mouth through to skin, depending on the anatomical site involved. Because of the potential respiratory obstruction, trismus and the possibility of abscess rupture with inhalation of pus, general anaesthetic induction and intubation are hazardous. Tracheostomy may be life-saving on occasions.

INFECTIONS OF WOUNDS AND BURNS

Wounds may be infected with a range of organisms. Oral wounds tend to be infected mainly with bacteroides, fusobacteria and streptococcal species; skin wounds mainly with *Staphylococcus aureus* and *Escherichia coli*. The source of infection can be endogenous from the local flora, or exogenous from the operator, a member of staff, another patient, from inanimate objects, or by the airborne route. Wound infection is increased by:

(a) surgery that is excessively traumatic or with poor asepsis,

(b) overcrowding and poor hygiene,

(c) poor host resistance,

(d) duration of surgery,

(e) 'dirty' surgery, e.g. neck resection plus intra-oral dissection.

Burns can be invaded by any micro-organism but especially mixed infections of *Staphylococcus aureus*, Gram-negative bacilli including *Pseudomonas aeruginosa* (*pyocyaneus*), and/or beta haemolytic streptococci (*Streptococcus pyogenes*). Sources of infections are as for surgical wounds but some burns units have resident pathogens that can cause infection (**nosocomial** infections).

Burns should be swabbed for culture at each change of dressing or where there is evidence of infection in view of the danger of deep invasion and septicaemia. Local cleansing with appropriate antiseptics, and systemic antimicrobials are usually indicated (page 228).

Infections of wounds after 'clean' surgery (see above (e)), and burns may well suggest poor aseptic techniques—which should then be reviewed.

SUPPURATIVE SIALADENITIS

This is discussed in Volume 2.

NON-ODONTOGENIC BACTERIAL INFECTIONS IN THE HEAD AND NECK

Children may occasionally develop cervico-facial bacterial abscesses without evidence of a dental source. These are usually abscesses in the submandibular lymph nodes, secondary to haematogenous spread of bacteria (Fig. 9.27). Since these infections are usually caused by penicillin-resistant *Staphylococcus aureus*, flucloxacillin is the antibiotic of choice. Rarely, abscesses are related to immune deficiency such as chronic granulomatous disease (Volume 2), to mycobacterial infection such as tuberculosis and atypical mycobacteria (see Fig. 2.13, p. 22; and Volume 2), to cat-scratch fever or mucocutaneous lymph node syndrome (Volume 2).

Buccal cellulitis is an uncommon infection of buccal tissues in pre-school children, usually caused by *Haemophilus influenzae* type B.

ACTINOMYCOSIS

Cervico-facial actinomycosis is caused by *Actinomyces israelii*, a bacterium showing some features of a fungus. The organism is an intra-oral commensal but may rarely give rise to bony or, more usually, soft tissue infections after tooth extraction or jaw fracture. Clinically a brawny, purple swelling over or below the angle of the mandible

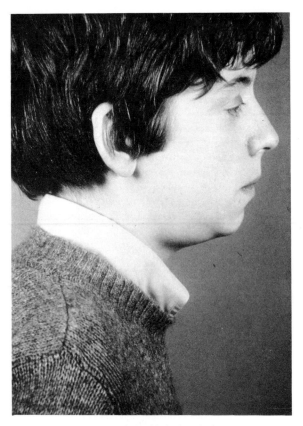

Fig. 9.27 Submandibular lymphadenitis.

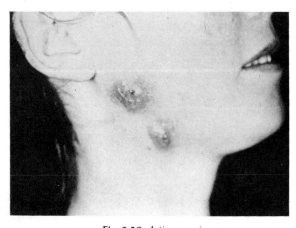

Fig. 9.28 Actinomycosis.

with multiple sinuses is classical (Fig. 9.28). Drainage of the swelling may produce pus containing 'sulphur granules' which are colonies of the organisms. Gram staining and microscopy of these granules show typical hyphae and clubs. The organisms excite a response showing features of both acute and chronic inflammation. The importance of actinomycosis is that prolonged antibiotic therapy for 6–8 weeks with penicillin or amoxycillin is needed. Minocycline (a tetracycline) is the antimicrobial of choice in patients allergic to penicillin.

Viral, fungal and protozoal infections

These are considered in Chapter 2 and Volume 2.

TREATMENT OF BACTERIAL INFECTIONS
(Table 9.8)

As indicated above, *removal of the cause of infection and drainage of pus* are the prime means of treatment of these infections.

Antibacterials

Antibacterials are indicated in the following circumstances (Tables 9.8 and 9.9; see also Chapter 5 and Table 8.1).

1. *Bacterial infections* (together with appropriate surgical or other measures).
    Infections of fascial spaces of neck.
    Osteomyelitis.
    Odontogenic infections in ill or immunocompromised patients.
    Acute ulcerative gingivitis.
    Suppurative parotitis.
    Suppurative lymphadenitis.
    Actinomycosis.
    Tuberculosis.
    Syphilis.
2. *Prophylaxis.*
    Of infective endocarditis (Chapter 2).
    In cerebrospinal rhinorrhoea (Volume 2): however, many units do not now give prophylaxis for this.
    In facial fractures or compound skull fractures (Volume 2).
    In major oral and maxillofacial surgery (e.g. osteotomies and 'dirty' cancer surgery).
    Possibly surgery in patients with ventriculo-atrial shunts and prosthetic hip replacements (Chapter 2).

Table 9.9

Antibacterials useful in dentistry

Infection	Common choices of antimicrobials in UK*	
	First choices	Alternative if patient is allergic to first choice or if that drug is otherwise contraindicated
Dental abscess	Penicillin V Metronidazole	Erythromycin Tetracyclines
Fascial space infection	Benzylpenicillin (i.m. or i.v.) Metronidazole (i.m. or i.v.)	Erythromycin Tetracyclines
Pericoronitis	Penicillin V Metronidazole	Erythromycin Tetracyclines
Osteomyelitis	Benzylpenicillin (i.m.) Metronidazole (i.m.)	Clindamycin Erythromycin Tetracyclines
Wound infection	Penicillin V Metronidazole	Erythromycin Tetracyclines
Sinusitis/oroantral fistula	Co-trimoxazole Ampicillin	Erythromycin Tetracyclines
Suppurative sialadenitis	Flucloxacillin	Erythromycin
Actinomycosis	Benzylpenicillin (i.m.) Amoxycillin	Minocycline

* Culture and sensitivity of bacteria may indicate alternative drugs. Table based on a survey of UK oral and maxillofacial surgeons, 1986 (Y. Gill and C. Scully; unpublished).

In surgery in immunocompromised patients or where there has been local irradiation (Chapter 2).

3. Antibacterials are also indicated in some instances of:

pericoronitis
dental abscess
dry socket
minor oral surgery.

Oral antimicrobials should be used in most instances. Topical antimicrobials should be avoided since they may produce sensitization and may cause the emergence of resistant strains of micro-organisms.

Parenteral administration of antimicrobials may be indicated where:

(a) high blood levels are required rapidly (e.g. in serious infections);

(b) the patient can or will not take oral medications (e.g. an unconscious patient);

(c) the patient is to have a general anaesthetic within the following 4 hours (stomach should be kept empty);

(d) no oral preparation is available (e.g. there is no oral preparation of vancomycin—an antibiotic sometimes needed for endocarditis prophylaxis; Chapter 2).

Failure of an infection to respond to an antimicrobial within 48 hours should prompt reconsideration of:

(a) adequacy of drainage of pus;

(b) appropriateness of the antimicrobial;

(c) antimicrobial sensitivities of the micro-organism (staphylococci are now frequently resistant to penicillin);

(d) patient compliance;

(e) possible local factors (e.g. foreign body);

(f) possibility of unusual type of infection;

(g) possibility of impaired host defences (unusual and opportunistic infections are increasingly identified, particularly in the immunocompromised patient);

(h) *whether the lesion is actually an infection.*

In serious or unusual infections consult the clinical microbiologist.

Penicillins

Penicillins are useful bactericidal antibiotics that contain a beta-lactam ring in the molecule which interferes with bacterial cell wall synthesis. Unfortunately some micro-organisms, especially some staphylococci and Gram-negative rods, produce enzymes (lactamases or penicillinases) that destroy the beta-lactam bond and thereby render the antimicrobial ineffective. Antibiotic resistance may also be to methicillin (an increasing problem in *Staphylococcus aureus*) and some staphylococci are penicillin tolerant by a third, unidentified, mechanism.

Most oral infections respond to penicillins but these are contraindicated if:

(a) the patient is allergic to penicillin, since he may then develop at least an allergic rash and possibly anaphylaxis (Chapters 2, 4 and 5; Fig. 4.8, p. 110).

(b) the patient has received penicillin within the previous month, since then penicillin-resistant microorganisms may be present;

(c) the infection is likely to be resistant to penicillin or fails to respond to penicillin.

Amoxycillin is an orally active broad-spectrum penicillin whose absorption is better than that of ampicillin. It is not resistant to penicillinase and *Staphylococcus aureus* and bacteroides are often resistant. Amoxycillin is currently the first choice for the antimicrobial prophylaxis of infective endocarditis (see Fig. 2.12, p. 19); Chapter 2), but because of expense it is not the first choice for other oral infections (see Table 9.9). It is contraindicated in penicillin-hypersensitive patients, and may also cause rashes in patients with infectious mononucleosis, lymphoid leukaemia, or in those who are on allopurinol. Augmentin is a mixture of amoxycillin and potassium clavulanate: the latter inhibits some penicillinases. Augmentin is therefore active against most *Staphylococcus aureus* and against some Gram-negative bacteria.

Ampicillin is similar to amoxycillin. The many analogues have few if any advantages. Ampicillin is less well absorbed after oral administration than amoxycillin but is cheaper.

Benzylpenicillin is the prototype penicillin. It is not orally active, since it is destroyed by gastric acid, but it is the most effective penicillin where the organism is sensitive. Benzylpenicillin is effective mainly against Gram-positive cocci, especially streptococci (including oral streptococci). It is not resistant to penicillinase and is therefore ineffective against most *Staphylococcus aureus*. It is contraindicated in penicillin-hypersensitive patients.

Flucloxacillin is an orally active narrow-spectrum penicillin derivative which is penicillinase resistant and therefore effective against penicillin-resistant staphylococci. It is contraindicated in penicillin-hypersensitive patients. Cloxacillin is related but less well absorbed after oral administration. Both cloxacillin and flucloxacillin have low activity against streptococci.

Phenoxymethyl penicillin (penicillin V) is an acid-resistant orally active analogue of benzylpenicillin which is not resistant to penicillinase. The spectrum is similar to that of benzylpenicillin; it is cheaper than amoxycillin. It is contraindicated in penicillin-hypersensitive patients.

Procaine penicillin is a depot penicillin, not resistant to penicillinase, and is contraindicated in penicillin-hypersensitive patients. Rarely, a psychotic reaction results from procaine penicillin.

Cephalosporins

Cephalosporins are broad-spectrum antibiotics that have a beta-lactam ring structure. There are few absolute indications for their use in dentistry. Hypersensitivity is the main side-effect but some cause a bleeding tendency, some are nephrotoxic and most are expensive. About 10% of penicillin-allergic patients will also react to the cephalosporins. Cefuroxime and cephamandole are less affected by penicillinases than other cephalosporins and currently are the preferred drugs of this group. Cephamandole causes an Antabuse-type (disulfiram-type) reaction with alcohol (see below under Metronidazole).

Cephamandole is not orally active and is contraindicated if there is a history of anaphylaxis to penicillin.

Cefuroxime is not orally active and is contraindicated if there is a history of anaphylaxis to penicillin. Cefuroxime is not nephrotoxic.

There are only four orally active cephalosporins available (cephalexin, cephradine, cefadroxil and cefaclor). They are similar in activity to flucloxacillin but are also effective against some Gram-negative organisms.

Erythromycin

Erythromycin is an antibiotic with a similar antibacterial spectrum to penicillin, but is active against penicillinase-producing organisms. It is used in penicillin-allergic patients. It is bacteriostatic. Erythromycin estolate may cause liver disease and, therefore, the stearate should be used.

Erythromycin stearate is orally active and useful in those patients hypersensitive to penicillin since it is effective against most staphylococci and streptococci (Chapter 2) but there is rapid development of bacterial resistance.

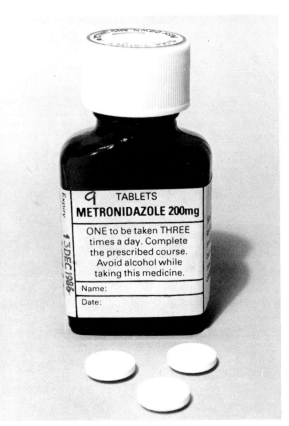

Fig. 9.29 *Metronidazole: an effective alternative to penicillin for many odontogenic infections.*

Metronidazole

Metronidazole is a nitroimidazole antimicrobial which interferes with the synthesis of nucleic acids by anaerobes and therefore is effective against them (Fig. 9.29). It should be used for less than 7 days (or peripheral neuropathy may develop, particularly in patients with liver dysfunction). Patients taking metronidazole should avoid alcohol, which causes an unpleasant disulfiram-type (Antabuse-type) reaction with flushing, vomiting and headaches. Metronidazole is contraindicated in pregnancy.

Metronidazole is commonly used in the treatment of acute ulcerative gingivitis and acute pericoronitis.

Sulphonamides

Sulphonamides compete for the bacterial enzymes that convert para-aminobenzoic acid to folic acid. They are bacteriostatic. The main indications for sulphonamides in dentistry were in the prophylaxis of post-traumatic meningitis but meningococci (*Neisseria meningitidis*) are increasingly resistant and many units now give no prophylaxis. Sulphonamides are contraindicated in pregnancy and in renal disease. In other patients adequate hydration must be ensured to prevent the (rare) occurrence of crystalluria. Other adverse reactions include erythema multiforme, rashes, and blood dyscrasias.

Co-trimoxazole, a combination of trimethoprim and sulphamethoxazole, is orally active, has a broad spectrum, and can be useful especially in the treatment of sinusitis. Co-trimoxazole is contraindicated in pregnancy since it interferes with folate metabolism.

Tetracyclines

Tetracyclines have a broad antibacterial spectrum and are bacteriostatic by interfering with bacterial protein synthesis. There are many preparations with little to choose between them, but doxycycline is useful since a single daily dose is adequate, while minocycline, which is given twice daily, is effective against meningococci—and both are safer for patients with renal failure since most other tetracyclines are nephrotoxic. In children below the age of 8 years, and pregnant and nursing mothers, tetracyclines are contraindicated since they cause intrinsic dental discoloration (Fig. 5.4, p. 24). Minocycline may cause superficial tooth staining in adults. Tetracyclines also predispose to oral candidosis.

Other antibacterials less commonly used in dentistry

Rifampicin is reserved mainly for treatment of tuberculosis, but may be used in prophylaxis of meningitis after head injury since *Neisseria meningitidis* may be resistant to sulphonamides. Although rifampicin is safe and effective, bacterial resistance rapidly occurs. Body secretions including saliva may turn red, and rifampicin may cause occasional rashes, jaundice or blood dyscrasias.

Gentamicin, since it can cause vestibular and renal damage, is reserved for prophylaxis of endocarditis under certain conditions (Chapter 2) or for the treatment of serious infections.

Vancomycin is also reserved for serious infections, prophylaxis of endocarditis under certain conditions (Chapter 2), and treatment of pseudomembranous colitis (see below). Vancomycin has to be given slowly intravenously and any extravenous extravasation may cause pain. Vancomycin may also cause nausea, rashes, tinnitus and deafness, and patients may turn red transiently (redneck syndrome). Vancomycin is contraindicated in renal disease.

Clindamycin has similar activity to erythromycin but is also active against anaerobes. It is said to be especially effective in bone infections but is rarely used since it may, especially in the elderly, produce a pseudomembranous colitis caused by colonization with *Clostridium difficile*.

FURTHER READING

Dinsdale R. C. W. (1985). *Viral hepatitis, AIDS and dental treatment*. London: British Dental Journal.

Finch R. G., Snider G. E., Sprinkle P. M. (1980). Ludwig's angina. *JAMA* **243**: 1171–1173.

Heimdahl A., Von Konow L., Satoh L., Nord C. E. (1985). Clinical appearance of orofacial infections of odontogenic origin in relation to microbiological findings. *J. clin. Microbiol.* **22**: 299–302.

Kirkpatrick B., Wise R. (1986). Man bites dog. *Br. med. J.* **293**: 1522–1523.

Kondell P. A. (1984). *Staphylococcus aureus in oral surgery*. Stockholm: Karolinska Institute.

Labriola J. D., Mascaro J., Alpert B. (1983). The microbiologic flora of orofacial abscesses. *J. oral Maxillofacial Surg.* **41**: 711–714.

McCracken A. W., Cawson R. A. (1983). *Clinical and oral microbiology*. New York: McGraw-Hill.

Porter S. R., Scully C., Cawson R. A. (1986). AIDS: update and guidelines for general dental practice. *Dent. Update* **14**: 9–17

Scully C. (1985). Hepatitis B: an update in relation to dentistry. *Br. dent. J.* **159**: 321–328.

Scully C., Cawson R. A. (1987). Medical problems in dentistry, 2nd edn. Bristol: Wright.

Shovelton D. S. (1982). The prevention of cross-infection in dentistry. *Br. dent. J.* **153**: 260–264.

Workshop report on the control of cross-infection (1986). *Br. dent. J.* **160**: 131–134.

Hazards in dentistry

HAZARDS TO PATIENTS

The main principle of any form of treatment is 'first do no harm'. Virtually any form of drug treatment or surgical procedure carries some risk to the patient, albeit often only a very low level of risk. The decision to treat, how to treat, or not to treat, is therefore based on a balanced judgement of risk that depends on a multitude of factors. For example, it is clearly essential to treat a patient with a life-threatening disease such as oral cancer. On the other hand, it is quite unnecessary to treat an asymptomatic benign condition such as white sponge naevus (Volume 2). Most conditions are intermediate, i.e. if not treated, there is some risk of complications. Unerupted wisdom teeth are common and may present a dilemma when the need for treatment to prevent possible complications such as pericoronitis may or may not exceed the risk of possible sequelae of operation such as inferior alveolar nerve or lingual nerve anaesthesia. Age, systemic disease, and social factors may also influence the decision to treat or perhaps the timing of the treatment. What, for example, is a simple extraction in a healthy patient may prove life-threatening to a haemophiliac or may produce chronic pain from osteoradionecrosis in a person who has received radiotherapy to the jaws. The replacement of a discoloured anterior restoration is hardly a priority for a wife caring for her dying husband but may well be a priority for a bride-to-be.

Many of the possible hazards to patients are outlined in the previous chapters in this volume or below, or are discussed in the other volumes of this series. Indeed, most chapters include some reference to hazards. Many 'accidents' can be avoided or the damage reduced in the following ways (Fig. 10.1). *Prevention is better than cure.*

1. Careful taking and documentation of the dental and medical histories, i.e. *history taking and note keeping.*

2. Full discussion with the patient about his or her condition and the likely complications of treating or not treating it, i.e. *informed consent—check always that what you intend to do concurs with the expectations of patients.*

3. Use of high-quality, well-maintained equipment and materials, i.e. *equipment maintenance; control of cross-infection; safety standards.*

4. Education of staff in principles of dentistry, management of emergencies, instrument maintenance, hygiene, control of cross-infection, use and disposal of toxic products, radiation protection, etc., i.e. *staff education and safety training—always work with a third party present.*

5. Undertaking only those forms of treatment and anaesthesia in which you have adequate competence and treating patients only with systemic disease with which you are competent to deal, i.e. *knowing your abilities and limitations—postgraduate education.*

6. Adopt a cautious approach to treatment: consider medical treatment before surgical, use only drugs with which you are familiar, and use the simplest procedure commensurate with the needs of the patient if surgery is indicated. Take especial care with general anaesthesia (Chapter 6) and, in general, be gentle with tissues (Chapter 8), i.e. *avoid unnecessary treatment or overprescribing—avoid unnecessary general anaesthesia; do not act as operator–anaesthetist.*

If an incident does occur:

(a) *do* treat the patient or refer as appropriate;

(b) *do* record everything accurately in the notes with details of the incident, and signed by any third party present;

(c) *do* report, in writing, full details to your Medical Defence Society;

(d) *do not* admit liability nor reply directly to threats of proceedings or compensation claims (see Further Reading).

Some of the hazards to patients are discussed elsewhere in the text or series and are summarized in Table 10.1; others are outlined in Table 10.2 and below.

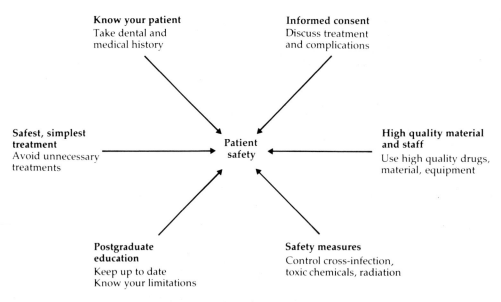

Fig. 10.1 *Reducing hazards to patients.*

Physical damage

Trauma

Much of the equipment used in dental practice constitutes some hazard to the patient. Obvious dangers are the trapping of fingers or limbs when moving the dental chair; and damage from the drill or sharp instruments. Particularly disconcerting are eye injuries and, for this reason, patients should always be protected with eye-shields when undergoing procedures using dental drills or wires, or procedures under general anaesthesia (Chapter 9).

Damage to the mouth is especially possible when rotating instruments are used (particularly discs without guards), or during general anaesthesia—too many incisors are damaged by careless use of a laryngoscope, and too many lips bruised or lacerated by careless retracting (Fig. 10.2; see also Chapter 8).

Extraction of the wrong teeth is an ever-present hazard which will only be avoided by careful history-taking and examination, careful documentation, and careful attention to detail and cross-checking by all concerned. Iatrogenic jaw fractures and temporomandibular joint dislocation are rare complications.

Since disposable needles and scalpels are now used almost universally, and the quality of equipment has improved, breakages and loss into the tissues in the course of normal use are now rare. Of course, if the instrument is mishandled or the patient moves violently, accidents can happen. A particular problem is the breakage of a local

Table 10.1
*Some hazards to dental patients discussed elsewhere**

Hazards	Chapters
Infections	2, 9
Drug reactions	2, 5
Inhaled foreign bodies	4, 6, 7
Emergencies in the dental chair	4
Complications of surgery	8

* See also other volumes in this series.

Table 10.2
Other potential hazards to dental patients

Physical injury, including nerve injury

Chemical injury, including mercury toxicity

Radiation

Psychological damage

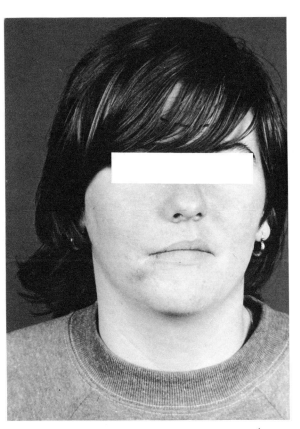

Fig. 10.2 *Blistering at the right commissure after careless handling of the tissues.*

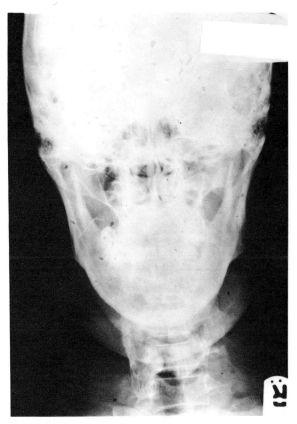

Fig. 10.3 *Needle fractured after inferior alveolar local anaesthetic injection.*

analgesic needle—especially when giving an inferior alveolar nerve block. Needles break at points of stress, e.g. at points of bending or at the hub if inserted that far—which, anatomically, is unnecessary (Fig. 10.3; Chapter 6), and a set of mosquito forceps should be at hand to grasp the fractured end and remove the needle. However, the main danger with fractured instruments is that of inhalation (see below).

Asphyxia

Protection of airway patency is of paramount importance since brain damage soon follows hypoxia, and death can occur rapidly. Three minutes of cerebral hypoxia is usually regarded as sufficient to produce irreversible brain damage.

Airway obstruction is usually produced by laryngeal spasm or a foreign body in the airway but may be caused by oedema or haematoma formation around the larynx. If

treatment of the cause does not almost immediately clear the airway, tracheostomy may well be required (Chapter 8).

1. *Laryngeal spasm.* Laryngeal spasm is especially likely to occur if there is laryngeal irritation by, for example, mucus or saliva, particularly during induction of general anaesthesia with an intravenous barbiturate such as methohexitone (Chapter 6), or by fluid or debris during recovery. The airway should be sucked clear and oxygen given; suxamethonium may be required and the patient then must be ventilated.

2. *Inhalation or ingestion of foreign bodies.* Extreme caution must be exercised when small objects are introduced into the mouth, lest they be inhaled or ingested (Fig. 10.4). Particular dangers are posed by endodontic instruments, dental burs that are inadequately secured in the handpiece, and restorations such as inlays and crowns. The patient most at risk, of course, is the one who is

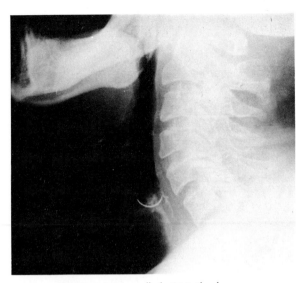

Fig. 10.4 *Suture needle 'lost' into the pharynx.*

having a general anaesthetic since then the protective cough reflex is depressed. The occasional particularly dangerous anaesthetist has even pushed a denture he had forgotten to remove into the larynx!

Patients treated without general anaesthetics should have restorative treatment under rubber dam or, if that is impossible, endodontic instruments should be secured on a 'parachute chain' (Figs. 4.11, 4.15, pp. 113–15; Volume 3).

3. *Laryngeal oedema/haematoma.* Trauma or infection in the neck or tongue; infection spreading from the floor of the mouth (Chapter 9), non-infective oedema such as in angioedema (Chapter 2), and haemorrhage as in patients with a bleeding tendency (Chapter 2) can all hazard the airway.

Surgical emphysema (see also Chapter 8)

A somewhat disconcerting but innocuous complication of dental treatment is surgical emphysema, in which there is rapid accumulation of air in the subcutaneous or submucosal tissues. Palpation produces a crackling sound, or crepitus. The cause is usually the use of the air rotor or compressed air syringe during endodontics; occasionally it can be other incidents such as air rotor soft tissue wounds. Most cases resolve spontaneously within a week.

Burns

Heat, cold, chemicals or radiation can burn patients.

Heat burns

Obvious causes of heat burns to be avoided are instruments just removed from the autoclave or hot-air oven since it is difficult to gauge their temperature through rubber gloves. Extraction forceps and metal mouth gags in particular retain heat for very many minutes and have caused severe orofacial burns. High-speed handpieces are water cooled and if working efficiently cannot burn tissues; if there is inadequate cooling, the dental pulp is easily damaged or destroyed. Prolonged use of handpieces may lead to overheating and burns from the hot shank may be produced.

Other occasional causes of thermal burns are from hot impression compound, naked flames and from electrical diathermy.

Cold burns

Cold burns are rare in dentistry, but spillage of liquid nitrogen is a problem attendant on use of certain types of cryosurgical equipment.

Chemical burns

Chemical burns are all too common. Acids, such as phosphoric acid, chromic acid and trichloracetic acid, and corrosives, such as paramonochlorphenol, continue to be spilt in patients' mouths or, worse, on their skin or eyes. The occasional practitioner has even managed to force caustic endodontic materials through the root apex and into the inferior alveolar nerve canal, with disastrous consequences (Fig. 10.5).

Radiation burns

Radiation burns from diagnostic radiation should now be unheard of, but radiation mucositis is common after therapeutic radiotherapy to the head and neck (Volume 2) and burns may occur during laser treatment. The hazards of ultraviolet and blue lights are discussed below.

Dental amalgam

Mercury is a potent neurotoxin. Though spilt mercury is a clear hazard to those in the environment, far less clear-cut is any risk from mercury in amalgam restorations. According to the American Dental Association, the British Dental Association, the Department of Health and the National Institute of Dental Research, *there is no evidence that amalgam fillings are dangerous to patients* (see *Journal of American Dental Association* (1983) **106**: 519).

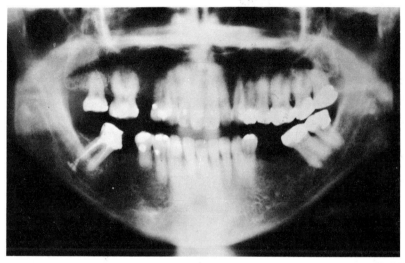

Fig. 10.5 *Root-filling material introduced into the right inferior dental canal during root treatment of the lower second molar.*

Radiation

Ionizing radiation such as x-rays are a hazard mainly where the individual is developing, such as the fetus or young child, or where cells are proliferating, such as in the gonads and bone marrow. Because of the capacity of ionizing radiation to induce genetic mutations in the germinal tissues (teratogenic effect) or to induce malignant tumours in other tissues (oncogenic effect), exposure must be kept to the very minimum.

The best way to reduce exposure is to take radiographs only where and when they are absolutely required for diagnosis or treatment.

Lead aprons

Plastic or rubber aprons with incorporated lead salts are available for protecting especially radiosensitive tissues (i.e. fetus, gonads, bone marrow, thyroid) from scattered radiation.

An apron of lead equivalent of 0.25 mm is adequate for dental use. For panoramic radiation and cephalometry, a double-sided apron that covers the patient's back and front as well as sides should be used.

Cassettes and intensifying screens

Extra-oral radiography uses cassettes containing intensifying screens. These are thin metal light-tight containers for light-sensitive film containing sheets of card covered with calcium tungstate crystals which emit light when struck by x-radiation—thereby exposing the film.

Cassettes reduce the radiation to about one-tenth of that necessary to produce an image of the same density on wrapped packet film, but the detail is not as good as intra-oral film, due to the very poor edge definition resulting from the crystals' diffuse light emission. The larger the crystals the poorer the definition—but the faster the film.

Dental x-ray sets are suitable for taking extra-oral lateral oblique views of the jaws using cassettes and intensifying screens.

OCCUPATIONAL HAZARDS TO DENTAL STAFF

All occupations are associated with some hazards and many are *far* more hazardous than dentistry. The various hazards that may arise in the practice of dentistry are outlined in Table 10.3 and Figure 10.6, but in most instances the level of risk is extremely low. Some of the hazards apply to staff and patients.

Certain organs are more prone to damage than others during dentistry: the eyes, respiratory system and skin are mainly at risk but dentists seem, in general, more concerned with hazards from infections and from mercury.

Table 10.3
Occupational hazards in dentistry

Infections

Allergies and toxic substances: mercury, methacrylates anaesthetic gas pollution etc.

Postural and other work-related injuries, including eye injuries, hearing loss etc.

Radiation, electrical and ultrasonic hazards

Hostile patients

Laboratory hazards: dusts, formaldehyde, solvents, contact dermatitis, burns etc.

Drug dependence

Medico-legal hazards

Stress and psychogenic disease

Socio-economically related problems

The eyes

Good eyesight is essential to the practice of dentistry and every care should be taken to protect the eyes from damage.

Foreign bodies

With drill speeds of 250 000 r/min small particles may be projected at velocities of up to 10 m/s and may cause conjunctivitis, corneal abrasions or even dangerous penetrating wounds. Particular care should also be taken when using or cutting wire. Patients or staff may be wounded.

Damage from instruments

Blunt injury may cause a subconjunctival haemorrhage— usually trivial, but this may conceal a deeper injury. Penetrating injuries can be caused by any sharp instrument such as a dental probe. Patients or staff may be wounded.

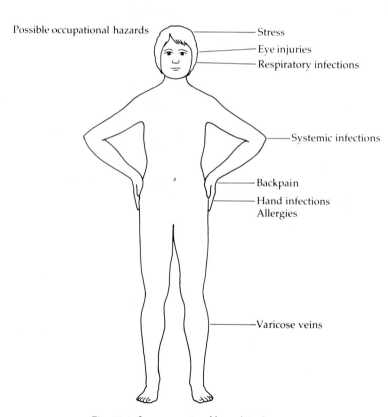

Fig. 10.6 *Some occupational hazards in dentistry.*

Damage from chemicals

Chemicals used in dentistry, particularly phosphoric acid, sodium hypochlorite, trichloracetic and chromic acids, can all cause serious chemical burns. Patients or staff can be wounded.

Cross-infection

Herpes simplex is one of the worst ocular infections that can be contracted by the dental surgeon, but bacterial conjunctivitis caused by *Staphylococcus aureus* is more common.

Ultraviolet light (315–400 nm) (Fig. 10.7)

Ultraviolet light (which is used for curing some dental resins) is damaging especially to the anterior segment of the eye, but the shorter wavelength component also damages the retina.

Blue light (400–500 nm)

Repeated viewing of blue-light sources used for curing filling materials may lead to visual fatigue and the light of short wavelength could damage the retina, thermally and photochemically.

Lasers

Lasers are used in some surgical procedures. Laser energies of different wavelengths have specific absorptive characteristics in tissues. The argon and neodymium-YAG lasers have wavelengths in the spectrum of visible light and are absorbed preferentially by pigmented tissues (such as the retina if shone in the eye). The CO_2 laser emits energy in the infrared zone, invisible but damaging because it produces heat. It is absorbed by all soft tissues. The helium–neon laser is less damaging but still must be used with care (Volume 2).

No laser should be shone into the eyes or in unintended directions.

Radiation (see page 243)

Surgery lighting

Correct illumination of the surgery is of prime importance. Colour-corrected tube lighting is now readily available, but additional illumination is necessary when operating, particularly in conservative dentistry. Most lights now employ quartz–halogen low-voltage (40 V) bulbs. The patient should be protected against bulb splintering by a safety glass front to the lamp, which can also be readily cleaned.

Recently, dicroic lighting has been used with success. This incorporates up to six focused spotlights, so switched that four are used at any one time, depending on the working position. Lights may be mounted on the ceiling so as to leave the operating area clear.

Prevention of eye injury

Eyes should be protected from foreign bodies, infected material, chemicals, and various forms of radiation.

The simplest and most effective method of preventing eye injury is the use of protective spectacles, preferably with plastic lenses and side shields, and the avoidance of excessive exposure to hazards. Close-viewing, fixing the eye on a light spot and treating anterior teeth increase the exposure to light. Exposures to wavelengths shorter than 500 nm are cumulative and the potential for injury increases the shorter the wavelength. The greatest retinal hazard is from light of wavelengths about 400 nm.

Protective glasses with coloured lenses of sufficient

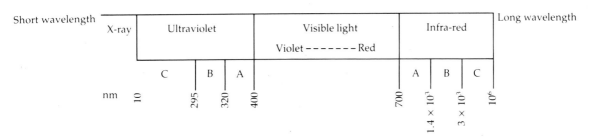

Fig. 10.7 *Optical radiation.*

optical density are indicated when using blue or ultra-violet light. Ordinary dark glasses do *not* filter the offending wavelengths but, by absorbing visible light, cause pupil dilatation, and exacerbate the problem. Red or yellow lenses are required.

The respiratory system

The respiratory system can be infected, or can be damaged by various dusts.

Infections

A range of infectious agents can be found in sputum or saliva, particularly if this is contaminated with blood. Those of most concern are the viral infections with high morbidity or mortality (Chapters 2 and 9) and bacterial infections such as syphilis and tuberculosis, but far more prevalent are upper respiratory viral infections (Table 10.4).

Aerosols from dental instruments

Water is delivered from the mains via an in-line system to cool the burs of high-speed handpieces. Water is warmed in the dental unit, for delivery by the air–water syringe.

The water supply tends to be contaminated—usually with oral micro-organisms including *Actinomyces* species, *Staphylococcus aureus*, *Pseudomonas* species and a range of other organisms. Such contamination appears to originate from the environment of the dental surgery, and enter the unit retrogradely, particularly through dental handpieces. Air rotors and ultrasonic scalers produce an aerosol containing micro-organisms originating from both the water supply and the mouth. Concern is often expressed about the possible spread of infection by aerosols. Although there is no reliable evidence for the transmission of infections by this route, ultrasonic scalers produce an aerosol containing micro-organisms. There is at least a theoretical possibility of transmission of *Legionella* species (Chapter 9) in this way. Aerosols remain suspended for as long as 35 minutes after production.

Dust

Dust can be created during various dental procedures and might constitute a hazard, particularly in the laboratory.

The drilling of tooth and old amalgams creates dust if adequate water cooling is not used (see page 242), but there is little evidence of occupational lung disease in clinical dental staff.

There are, however, reports of pneumoconioses and occupational asthma in dental technicians (Table 10.5). Materials such as beryllium, silica, hard metal and cobalt are the best recognized causes of pneumoconiosis in technicians, and lung biopsies from technicians have sometimes revealed deposits of silica, cobalt, chromium, aluminium, iron and molybdenum.

Occupational asthma has been precipitated in dental technicians by methyl methacrylate and cyanoacrylates; cobalt, nickel and chromium are other potential causes.

Many alginates contain fluoride salts, zinc oxide, or barium sulphate and various filler particles. These might

Table 10.4
Some micro-organisms that might be transmitted in the dental surgery

Bacteria	Viruses	Fungi
Streptococcus species Mycobacteria	Childhood fevers, e. g. mumps virus	Candida species
Treponema pallidum *Legionella* species	Upper respiratory tract viruses, e.g. common cold, tonsillitis	
	Coxsackie viruses, e.g. Herpangina	
	Hepatitis viruses: hepatitis A; hepatitis B; non-A, non-B hepatitis; delta agent	
	Human immunodeficiency viruses (HIV)	
	Herpesviruses: Epstein–Barr virus; cytomegalovirus; herpes simplex virus; varicella–zoster virus	

Table 10.5
Lung disease in dental technicians

Disease	Materials implicated
Pneumoconioses	Beryllium Silica Cobalt
Asthma	Cobalt Nickel Chromium

be inhaled, especially during dispensing and mixing, and produce a hazard either because of the metal salt or siliceous fibres—though the evidence for a real hazard from these is very slender. However, these particles may be less than 3 μm in diameter and 20 μm long and might constitute a hazard similar to that of asbestos fibres. Some impression materials such as 'Blueprint' are virtually dust free during mixing.

Asbestos is the generic term for various hydrated fibrous silicate minerals which break down to fibres often less than 1 μm wide and 10 μm long. Asbestos is used as a liner for casting rings and melting crucibles, and in some fire-resistant gloves. The use of asbestos should be avoided wherever possible because of the dangers, if it is inhaled or ingested, of asbestosis, carcinomas or mesothelioma.

One air-polisher system uses sodium bicarbonate powder (Prophy-Jet) which creates a dust cloud around the operator. Whether this is or is not harmful is unclear.

Prevention of respiratory injury

The most important preventive measures are the avoidance of the production of aerosols and dusts; prevention of inhalation of aerosols, dusts, vapours or fumes; and adequate room ventilation. The wearing of face masks, with adequate aspiration of the working area, and adequate room ventilation will reduce these risks.

Face masks rarely filter particles smaller than 5 μm (such as viruses) in diameter and the filtering efficiency of face masks varies from 14% to 99%. Nevertheless, they filter a great deal of debris. In any event, masks should preferably be changed every hour.

The ears

High-speed drills, especially those with ball-bearing endpieces (from the 1950s and 1960s), produced sufficient noise to constitute a slight hazard to hearing. Modern handpieces produce no significant hazard unless noise levels are above about 85 decibels.

Ultrasonic scalers may produce a small degree of tinnitus after prolonged use, but this is rarely clinically significant.

The skin

The main cutaneous problems in dental practice are maceration and dermatitis from repeated hand-washing, with occasional subsequent candidosis and other infections.

Maceration

The wearing of gloves reduces maceration (Chapters 2 and 9).

Infections

Local infections such as herpetic whitlow (Fig. 2.28; Volume 2) can be painful and incapacitating. Wearing of gloves will reduce the risk of infection. The skin, especially if broken or punctured by needlestick injury, may be the route for transmission of other viral infections such as hepatitis B or HIV (Chapters 2 and 9).

Burns

Hot composition in particular can cause burns, but any hot material or instruments or caustics can be responsible. Patients or staff may be wounded, and fire is a risk in the laboratory.

Dental amalgam dermatitis

An erythematous rash is a rare sequel to the placing or removal of an amalgam restoration in patients who appear to be hypersensitive to mercury. Occasionally, dental personnel develop contact allergy to mercury.

Contact dermatitis

Allergic contact dermatitis is uncommon in dentists but the following are possible causes.

1. Topical anaesthetics containing benzocaine.
2. Local analgesics containing para-aminobenzoic acid esters (procaine).
3. Methyl methacrylate monomer: sensitivity is predominantly to the hydroquinone stabilizer.
4. Essential oils (eugenol, cinnamon, peppermint, aniseed, spearmint, eucalyptol, menthol and thymol) and related substances such as balsam of Peru, benzoin, rosin, vanilla and perfumes in soaps, etc. Bacteriostatic agents in soaps and cleansers may induce allergies.
5. Nickel, in chrome-plated dental instruments.
6. Mercury.

Prevention of skin disorders

Direct contact with chemicals and drugs should be minimized and gloves worn wherever possible.

Gloves

Gloves protect against many physical, chemical and microbial agents. They will not, of course, prevent inoculation injuries and may be permeable to some organic solvents. A small proportion of some new gloves are supplied faulty.

Operating gloves vary in their durability, but most can be re-used if the external surface is cleaned with an antiseptic, such as chlorhexidine or povidone-iodine, that fairly effectively removes microbial contaminants. Ideally, gloves should be changed for each patient.

Systemic disease

Systemic complications result mainly from the following.

1. *Infections* (Chapters 2 and 9). Control of cross-infection to patients and staff is clearly the legal responsibility of the dentist. In the UK, dental practitioners are covered for illness related to infections by National Health Service Industrial Injury Regulations (S1 1974 No. 1547) which can give up to 85% of normal income during illness or injury. Such a claim is more likely to be successful if the dentist has been vaccinated against HBV, and has adequate cross-infection control in the practice. Current recommendations are that all clinical dental staff should be immunized against HBV.

Gloves should be worn by all staff handling teeth, mucous membranes, saliva or blood, or instruments that have been in contact with these.

2. *Drugs and dental materials.*

(a) *Mercury.* Mercury can present a hazard mainly if handled without due precaution, but a recent study of 193 dental personnel showed that 55% had levels of mercury in their hair similar to those found in non-dental controls. Nevertheless, a small proportion of dentists and surgery assistants have suffered from chronic mercury toxicity with tremor, inco-ordination, polyneuropathies, and accelerated senility. Rarely, deaths have been reported.

The greatest hazard from mercury arises when free mercury is spilt or comes into contact with the skin (such as in hand trituration). Mercury spilt near to hot areas (such as sterilizers), or accumulating in nooks and crannies, gives rise to mercury vapour, as do other sources (Table 10.6). Removal of old amalgams from teeth with an air rotor does not produce significant mercury vapour if adequate water cooling and aspiration are used. Apart from avoiding sources of mercury contamination, positive methods to reduce levels of mercury vapour in the surgery include adequate room ventilation, and the use of pre-portioned mercury capsules (Table 10.7).

Table 10.6
Potential sources of mercury exposure in dentistry

Accidental spills

Poor mercury hygiene

Manual mulling (trituration)

Mechanical amalgamators

Ultrasonic amalgam condensers

Heating amalgam carriers to dislodge debris

Failure to use water spray when removing old amalgams

Failure to use high-vacuum suction when removing old amalgams

Dry-heat sterilization of amalgam-contaminated instruments

Storage of waste amalgam improperly

Table 10.7
Reduction of mercury hazards in dental surgery

Avoiding sources (see Table 10.6)

Using capsulated amalgams

Adequate surgery ventilation

Monitoring of mercury levels

(b) *Anaesthetic gases.* Chronic exposure to trace anaesthetic gases has been reported to produce increased rates of various disorders in anaesthetists and operating room nurses. Dental personnel may be exposed to higher concentrations of these gases than are hospital operating room personnel, though usually for shorter periods of time. Up to 6800 p.p.m. nitrous oxide has been recorded in dental theatres.

Dental personnel exposed to inhalational anaesthetics appear to be predisposed to a range of general health problems and reproductive difficulties: male dentists have more liver, kidney and neurological disorders than controls, while their wives have an increased rate of spontaneous abortions. Dental surgery assistants can suffer from similar problems.

Nitrous oxide appears to be the agent predominantly responsible for these complications, especially a myeloneuropathy related to the interference by nitrous oxide with vitamin B_{12} metabolism. Exposed persons may also develop megaloblastic erythrocytes.

Inhalational anaesthetics should therefore be used only in a well-ventilated environment with a system (scavenger system) to absorb exhaled gases (Chapter 6). Scavenger systems can reduce nitrous oxide contamination by 97%.

Self-administration of these agents should also be avoided.

(c) *Controlled drugs.* Clearly there is a danger of drug abuse in clinical staff (Chapters 2 and 5).

3. Radiation (see also above).

Health and Safety at Work Act 1974 in relation to radiation protection

The dentist must ensure that he or she, staff and patients are not exposed to unnecessary radiation. All x-ray sets must conform to certain safety standards (Table 10.8); all involved in their use should be aware of the hazards; all should adopt practices that minimize the dangers; and safety should be monitored with the use of a special pack obtainable from the Nuclear Inspectorate (UK). The Nuclear Inspectorate has the responsibility for monitoring radiation safety and the right to inspect dental surgeries where there is x-ray equipment (see page 244).

Most modern x-ray equipment in the UK complies with safety standards since the Health and Safety at Work Act places an obligation on manufacturers, importers and suppliers in this respect.

Ionizing Radiations Regulations 1985 (IRR85)

An employer (including a self-employed person) must comply with these regulations and must co-operate with other employers if there is any possibility of radiation of any employee of the other party. The employer must notify the Health and Safety Executive 28 days before he or she intends (for the first time) to work with ionizing radiation. He must also inform the Executive of any change in the name and address of the practice.

Employers must restrict the exposure of employees and other persons to ionizing radiation and must designate as a controlled area, any area where an employee can be exposed. Local operating rules such as the Family Practitioner Committee's *Basic rules in dental radiography* should be displayed; a named person with appropriate knowledge must take day-to-day responsibility for ensuring compliance with the regulations and for overseeing radiation safety (usually this will be the dentist); and anyone using an x-ray set should be appropriately trained. Women should be warned of the possible hazard to a fetus.

Details of relevant literature are given in the Further reading section at the end of this chapter.

Walls

Solid structural walls of brick or concrete, but not thin partition walls, will attenuate ionizing radiation.

Monitoring

The current permissible limit for whole-body radiation in the UK in the course of occupational exposure is 50 milliSieverts/year. If the dose is unlikely to exceed 15 mSv/year, health surveillance and monitoring are not required by law; most dentists and their staff fall into this category.

However, monitoring by film badge is convenient and cheap and, if nothing else, is a reassuring way of demonstrating the low level of exposure. X-ray equipment should be checked annually. The National Radiation Protection Board (NRPB), Personnel Monitoring Service, Harwell, Didcot, Oxon, can provide details on monitoring.

Table 10.8
Radiation protection

Patients	Staff
Only take radiographs if necessary Reduce or avoid x-ray use in pregnancy	
Use fastest films that will give diagnostic result	Use only safe equipment
Use intensifying cassettes where otherwise excessively long exposures would be needed	Only staff over 16 years of age can work with radiation
Do not direct x-ray beam at gonads or thyroid or eyes; use lead shield for gonads	Only have essential staff in room
	Stand as far as possible away from x-ray machine, and out of line of primary beam
	Never manually hold films in the mouth
	Do not delegate radiography to staff unqualified in its use
	Use National Radiological Protection Board (NRPB) monitoring service
	Abide by *Ionising Radiations Regulations* 1985, No. 1333 (1985). London: HMSO

4. *Mental health.* Dentistry appears to be stressful and dentists seem to have rates of cardiovascular disease, drug and alcohol abuse and divorce above those of the general population, at least in the USA. Nearly one-third of UK dentists have job dissatisfaction, and male dentists have higher indices of anxiety and Type A coronary artery disease-prone behaviour than the general population. Perceived culpable aspects of practice include the NHS system of piecework remuneration and a bad public image of dentistry.

Death rates for dentists

The standardized mortality ratio (SMR) used to assess death rates is the ratio of observed deaths in an occupation to the national average death rate for age and sex. An SMR of less than 100 indicates a reduced death rate; an SMR of over 100 indicates an increased rate. In 1981, UK male dentists had an SMR of 59 which is far better than that for many other professions and for others in the same social class I. Single women dentists, however, had an SMR of 123. The reasons for the discrepancies are unclear.

General legislation related to hazards (UK)

Health and Safety at Work Act, 1974

Apart from those in private domestic employment, this act applies to all employers, employees and the self-employed, and provides statutory protection over and above common law protection.

Objectives

The Act aims to secure the health, safety and welfare of those at work, and also to protect the general public from risks to their health and safety arising from the activities of workpeople; to control the safekeeping, use and handling of dangerous substances; and to control the emission into the atmosphere of noxious and offensive substances from work premises.

Administration

The Secretary of State for Employment is empowered by the Act to make health and safety regulations and either to replace or extend existing regulations made under other statutes. He is advised by the Health and Safety Commission, and though he may act on his own initiative, he must consult the commission before enacting any new regulations or adopting codes of practice. Both he

and the Commission must consult with appropriate bodies such as trade unions or employers' associations before framing proposals for new or revised legislation.

The Health and Safety Executive is the control arm of the Commission responsible for enforcing the Act's provisions, though certain of these duties have devolved on local authorities. The Health and Safety Inspectorate is responsible for ensuring these regulations are observed. More detailed information can be obtained from leaflets, which are free of charge, from the Health and Safety Executive, Baynards House, 1 Chepstow Place, London W2 47F (Telephone 01 229 3456), or from any local office of the executive.

HSC1 Some legal aspects and how they affect you.
HSC2 The Act outlined.
HSC3 Advice to employers.
HSC4 Advice to the self-employed.
HSC5 Advice to employees.
HSC6 Guidance notes on employers' policy statements.
HSC7 Regulations, approved codes of practice and guidance literature.

Employers

An employer is obliged to ensure *as far as is reasonably practicable* the health, safety and welfare of his or her employees whilst at work. Employers have a similar duty to anyone who may be affected by the activities or disposition of their business.

In more specific terms, the dentist is obliged to undertake the following.

1. Provide and maintain a 'plant and system of work that is safe and without risk to health and safety', i.e. dental equipment such as the dental chair, dental unit, autoclave, x-ray units and items such as the receptionist's chair or electric typewriter.

2. Arrange a safe system of using, handling, storing and transporting substances. This includes substances in solid, liquid or gaseous form, such as chemicals, drugs, mercury and anaesthetic gases.

3. Provide all necessary information, instruction, training and supervision as is required to ensure the health and safety at work of employees. The employees should, for example, know about risks of cross-infection, radiation and of the use of drugs and chemicals.

4. Maintain any place of work under his or her control in a condition that is safe and without risk to health, and to provide a safe way in and out.

5. Provide and maintain a safe working environment.

6. Conduct the practice in such a way as to ensure that those not in his employment are not subjected to risks to their health and safety. This includes patients, visitors, anyone employed to undertake repairs or maintenance, and all who may be reasonably considered to be at risk, such as those who pass by the premises.

7. Give information as may be necessary to persons not in his or her employment of any aspect of the way the practice is conducted that might adversely affect their health or safety. For example, contractors should be warned about the disposal of sharps, infected waste, etc.

Safety policies

A dentist who employs five or more employees must formulate a safety policy and bring it to the personal notice of all staff. Ideally, each employee should be given a copy and sign a receipt that it has been received and understood.

The first part of the safety policy should be a general declaration of the employer's intention to provide a safe and healthy working environment suitably amplified by his duties under the Act. The name of the person ultimately responsible for the fulfilling of the policy (usually the principal or a designated partner) must be noted. Employees must also be reminded of *their* obligations under the Act, and it may be sensible to give each a copy of the leaflet HSC5 (see above).

The second part of the safety policy statement should be more specific and relate to particular hazards connected with cross-infection control, drug safety, radiography, handling of mercury, service supplies to dental equipment, and so on.

The employer is responsible for the training of staff so that all can participate satisfactorily in the implementation of the policy document. In-service training may be the most practicable and appropriate arrangement.

Employees

An employee must take reasonable care of himself and others who may be affected by his work activity. He must also co-operate with the employer and any other person upon whom the Act imposes a duty to see this is complied with. The employee must not intentionally or recklessly interfere with, or misuse, anything provided in the interest of health and safety.

Manufacturers and suppliers

Designers, manufacturers, suppliers or importers of equipment or substances must ensure, as far as is reasonably practicable, that there is no risk to safety or health. They must carry out appropriate testing and inspection and provide all necessary information relating to the purpose for which the equipment is intended, along with instructions regarding its safe use. Those who install and maintain equipment have a similar obligation.

Enforcement of the Act

A Health and Safety Inspector may enter work premises at any reasonable time and, if he considers that a dangerous situation exists, he can enter at *any* time. It is an offence to obstruct an Inspector in the course of his statutory duties. He has the right to examine premises, documents, substances, systems of work and equipment. He may seize equipment or render it harmless, as well as take measurements, samples, photographs and seek information. An Inspector can, where necessary, serve either an improvement notice or a prohibition notice.

An improvement notice is served upon the person who, in the opinion of the inspector, is contravening a relevant statutory provision. It specifies the provision that is being infringed, the reasons why the Inspector believes this to be so, and the time allowed for remedial action.

A prohibition notice is used when there is risk of serious personal injury. It is served upon the person performing or controlling a dangerous activity. Its effect is either immediately to stop the activity until remedial action has been taken, or, if the Inspector considers there is no immediate danger, time will be allowed to remedy the situation.

Those who have been served with either an improvement or a prohibition notice have right of appeal to an industrial tribunal provided the appeal is lodged with the Central Office of Tribunals within 3 weeks of the notice being served. Upon the lodging of an appeal, the operation of an improvement notice is suspended until the matter is decided, but a prohibition notice can only be suspended if the tribunal so orders at a specially convened sitting before the main hearing.

Penalties

It is an offence liable to prosecution to contravene any of the general duties under the Act or any regulations made under it, or to ignore the serving of any notices.

Summary conviction (trial before a Magistrate's Court) attracts a fine of up to £1000. Conviction on indictment (before a Crown Court) can result in a fine of unlimited amount or imprisonment up to a term of 2 years, or both.

If having been convicted of an offence the perpetrator allows it to continue, he is liable to a fine of up to £50 for each day of its continuation.

Whilst a civil action cannot be taken solely as a result of the Act being infringed, a person who suffers injury or damage may still sue for negligence.

Safety representatives and committees

Recognized trade unions have the right to appoint safety representatives from among the employees at a place of work, and the recognized unions include the British Dental Association, National and Local Government Officers' Association and Union of Shop, Distributive and Allied Workers. Safety representatives should have been in the practice's employ for a minimum of 2 years, or have been in similar employment for that time, and be at least 18 years of age. No statutory liability additional to that of an employee falls upon safety representatives.

Safety representatives should, among other things, investigate potential hazards, make representations to employers and represent the staff in dealing with the inspectorate. The safety representatives may request an employer to establish a safety committee, which acts as a focus both for staff participation in the prevention of hazards and for staff and employer co-operation. Employers must consult safety representatives on matters relating to the implementation of the appropriate health and safety regulations.

The extent to which the unions will apply their rights in the case of dental practice is unclear. Detailed regulations are found in the Statutory Instrument, HMSO 1977 No. 500.

Factories Act 1961

Heating, ventilation and extraction

An adequate room temperature (60°F or 15.5°C after the first hour) must be maintained. Air conditioning will keep the temperature constant, heating it during the winter and cooling it in the summer. Good ventilation is essential, as surgeries tend to get steamy because of the autoclave and may be contaminated with mercury vapour and anaesthetic gases as well as the typical dental practice smells of eugenol, etc. Laboratories tend to get steamy or smoke filled, and all burn-out furnaces should have smoke extractors. Dust extraction is necessary wherever there is a hazard such as metal, plaster, ceramic or pumice dust.

Overcrowding

A minimum of 11 cubic metres (400 cubic feet) of space per worker is needed, not counting any area more than 4.3 metres (14 feet) from the floor, and rooms must not become so overcrowded as to endanger health.

Staff facilities

Adequate staff facilities, such as a cloakroom for hanging outdoor clothes (coats, jackets, etc.), lockers for personal effects, and a room in which to make hot drinks and eat refreshments, must be made available. Within a small practice, employing perhaps only one technician, a shared facility with the dental surgery assistant will suffice.

Dangerous materials and equipment

All dangerous equipment and materials must be clearly marked. The onus is on the employer to ensure that every

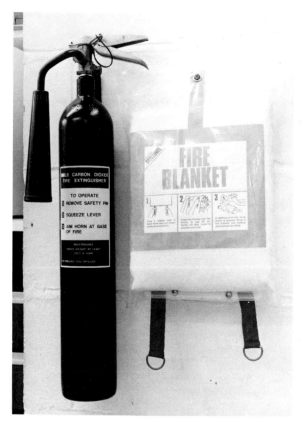

Fig. 10.8 *Safety equipment for fire hazards.*

member of staff is trained to use the machinery and dangerous materials and that these must be safe, and without risk to health, as far as possible. All machinery should be fenced; this applies in particular to centrifugal casting apparatus. Gas bottles must be stored outside the working area; acids and cyanide solutions should be kept apart and stored in a fume cupboard. Dangerous drugs must be stored in an appropriate locked receptacle (Chapter 5).

Accidents

A record must be kept of any major accident or dangerous occurrence, which must also be reported to the Factories Inspector. It may also be wise to keep an unofficial record of minor accidents.

Notices

The Factories Inspector will advise about the various notices that have to be displayed under the Act.

Fire precautions

There must be an adequate means of fire escape and fire extinguishers for inflammables, such as polymers and monomers, and for electrical and general combustibles (Fig. 10.8). A fire certificate will be necessary if more than 20 persons are employed, or more than 10 persons working on other than the ground floor.

First aid

A first aid box must be kept and maintained—minimum contents are laid down in the Factories Order.

Cleanliness

The surgery and laboratory must be kept clean of dirt, wax, plaster, etc. (all benches and floors should be swept and cleaned each evening). The walls and ceilings should be washed every 14 months and redecorated every 7 years, according to the Act.

An adequate supply of drinking water and cups must be provided as well as reasonable washing facilities and adequate sanitary conveniences, with separate facilities for each sex if there are more than five male and female employees.

FURTHER READING

Cooley R. L., Barkmier W. N. (1982). Techniques and devices for recovering mercury and preventing contamination. *Gen. Dentistry*, **30**: 36–41.

Cooley R. L. *et al.* (1978). Ocular injuries sustained in the dental office. *JADA*, **97**: 985–988.

Forman-Franco D. *et al.* (1978). High-speed drill noise and hearing: audiometric survey of 70 dentists. *JADA*, **97**: 479–482.

HMSO (1985). *The Ionising Radiations Regulations*, No. 1333. London: HMSO.

HMSO (1985). *The Approved Code of Practice for the protection of persons against ionising radiation arising from any work activity.* London: HMSO.

HMSO (1988). *Guidance notes for the protection of persons against ionizing radiations arising from medical and dental use.* London: HMSO.

Scully C., Cawson R. A. (in preparation). *Occupational hazards in dentistry.* London: Butterworth.

Seear J. (1981). *Law and ethics in dentistry*, 2nd edn. Bristol: Wright.

Smith N. J. D. (1986). *Brit. dent. J.*, **135**: 135–137.

Index